Optimizing Antimicrobial Therapy of Sepsis and Septic Shock

Guest Editor

ANAND KUMAR, MD

CRITICAL CARE CLINICS

www.criticalcare.theclinics.com

Consulting Editor
RICHARD W. CARLSON, MD, PhD

January 2011 • Volume 27 • Number 1

SAUNDERS an imprint of ELSEVIER, Inc.

W.B. SAUNDERS COMPANY
A Division of Elsevier Inc.

Elsevier Inc. ● 1600 John F. Kennedy Blvd., ● Suite 1800 ● Philadelphia, Pennsylvania 19103-2899

http://www.theclinics.com

CRITICAL CARE CLINICS Volume 27, Number 1
January 2011 ISSN 0749-0704, ISBN-13: 978-1-4557-0431-6

Editor: Patrick Manley

Critical Care Clinics (ISSN: 0749-0704) is published quarterly by Elsevier Inc., 360 Park Avenue South, New York, NY 10010-1710. Months of issue are January, April, July, and October. Business and Editorial Offices: 1600 John F. Kennedy Blvd., Suite 1800, Philadelphia, PA 19103-2899. Customer Service Office: 6277 Sea Harbor Drive, Orlando, FL 32887-4800. Periodicals postage paid at New York, NY and additional mailing offices. Subscription prices are $179.00 per year for US individuals, $435.00 per year for US institution, $87.00 per year for US students and residents, $222.00 per year for Canadian individuals, $539.00 per year for Canadian institutions, $257.00 per year for international individuals, $539.00 per year for international institutions and $127.00 per year for Canadian and foreign students/residents. To receive student/resident rate, orders must be accompanied by name of affiliated institution, date of term, and the *signature* of program/residency coordinator on institution letterhead. Orders will be billed at individual rate until proof of status is received. Foreign air speed delivery is included in all *Clinics* subscription prices. All prices are subject to change without notice. POSTMASTER: Send address changes to *Critical Care Clinics*, Elsevier Periodicals Customer Service, 11830 Westline Industrial Drive, St. Louis, MO 63146. **Customer Service: 1-800-654-2452 (US). From outside of the US, call 1-314-447-8871. Fax: 1-314-447-8029. E-mail: journalscustomerservice-usa@elsevier.com (for print support) or journalsonlinesupport-usa@elsevier.com (for online support).**

Reprints. For copies of 100 or more of articles in this publication, please contact the Commercial Reprints Department, Elsevier Inc., 360 Park Avenue South, New York, NY 10010-1710. Tel.: 212-633-3813; Fax: 212-462-1935; E-mail: reprints@elsevier.com.

Critical Care Clinics is also published in Spanish by Editorial Inter-Medica, Junin 917, 1er A, 1113, Buenos Aires, Argentina.

Critical Care Clinics is covered in *MEDLINE/PubMed (Index Medicus)*, *EMBASE/Excerpta Medica*, *Current Concepts/Clinical Medicine*, *ISI/BIOMED*, and *Chemical Abstracts*.

Printed and bound in the United Kingdom
Transferred to Digital Print 2011

Contributors

CONSULTING EDITOR

RICHARD W. CARLSON, MD, PhD
Chairman Emeritus, Department of Medicine, Maricopa Medical Center and Director, Medical Intensive Care Unit; Professor, University of Arizona College of Medicine; and Professor, Department of Medicine, Mayo Graduate School of Medicine, Phoenix, Arizona

GUEST EDITOR

ANAND KUMAR, MD
Attending Physician, Section of Infectious Diseases, Section of Critical Care Medicine, Medical Microbiology and Pharmacology/Therapeutics, Sections of Critical Care Medicine, and Infectious Diseases, University of Manitoba, Manitoba, Canada; Robert Wood Johnson Medical School, University of Medicine and Dentistry, Camden, New Jersey

AUTHORS

DAVID ANDES, MD
Associate Professor, Departments of Medicine and Microbiology and Immunology, University of Wisconsin, Madison, Wisconsin

WILLIAM A. CRAIG, MD
Emeritus Professor of Medicine, Department of Medicine, University of Wisconsin School of Medicine and Public Health, Madison, Wisconsin

JARED L. CRANDON, PharmD, BCPS
Associate Director, Clinical and Experimental Pharmacology, Center for Anti-Infective Research and Development, Hartford Hospital, Hartford, Connecticut

G.L. DRUSANO, MD
Co-Director, Ordway Research Institute, Albany, New York

HENRY S. FRAIMOW, MD
Associate Professor of Medicine, Division of Infectious Diseases, UMDNJ-Robert Wood Johnson Medical School, Cooper University Hospital, Camden, New Jersey

DUANE J. FUNK, MD, FRCP(C)
Assistant Professor, Section of Critical Care Medicine, Department of Anesthesia, University of Manitoba, Manitoba, Canada

ANAND KUMAR, MD
Attending Physician, Section of Infectious Diseases, Section of Critical Care Medicine, Medical Microbiology and Pharmacology/Therapeutics, Sections of Critical Care Medicine, and Infectious Diseases, University of Manitoba, Manitoba, Canada; Robert Wood Johnson Medical School, University of Medicine and Dentistry, Camden, New Jersey

ALEXANDER LEPAK, MD
Infectious Disease Fellow, University of Wisconsin, Madison, Wisconsin

JEFFREY LIPMAN, MBBCh, FCICM, MD
Department of Intensive Care Medicine, Royal Brisbane and Women's Hospital; Burns, Trauma and Critical Care Research Centre, The University of Queensland, Royal Brisbane and Women's Hospital, Herston, Brisbane, Queensland, Australia

THOMAS P. LODISE, PharmD
Associate Professor, Albany College of Pharmacy and Health Sciences; Visiting Professor, Ordway Research Institute, Albany, New York

JOAN R. MASCLANS, MD, PhD
Critical Care Department, Vall d'Hebron University Hospital, Vall d'Hebron Research Institute, Universitat Autònoma de Barcelona, Barcelona, Spain

ROBERT G. MASTERTON, FRCPath, FRCP [Edin & Glas]
Department of Microbiology, Ayrshire & Arran NHS Board, The Ayr Hospital, United Kingdom

DAVID P. NICOLAU, PharmD, FCCP, FIDSA
Director, Center for Anti-Infective Research and Development; Division of Infectious Diseases, Hartford Hospital, Hartford, Connecticut

XAVIER NUVIALS, MD
Critical Care Department, Vall d'Hebron University Hospital; Vall d'Hebron Research Institute, Universitat Autònoma de Barcelona, Barcelona, Spain

MERCEDES PALOMAR, MD, PhD
Critical Care Department, Vall d'Hebron University Hospital; Vall d'Hebron Research Institute; School of Medicine, Universitat Autònoma de Barcelona, Barcelona, Spain

JORDI RELLO, MD, PhD
Critical Care Department, Vall d'Hebron University Hospital, Barcelona; Vall d'Hebron Research Institute; Centro de Investigación Biomédica En Red de Enfermedades Respiratorias; School of Medicine, Universitat Autònoma de Barcelona, Barcelona, Spain

JASON A. ROBERTS, PhD, BPharm (Hons), FSHP
Departments of Intensive Care Medicine and Pharmacy, Royal Brisbane and Women's Hospital; Burns, Trauma and Critical Care Research Centre, The University of Queensland, Royal Brisbane and Women's Hospital, Herston, Brisbane, Queensland, Australia

JOHN C. ROTSCHAFER, PharmD
Professor, Department of Experimental and Clinical Pharmacology, College of Pharmacy, University of Minnesota, Minneapolis, Minnesota

CHRISTOPHER J. SULLIVAN, MD
Critical Care, Fairview Hospital System, Minneapolis, Minnesota

CONSTANTINE TSIGRELIS, MD
Assistant Professor of Medicine, Division of Infectious Diseases, UMDNJ-Robert Wood Johnson Medical School, Cooper University Hospital, Camden, New Jersey

MARTA ULLDEMOLINS, PharmD
Critical Care Department, Vall d'Hebron University Hospital; Vall d'Hebron Research Institute, Universitat Autònoma de Barcelona, Barcelona; Centro de Investigación Biomédica En Red de Enfermedades Respiratorias, Spain

MARY A. ULLMAN, PharmD
Department of Clinical Pharmacy, Regions Hospital, St Paul, Minnesota

JULIE M. VARGHESE, BPharm (Hons)
Burns, Trauma and Critical Care Research Centre, The University of Queensland, Royal Brisbane and Women's Hospital, Brisbane, Queensland, Australia

Contents

This article reviews the principles of antimicrobial pharmacokinetics and pharmacodynamics in the context of the ICU for the most commonly used antibiotics. For therapy to truly be efficacious, the regimen must be effective against the organism, but not harmful to the patient. We review how optimization of chemotherapy requires a careful balancing of efficacy against toxicity when selecting dose and dose schedules. In addition, we discuss the importance of considering concentrations at the site of infection and how dose optimization can help suppress resistance emergence and preserve our antimicrobial armamentarium for the future. Finally, we examine combination chemotherapy and strategies for optimizing the administration of multiple agents.

Antimicrobial pharmacokinetics (PK) and pharmacodynamics (PD) are important considerations, particularly in critically ill patients with severe sepsis and septic shock. The pathophysiologic changes that occur in these conditions can have a major effect on pharmacokinetic parameters, which in turn could result in failure to achieve pharmacodynamic targets for antimicrobials thus adversely affecting clinical outcome. This paper discusses the pathophysiologic changes that occur during severe sepsis and septic shock and the consequent effects on antimicrobial PK and PD. The effect of PK/PD on specific antimicrobial classes is discussed and a rational framework for antimicrobial dosing is provided. Knowledge of PK/PD properties of antimicrobials can be used to personalize dosing regimens not only to maximize antimicrobial activity but also to minimize toxicity and reduce the development of antimicrobial resistance.

Inappropriate empirical antibiotic therapy for severe infections in the intensive care unit is a modifiable prognostic factor that has a great effect on patient outcome and health care resources. Inappropriate treatment is usually associated with microorganisms resistant to the common antibiotics, which must be empirically targeted when risk factors are present. Previous antibiotic exposure, prolonged length of hospital stay, admission category, local susceptibilities, colonization pressure, and the presence of invasive devices increase the likelihood of infection by resistant pathogens. Consideration of issues beyond in vitro susceptibility, such as antibiotic physicochemistry, tissue penetration, and pharmacokinetic/pharmacodynamic-driven dosing, is mandatory for the optimization of antibiotic use.

For decades, health care workers faced the challenge of how to adequately treat life-threatening infections. To a great extent, the primary focus on improving outcomes has centered on improvement in resuscitation, deployment of antimicrobials of increasing potency, and development of novel adjunctive therapies. However, the current studies conclusively show that early recognition of life threatening infection and rapid initiation of appropriate antimicrobial therapy is the critical element in reducing mortality. If "Time is tissue" when it comes to thrombolytic therapy for acute myocardial infarction and thrombotic stroke, then an appropriate rule for life-threatening infections, particularly septic shock, is "Speed is life."

Given their popularity and favorable safety profile, it is no wonder that there has been considerable interest in developing strategies to most effectively use beta-lactam therapy. Dating back to the first days of penicillin, it was noted that there was an observed benefit to prolonging the infusion time or dosing more frequently. Since that time, considerable research has been performed to help understand and justify these dosing strategies. This article discusses the pharmacology behind these dosing strategies and presents some of the contemporary literature describing the perceived and observed clinical benefits.

Fluoroquinolones have become a staple antimicrobial in a variety of settings for a wide spectrum of infectious diseases. Although fluoroquinolones have been associated with a broad spectrum of adverse events, the side effect profile is generally acceptable. Their use in the intensive care unit as empiric therapy is becoming compromised due to the development of multiple drug resistant gram negative pathogens and collateral damage with C difficile & MRSA. Fluoroquinolones should be used along with another antibiotic of different chemical structure, mechanism of action, and pharmacodynamic profile to ensure adequate initial antimicrobial coverage and maximize the likelihood of a favorable clinical and microbiologic response.

The appearance of new third- and fourth-generation cephalosporins, carbapenems, and fluoroquinolones have decreased the use of aminoglycosides as monotherapy for most gram-negative infections. Historically, aminoglycosides were used in combination with other antibiotics to enhance bacterial killing and improve overall efficacy. However, most studies have failed to demonstrate improved outcomes in patients treated with antibiotic combinations over those receiving monotherapy. Only recently has early combination therapy been associated with reduced mortality in septic shock. This article reviews the pharmacokinetics, pharmacodynamics, and toxicodynamics of aminoglycosides, describing dosing strategies and other effects to improve outcomes in critically ill patients with serious infections.

THE CLINICS ARE NOW AVAILABLE ONLINE!

Access your subscription at:
www.theclinics.com

Preface

Optimizing Antimicrobial Therapy of Sepsis and Septic Shock

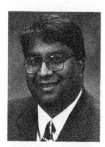

Anand Kumar, MD
Guest Editor

Since the advent of modern antimicrobial therapy with the introduction of penicillin over 50 years ago, the focus of the pharmaceutical scientists and clinicians has primarily been on the development of ever more potent and broad spectrum agents to counter the inevitable and inexorable expansion of antimicrobial resistance. In that regard, pharmaceutical science has been tremendously successful with dozens of classes of antimicrobials and hundreds of individual agents now available around the globe. Yet, the problem of resistance has continued unabated to the point that some pathogens appear impervious to virtually every known antimicrobial.

New antimicrobial agents in the pipeline have slowed dramatically. While this may be a serious concern if sustained in the long term, in the short term it provides an impetus for alternative approaches. Among these are learning how to use the antimicrobials we already have in a more effective manner. This issue of *Critical Care Clinics* is dedicated to that question. Rather than focusing on the newest drugs in development, the articles in this collection are dedicated to addressing the issue of how we can use the drugs that we already have in a fashion that maximizes their effectiveness. Although this question is always of importance, critically patients, particularly those with septic shock, represent the group in which optimal antimicrobial therapy may have the greatest impact. Fundamentally, optimization of antimicrobial therapy (whether choosing a microbiologically appropriate drug, using a multi-drug strategy for a single pathogen, optimizing pharmacokinetic/pharmacodynamic indices, using a cidal rather than a static agent, or simply using larger doses) primarily involves more rapid elimination of the pathogen. Infections where an antimicrobial therapy delay-dependent risk of irreversible and irreplaceable organ failure exists (such as bacterial meningitis and septic shock) are the conditions most likely to show a clear benefit.

Crit Care Clin 27 (2011) xi–xii
doi:10.1016/j.ccc.2010.11.007
0749-0704/11/$ — see front matter © 2011 Elsevier Inc. All rights reserved.

Although not well known, the initial use of penicillin involved continuous infusion. Convenience combined with the exceptional efficacy of the compound drove the transition to intermittent dosing regimens without significant evidence of superior effect. In these times of increasing antimicrobial resistance, perhaps a rigorous re-evaluation of our clinical approach to antimicrobial administration in life-threatening infections can fill in the gap pending development of novel drugs, while resulting in improved outcomes for our patients.

Anand Kumar, MD
Section of Critical Care Medicine
Section of Infectious Diseases
Medical Microbiology and Pharmacology/Therapeutics
University of Manitoba Health Sciences Centre
JJ 399 700 William Avenue, Winnipeg
Manitoba R3E-0Z3, Canada

Robert Wood Johnson Medical School
University of Medicine and Dentistry
Camden, NJ, USA

E-mail address:
akumar61@yahoo.com

DEDICATION

For my wife, Aparna

Pharmacokinetics and Pharmacodynamics: Optimal Antimicrobial Therapy in the Intensive Care Unit

Thomas P. Lodise, PharmD[a,b], G.L. Drusano, MD[b,*]

KEYWORDS

• Antimicrobial therapy • Intensive care unit • Pharmacokinetics
• Pharmacodynamics

The life-saving benefits of prompt, appropriate therapy are well documented. Studies have consistently demonstrated that delivery of early, appropriate antimicrobials reduces the morbidity and mortality associated with serious infections among patients in the intensive care unit (ICU).[1–4] Although delivery of early therapy is of paramount importance, we show that appropriate antimicrobial therapy entails more than administering the drug with an "S" beside it on the microbiology laboratory report.

This article reviews the principles of antimicrobial pharmacokinetics and pharmacodynamics in the context of the ICU for the most commonly used antibiotics (β-lactams, quinolones, aminoglycosides, and vancomycin). For many antibiotics, the "pharmacodynamic" or the exposure variable linked with outcome has been identified. This linkage is derived from both pre-clinical and clinical data and informs drug selection, dosing, and the administration schedule. In addition, we will discuss the importance of considering concentrations at the site of infection and how dose optimization can help suppress resistance emergence and preserve our antimicrobial armamentarium for the future. We will also discuss combination chemotherapy and strategies for optimizing the administration of multiple agents. Finally, for therapy to truly be efficacious, the regimen must be effective against the organism, but not harmful to the patient. We will review how optimization of chemotherapy requires a careful balancing of efficacy against toxicity when selecting dose and dose schedules.

[a] Albany College of Pharmacy and Health Sciences, Albany, NY, USA
[b] Ordway Research Institute, 150 New Scotland Avenue, Albany, NY 12208, USA
* Corresponding author.
E-mail address: gdrusano@ordwayresearch.org

Crit Care Clin 27 (2011) 1–18
doi:10.1016/j.ccc.2010.11.003
0749-0704/11/$ – see front matter © 2011 Elsevier Inc. All rights reserved.

criticalcare.theclinics.com

PHARMACODYNAMICS: FROM BENCH TO BEDSIDE
Minimum Inhibitory Concentration

Although pharmacokinetics can be loosely defined as the impact of the body on the disposition of an administered drug, pharmacodynamics can be defined as the effect of that administered agent both for its intended purpose (bacterial cell inhibition and killing) as well as unintended consequences, such as drug-mediated toxicity. In the realm of antibacterial chemotherapy, the minimum inhibitory concentration (MIC) is the pharmacodynamic parameter most often used to describe the relationship between antimicrobial drug and physiologic activity. The MIC is defined as the lowest or minimum antimicrobial concentration that inhibits visible microbial growth in artificial media after a fixed incubation time.[5,6] The MIC provides a quantitative measure of drug activity against the bacterial pathogen in question and allows one to calibrate the drug exposure to its potency.[7–9]

Although useful as a quantitative measure of drug activity or potency, the MIC is not without limitations. The MIC does not mirror physiologic conditions. The MIC is a static measure and is not reflective of the fluctuating drug concentrations typically observed during the dosing interval. Because the MIC measures only growth inhibition, it does not reflect the rate at which bacteria are killed, nor can it identify if an exposure-kill response relationship exists for a particular antibiotic-pathogen pairing. Furthermore, the MIC quantifies net growth only over an 18- to 24-hour observation period. Killing and re-growth may well occur during this period, as long as the net growth is zero. Finally, the MIC does not account for the postantibiotic effects of antibiotics.[9]

Antimicrobial Pharmacodynamics: "The Shape of the Concentration–Time Profile Curve Makes a Difference"

Examination of the shape of the concentration-time profile curve in relation to the MIC surmounts many of the limitations of the MIC and provides much better prediction of antimicrobial effect than the MIC or exposure profile alone.[7–9] The observed effects of some antimicrobial classes are most closely associated with the peak concentration/MIC ratio (Peak/MIC ratio). For others, it is the index of drug exposure over a full dosing interval relative to the MIC (eg, area under the concentration-time curve/MIC ratio, or the AUC/MIC ratio) that is most predictive. In some cases, the time that drug concentration exceeds a threshold throughout a dosing interval (Time>MIC) is most closely associated with the outcome (**Fig. 1**).[7,8]

It should be clearly stated that in the vast majority of instances, it is the free or nonprotein drug that is microbiologically active.[7,8,10,11] There are occasional exceptions, mostly with the therapy of gram-positive infections. Daptomycin is one such example;

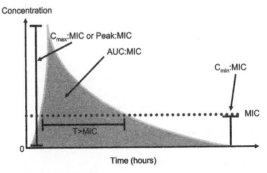

Fig. 1. Common pharmacodynamic indices.

protein binding is approximately 90% to 92% (free drug 8%–10%), but the agent behaves as if the drug is approximately 75% bound (25% free).[12] Nonetheless, the guiding principle is that protein binding can have an adverse impact on the pharmacodynamics (PD) and microbiological activity of an antibacterial agent.[10,11]

Because the shape of the drug exposure is examined in relation to the MIC, there is an inverse relationship between the concentration–time profile/MIC ratio and MIC value. Like all mathematical expressions, the denominator drives this relationship. The higher the MIC value, the lower the measure of drug exposure relative to the MIC (the time > MIC is shorter, and the AUC/MIC ratio and the peak/MIC ratio are reduced) and the lower the level of the expected microbiological effect. This was demonstrated in a granulocytopenic rat model of *Pseudomonas aeruginosa* sepsis by Drusano and colleagues.[13] In their investigation, the effect of lomefloxacin on survivorship was assessed. Two isogenic mutants of the parent strain were created that had higher MICs against lomefloxacin MICs; the MICs of the 3 strains (the parent and 2 mutant strains) for the drug were 1, 4, and 8 mg/L, respectively. With a standard dose of 80 mg/kg, survivorship decreased as the MIC increased. Furthermore, survivorship curves were virtually identical for the parent and mutant strain with an MIC of 4 mg/L when a 20-mg/kg drug dose was administered to the parent strain resulting in an AUC/MIC ratio that was identical to the AUC/MIC ratio observed for mutant strains (MIC of 4 mg/L) with the standard 80 mg/kg dose. This indicates that either the exposure or the MIC can be changed, but that the outcome is related to the pharmacodynamically linked variable, in this instance, the AUC/MIC ratio. Also, with the same drug exposure, increasing the MIC leads to reduced response rates.

Application of Pharmacokinetic/Pharmacodynamic Principles to Clinical Practice

With advances in mathematical modeling, it is possible to apply our understanding of antimicrobial PD into clinical practice. In particular, Monte Carlo simulation (MCS) can be used to integrate pharmacokinetic (PK), PD, and MIC data to design antibiotic regimens that have a high probability of achieving the PD target linked to effect against the range of pathogens likely to be encountered in clinical practice. MCS is a technique that incorporates the variability in PK among potential patients (between-patient variability) when predicting antibiotic exposures and allows calculation of the probability for obtaining a critical target exposure that drives a specific microbiological effect for the range of possible MIC values. If a number of volunteers or patients are given a specific drug dose or regimen, even on a mg per kg basis, there will be true variability in the observed concentration-time profiles among these patients. For example, the peak serum concentrations and AUC_{0-24h} will vary among individuals. In essence, MCS is a mathematical modeling technique that "simulates" the dispersion or full spread of concentration-time exposure values (eg, peak concentration, area under the curve) that would be seen in a large population after administration of a specific drug dose or regimen. Once the distribution in concentration-time profiles is determined, the probability of achieving the PD target at each MIC value for a given MIC range (ie, probability of target attainment [PTA] profile) is ascertained. Because the fraction of the organism collection at each MIC value likely to be encountered in clinical practice is known, an overall or weighted average (expectation) of the probability of target attainment rates can be calculated. This information can be used to judge how useful a specific drug dose will be for its intended population.[8,14–16]

A major consideration for MCS is the pharmacokinetic model used to estimate distributions in exposure profiles likely to be encountered in practice.[9,17] Caution should be exercised when employing a PK model derived from healthy volunteer studies. While healthy volunteer studies are often viewed as a conservative estimate of drug exposures, it is not always the case. For MCS, the measure of central tendency (high drug clearance, short half lives) is not of utmost importance. Because MCS calculations are explicitly creating a distribution, it is the measure of dispersion surrounding the measure of central tendency that is the driving factor. Secondary to the limited variability surrounding PK parameters from healthy volunteer studies, it is possible that they overestimate the PTA. This was observed in the pharmacodynamic profile of ceftobiprole; healthy volunteer data provided a more favorable probability of target attainment profile then that derived from actual patients.[18]

ADDITIONAL PK/PD CONSIDERATIONS
Concentrations at Site of Infection

Most clinical pharmacodynamic and Monte Carlo simulation studies have focused on free concentrations in plasma. When assessing the PK/PD of an antibiotic, it is also important to consider concentrations achieved at the site of infection. Free concentrations in plasma are often not acceptable proxies for free concentrations at the site of infection. For meropenem, median concentrations achieved in the epithelial lining fluid (ELF) concentrations were only 25% of those observed in the plasma among patients with VAP.[19] As one can imagine, this has a considerable effect on the PD profile at the site of infection. These data highlight the need to consider concentrations at the site of infection, particularly for difficult to penetrate sites like ELF, before designing dosing scheme for implementation into clinical practice.

Suppression of Resistance

Up to this point, this article has been focused on PD targets of clinical success. The next frontier in PK/PD is identifying antibiotic dosing scheme and drug combinations that minimize the emergence of resistance. Data available to date suggest that PD targets for resistance prevention are generally higher than PD targets for success. Jumbe and colleagues[20] demonstrated that resistance suppression in a mouse thigh infection model with *P aeruginosa* required an AUC/MIC ratio of 157. Tam and colleagues[21] also showed, with *Staphylococcus aureus* studied in a hollow fiber infection model using the quinolone garenoxacin, that 2 regimens (AUC/MIC ratio of 100 vs an AUC/MIC ratio of 280) produced identical rates of bacterial cell kill, but only the more intense regimen suppressed resistance emergence for the full 10 days of the experiment. Further study is still needed in the area of resistance suppression but the current data suggest that obtaining the PK/PD target against the range of MIC encountered clinically is not likely with conventional dosing and will most likely require more intensive regimens.[20,21]

Combination Chemotherapy

There are a number of advantages and disadvantages to combination chemotherapy. The spectrum of combination chemotherapy, if well chosen, may be markedly improved, so that "appropriate" chemotherapy will be on board from the beginning. The drugs may interact in a synergistic or additive manner, so that ultimately the clinician can achieve a higher probability of a good clinical outcome. Combination therapy is also highly likely to result in suppression of resistance, even if the drug interaction is antagonistic. Among the disadvantages, one bears both the toxicity and cost burden of more than one drug. In addition, if the drugs interact in a severely antagonistic fashion, there may not be sufficient control of bacterial replication to drive a good clinical outcome.

Oftentimes, people refer to drug interaction as being synergistic, additive, or antagonistic. Other somewhat meaningless terms such as "indifference" have also popped up in the infectious diseases literature. When thinking about drug interaction, there are 2 very important issues. The first is endpoint. In most instances, the endpoint is bacterial cell kill. However, other endpoints are possible, particularly suppressing the amplification of resistant organism subpopulations. The second issue is defining the reference condition. For instance, there are 2 common null reference models, Loewe Additivity and Bliss Independence (there are others). For Loewe Additivity, the idea is that additivity of interaction (the null reference model) is like adding a drug to itself, as it goes up the exposure-response curve. "Antagonism" is the occurrence of drug interaction that results in an effect (again, generally bacterial cell kill) that is statistically significantly less than additivity (the null reference model), whereas "synergy" is an interaction resulting in an effect significantly greater than additivity.

Our laboratory has examined the interaction between meropenem and tobramycin in vitro.[22] In **Table 1**, we display the half maximal inhibitory concentration (IC_{50}) values and α interaction values for meropenem and tobramycin for a wild-type *P aeruginosa* and its isogenic, efflux pump-overexpressed mutant. For the wild-type isolate, the interaction parameter is positive, but the confidence interval overlaps zero, making the interaction additive. For the mutant, the interaction term is very near zero, with a wide boundary crossing zero, again interpreted as additive interaction. This evaluation was for bacterial cell kill. We also examined resistance suppression in this experiment. The height of the mountain expresses the number of resistant colonies present for the two drugs. One can see in **Fig. 2**A, the number of meropenem-resistant isolates decrease with increasing concentration of either drug. However in **Fig. 2**B, increasing tobramycin concentrations have less effect in decreasing tobramycin-resistant isolates than does meropenem. Nevertheless, in both instances, the combination suppresses the amplification of resistant isolates and the interaction is quite valuable at that level.

This experiment was performed using static concentrations of both agents. In 2 other experiments, we used our in vitro hollow fiber system, where patient-like concentration-time curves can be generated to examine the interaction of antibiotics.[23,24] In our evaluation of meropenem plus levofloxacin against *P aeruginosa* in the in vitro hollow fiber system, we found that, somewhat surprisingly, the interaction of meropenem and levofloxacin was synergistic for cell kill. This was true for both a wild-type organism and a MexAB pump-overexpressed isogenic isolate. The

Table 1
Interaction parameters and respective IC_{50}s for meropenem and tobramycin for a wild-type isolate and its isogenic MexAB efflux pump-overexpressed mutant[a]

Isolate	Interaction Parameter α (Unitless)	IC_{50} (mg/L)	
		Meropenem	Tobramycin
Wild type	0.5665(-0.7525–1.884[b])	14.99(13.01–16.96)	4.678(3.919–5.437)
MexAB pump-overexpressed mutant	0.9545×10^{-6}(-0.671–0.671[b])	33.61(25.91–41.31)	3.803(3.498–4.107)

Abbreviation: IC_{50}, half maximal inhibitory concentration.
[a] The values in parentheses are 95% confidence intervals.
[b] Additive interaction.
Data from Drusano GL, Liu W, Fregeau C, et al. Differing effects of combination chemotherapy with meropenem and tobramycin on cell kill and suppression of resistance of wild-type *Pseudomonas aeruginosa* PAO1 and its isogenic MexAB efflux pump-overexpressed mutant. Antimicrob Agents Chemother 2009;53(6):2266–73.

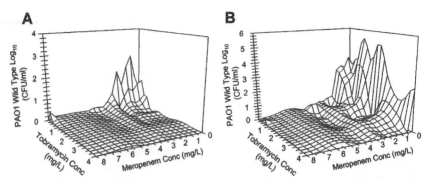

Fig. 2. Emergence of resistance to meropenem (A) and tobramycin (B) in the wild-type isolate *Pseudomonas aeruginosa* PA01. (*Reprint from* Drusano GL, Liu W, Fregeau C, et al. Differing effects of combination chemotherapy with meropenem and tobramycin on cell kill and suppression of resistance of wild-type *Pseudomonas aeruginosa* PAO1 and its isogenic MexAB efflux pump-overexpressed mutant. Antimicrob Agents Chemother 2009;53(6):2266–73 [Figure 2]; with permission.)

surprise comes from the fact that both meropenem and levofloxacin are both pumped by MexAB. Dogma indicates that drugs should be chosen for combination because of orthogonality of resistance emergence probability. In this case, however, we hypothesize that we saw increased cell kill *and* resistance suppression because the 2 drugs worked together to saturate the pump.

With rifampin plus moxifloxacin for *Mycobacterium tuberculosis*, we saw mild but significant antagonism with respect to cell kill, but synergy with respect to suppression of emergence of resistance.[24] The important message here is that whereas synergy is preferable for cell kill along with resistance suppression, some mild antagonism may be acceptable, so long as there is good interaction with regard to resistance suppression. Both endpoints (cell kill and resistance suppression) need to be considered when evaluating combination therapy.

β-LACTAM ANTIBIOTICS
Mechanism of Effect

These agents are relatively concentration-independent in their kill rate and have been referred to as concentration-independent or "time-dependent killers." For the time-dependent antibiotics like the β-lactams, concentrations do not have to remain above the MIC for the entire dosing interval. This phenomenon is also related to its mechanism of action, acylation of the β-lactam–binding proteins. The ability of β-lactams to achieve a particular level of acylation of the β-lactam–binding proteins does not occur instantaneously. This is a reaction that takes place over time. This explains why the drug concentrations do not need to exceed the MIC for the full dosing interval. The level of acylation that is required for stasis or maximal cell killing occurs over a period of time that is shorter than the dosing interval, and varies among different types of β-lactams. Craig's laboratory[7] has convincingly shown that to attain a static effect (ie, the number of organisms at the infection site are unchanged at 24 hours from time zero, when therapy is initiated), penicillins require approximately 30% free drug Time>MIC, whereas cephalosporins (and probably monobactams) require 40% free drug Time>MIC. Carbapenems require the lowest amount at about 20% free drug Time>MIC. For near-maximal bacterial cell kill, these numbers are approximately 50%, 60% to 70%, and 40%. There is variability attributable to both the strain examined and the drug examined for these percentages, but they are valuable guides to the microbiological effect that may be expected from a specific dosing regimen.

Clinical Correlation for β-lactams: Prolonged Infusion

Extending the infusion time is a β-lactam dose optimization strategy that is becoming increasing popular in clinical practice to protect against self-plagarism. Administering a dose of a β-lactam agent as an infusion longer than the conventional 0.5- to 1.0-hour infusion duration has 2 main effects. First, it produces a lower peak concentration of the drug. Because the bacterial kill rate for these agents is not concentration-dependent, this does not present a major disadvantage.[7,8,25–27] Second, the drug concentrations remain in excess of the MIC for a longer period of time. Because this is what drives antibacterial effect for β-lactams, this will yield a more favorable PTA profile, especially against organisms with high MIC values. It should also be noted that this can be done with less frequent drug dosing.[15]

Extending the infusion time can be accomplished by either administering continuously throughout the day (continuous infusion) or prolonging the infusion time for a major portion of the dosing interval (prolonged infusion). From a PD profiling viewpoint, the two infusion methodologies yield nearly identical PTA profiles as show in the study by Kim and colleagues (**Fig. 3**).[28] In this study PTA curves for prolonged and continuous infusions of piperacillin/tazobactam (TZP) were indistinguishable and both were superior to the intermittent infusion of TZP for MIC values greater than 4 mg/L.

The low PTA results observed with TZP intermittent dosing for MIC values in excess of 4 mg/L is concerning since the TZP Clinical Laboratory Standards Institute (CLSI) susceptibility breakpoint for non-lactose fermenting Gram-negative bacteria is 64/4 mg/L.[6] The clinical relevance of discordance is highlighted by a study that examined the efficacy of TZP in hospitalized patients with bacteremia due to P aeruginosa.[29] The

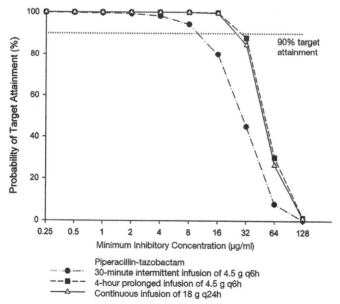

Fig. 3. Probability of achieving 50% fT>MIC for piperacillin/tazobactam regimens containing piperacillin 16 g/d. (*Reprint from* Kim A, Sutherland CA, Kuti JL, et al. Optimal dosing of piperacillin-tazobactam for the treatment of *Pseudomonas aeruginosa* infections: prolonged or continuous infusion? Pharmacotherapy 2007;27(11):1490–7 [Figure 2]; with permission.)

results showed that the 30-day mortality rate was significantly higher among patients treated with TZP versus patients treated with a non-TZP anti-pseudomonal β-lactam with isolates possessing an TZP MIC of either 32 or 64 mg/L (86% vs 22%, P = .004), while there was no significant difference between the 2 treatment groups for isolates with an MIC of up to 16 mg/L (30% vs 21%, P = .673). Collectively, these findings and the results of the TZP MCS studies highlight the importance of considering PTA data when evaluating the utility of an antibiotic dosing scheme. These data also reinforce the idea that appropriate antimicrobial therapy entails more than administering the drug with an "S" beside it on the microbiology laboratory report.

The benefits of prolonged β-lactam infusion among critically ill patients were highlighted by the study performed at Albany Medical Center Hospital.[9,15] Preliminary mathematical modeling and Monte-Carlo simulation demonstrated that a prolonged infusion of piperacillin/tazobactam would optimize the fraction of patients who attained a near-maximal rate of bacterial kill up to and including an MIC value of 16 mg/L of piperacillin. Based on these findings, an automatic switch order was then put in place at Albany Medical Center hospital. Any order for piperacillin/tazobactam 3.375 g every 4 or 6 hours would be automatically switched to an 8-hour dosing interval with a 4-hour prolonged intravenous (IV) infusion of 3.375 g. In a retrospective evaluation of outcomes following this switch, the short (half-hour) infusion was compared with the outcomes seen with the prolonged infusion in patients with infections caused by P aeruginosa.

The comparison groups were well matched, yet the outcomes were markedly different (**Fig. 4**). The outcome was dependent upon the morbidity of the patient,

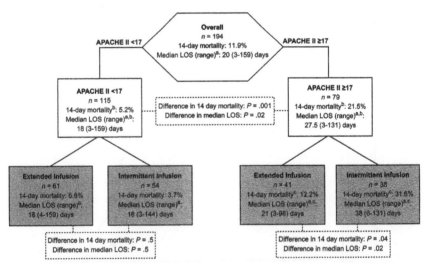

Fig. 4. Comparison of outcomes of patients with APACHE II scores ≥17 and patients with APACHE II scores <17 (the Classification and Regression Tree [CART]-derived breakpoint) who received either an extended infusion of piperacillin-tazobactam or an intermittent infusion of piperacillin-tazobactam. LOS, length of stay. [a]Excludes patients who died within 14 days of collection of P aeruginosa–positive culture sample. [b]Comparison between patients with an APACHE II score <17 and patients with an APACHE II score ≤17 was P<.05. [c]Comparison between the extended group and the intermittent infusion group was P<.05. (*Reprint from* Lodise TP Jr, Lomaestro B, Drusano GL. Piperacillin-tazobactam for *Pseudomonas aeruginosa* infection: clinical implications of an extended-infusion dosing strategy. Clin Infect Dis 2007;44(3):357–63 [Figure 2]; with permission.)

indexed by the Acute Physiology and Chronic Health Evaluation II (APACHE II) score. For the least ill patients, those with APACHE II scores lower than 17, prolonged infusion did not improve the outcome measures (all-cause 14-day mortality and hospital length of stay). In contrast, the most ill patients, those with APACHE II scores of 17 or higher, prolonged infusion contributed to significantly lower all-cause mortality (12.2% in the prolonged infusion group vs 31.6% in the short infusion group; P<.04) and hospital length of stay (median length of stay 21 vs 38 days, respectively; P<.02).[15] In summary, prolonged infusion, which optimizes target attainment for achieving near-maximal bacterial cell kill, provided better measured outcomes among the sicker patient group. Furthermore, the results highlight the importance of examining the influence of treatment within a population at greatest risk for the outcome of interest.

QUINOLONE ANTIMICROBIALS
Mechanism of Action

Quinolones are fully synthetic compounds and they exert their effect by interfering with DNA replication. Early quinolones, such as naladixic acid, had neither the potency nor rate of kill seen with more modern compounds and also suffered from rapid emergence of resistance. The modern quinolones have had a number of structural modifications that result in much greater potency across the spectrum of bacteria.

Quinolones are a classical example of concentration-dependent bacterial killing agent. Like aminoglycosides, as the drug concentration increases, the rate of kill increases. They also induce a moderate persistent or post-antibiotic effect (PAE). Generally, the driver for effect is the AUC/MIC ratio, although, on occasion peak concentration/MIC ratio has been linked to effect, mostly because there is a very tight correlation between these two indices. Interestingly, when one looks at suppression of drug resistance, the pharmacodynamically linked index may differ from that which is linked to rate of bacterial cell kill.[30]

Clinical Correlation for Quinolones

The first pharmacodynamic relationship generated for fluoroquinolones was a retrospective analysis of several studies with ciprofloxacin.[31] Patients mostly had lower respiratory tract infections (n = 58), but there was an admixture of patients with skin/skin structure infection (n = 9), bacteremias (n = 4), and complicated urinary tract infections (n = 3). A significant logistic regression relationship was observed between the AUC/MIC ratio and the probability of a good microbiological outcome. Analysis by a stratified Kaplan-Meier approach also displayed a relationship between the AUC/MIC ratio and the time to eradication of the pathogen. The breakpoints for organism clearance were an AUC/MIC ratio of 125 (main breakpoint) and 250 (secondary breakpoint). Interestingly, whereas the CLSI susceptibility breakpoint is 2 mg/L or less, the probability of maximal dose ciprofloxacin (400 mg IV every 8 hours) at the mean ciprofloxacin clearance in achieving an AUC/MIC ratio of 125 was suboptimal (<90%) for MIC values in excess of 0.5 mg/L. If the clearance at the mean value plus 1 standard deviation is simulated, probability of target attainment is only in excess of 90% for MIC values of 0.25 mg/L or less.

The first prospective pharmacodynamic clinical studies were performed by Drusano and colleagues.[32,33] This group studied the pharmacodynamics of levofloxacin in community-acquired infections and hospital-acquired pneumonia; analysis plans were prospectively filed for both with the Food and Drug Administration. In the community infection study, where a 500-mg levofloxacin dose was used, relationships were identified between outcomes (clinical and microbiologic) and both the AUC/MIC ratio and the peak/MIC ratio. For clinical response, the peak/MIC ratio and primary infection site were the major determinants of a successful outcome (**Fig. 5A**). All urinary tract infections were successfully treated, regardless of the peak/MIC ratio. In contrast, for respiratory tract infections, a 90% probability of a good clinical outcome was attained at a peak concentration/MIC ratio of 8.9, whereas skin and skin structure infections required a peak concentration/MIC ratio of 16.3 for a 90% success rate.[33]

In a nosocomial pneumonia study, levofloxacin AUC/MIC ratio (a 750-mg dose was used) and age were identified as the independent variables of microbiological response.[32] As age increased, the likelihood of eradicating the pathogen decreased (see **Fig. 5B**). In addition, failure to attain an AUC/MIC ratio of 87 had a major effect on eradication. At the median age of patients in the trial (53 years), patients attaining the levofloxacin AUC/MIC ratio of 87 or greater had an 81% probability of pathogen eradication, whereas those who did not had a 51% likelihood of pathogen eradication. It should also be noted that in this study, the probability of attaining the breakpoint value of 87 remained above 90% only at MIC values of 0.5 mg/L or less for levofloxacin 750 mg IV every 24 hours. Clearly, for both ciprofloxacin and levofloxacin, the CLSI sensitivity breakpoint values for gram-negative bacilli are set incorrectly and need to be decreased by several tube dilutions to come in line with these clinical observations. These results also highlight the importance of assessing the likelihood that the selected dosing regimen achieves the pharmacodynamic target of interest for organisms likely to be encountered in clinical practice.

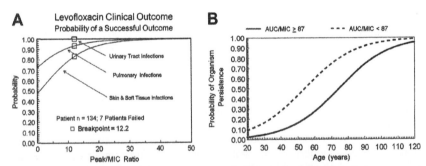

Fig. 5. (A) Levofloxacin clinical outcome probabilities of successful outcome (n = 134 patients; 7 clinical failures). The probability curve for successful clinical outcome versus the ratio of the peak plasma concentration to the minimum inhibitory concentration (peak/MIC) is shown. Breakpoints for the pharmacologic variables indicate the value for which there is a significantly increased probability of successful outcome as determined by classification and regression tree analysis. The figure illustrates the probability curves for successful clinical outcome including peak/MIC ratio and 3 infection sites. (*Reprint from* Preston SL, Drusano GL, Berman AL, et al. Pharmacodynamics of levofloxacin: a new paradigm for early clinical trials. JAMA 1998;279(2):125–9 [Figure 1]; with permission.) (*B*) Probability of eradication of the pathogen, as a function of age and whether the patient achieves an area under the curve (AUC):MIC ratio of ≥87. Patients with younger age and who achieve an AUC:MIC ratio of ≥87 have a significantly higher probability of achieving eradication of their pathogen. Classification and regression tree analysis identified the breakpoint for age as 67 years. (*Reprint from* Drusano GL, Preston SL, Fowler C, et al. Relationship between fluoroquinolone area under the curve: minimum inhibitory concentration ratio and the probability of eradication of the infecting pathogen, in patients with nosocomial pneumonia. J Infect Dis 2004;189(9):1590–97 [Figure 1]; with permission.)

AMINOGLYCOSIDE ANTIBIOTICS
Mechanism of Effect

These agents are the quintessential concentration-dependent killing agents. In contrast to β-lactams, as concentration rises, so does the kill rate, showing little tendency to flatten out. Aminoglycosides exert their concentration-dependent effect through several different distinct mechanisms. Aminoglycosides' primary site of action is the 30S ribosomal subunit in the cytoplasm.

Mechanism of Nephrotoxicity

Aminoglycosides have gone through a period of decreased use, mainly because of their toxic properties, particularly nephrotoxicity. In the ICU, loss of renal function caused by nephrotoxicity may increase mortality by as much as 40%.[34] The basic science behind this toxicity has been well reviewed by Mingeot-Leclercq and Tulkens' laboratory.[35] In brief, aminoglycosides are filtered at the glomerulus. The site of the nephrotoxicity is the proximal renal tubular epithelial cell (PRTE cell). A key factor is that the active transport process leading to nephrotoxicity is saturable. Because it is saturable, dosing of aminoglycosides on a daily basis results in a decreased uptake of the molecule into the PRTE cell. This, in turn, creates a window of opportunity for low likelihood of nephrotoxicity occurrence. In contrast, multiple daily dosing produces higher uptake into the PRTE cells and results in a more rapid manifestation of nephrotoxicity. It is important to note that once-daily or pulse dosing can result in substantial nephrotoxicity if it is administered long enough (typically longer than 7 days).[36,37]

Clinical Correlation for Aminoglycosides: Balancing Effect and Toxicity

Because peak concentrations and AUC are highly correlated, it has been possible to demonstrate that both peak concentration/MIC ratio and AUC/MIC ratio can be linked to outcome.[38] In a retrospective evaluation of patients with hospital-acquired pneumonia, Kashuba and colleagues[38] were able to demonstrate that the peak concentration/MIC ratio and the AUC/MIC ratio were both significantly linked to measures of clinical response (in this case, both temperature defervescence and white blood cell normalization). The response for temperature defervescence is displayed in **Fig. 6**. When examining **Fig. 6**, one can see by inspection that a 90% probability of attaining the endpoint by Day 7 of therapy (a duration driving a low probability of nephrotoxicity) is achieved with an AUC/MIC ratio of approximately 156.

With an understanding of the exposure profile required for maximal effect, it is possible to determine how much toxicity is likely to be induced in a given patient. Toxicity is related to directly to exposure and the degree of toxicity observed will depend on the drug exposure required to achieve an optimal effect. **Fig. 7**A–C shows the aminoglycoside exposure-nephrotoxicity relationship observed in a randomized, double blind comparison of once- versus twice-daily dosing of aminoglycosides.[36,37] There was a major shift in the probability of nephrotoxicity from once-daily to twice-daily dosing. Time to the occurrence of a nephrotoxic event was a function of days of therapy, stratified by whether patients received vancomycin concurrently (see **Fig. 7**A–C). In the absence of concurrent vancomycin use, there was a very small probability of a nephrotoxic event at day 7. In contrast, the likelihood of nephrotoxicity was exacerbated by concurrent administration of vancomycin. It should be pointed out that this Cox model was developed from the twice-daily dosing group. The once-daily dosing group had a low probability of nephrotoxicity even with the coadministration of vancomycin. Consequently, by administering the drug once daily, avoiding concurrent nephrotoxins and limiting duration of therapy to 7 days, these agents can be safely administered in the ICU setting.

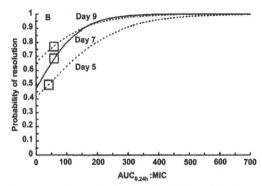

Fig. 6. Probability of temperature resolution by days 5, 7, and 9 of aminoglycoside therapy as determined by logistic regression analysis. Use of AUC_{0-24}/MIC as a predictor variable. Squares indicate breakpoints for the significant predictors as determined by CART analysis. (*Reprint from* Kashuba AD, Nafziger AN, Drusano GL, et al. Optimizing aminoglycoside therapy for nosocomial pneumonia caused by gram-negative bacteria. Antimicrob Agents Chemother 1999;43(3):623–29 [Figure 1]; with permission.)

Knowledge of the concentration-time profiles associated with effect and toxicity can be used to ascertain the overall utility of aminoglycosides in treating serious infections of varying MIC values.[36] **Table 2** displays the likelihood of attaining temperature defervescence at day 7 as a function of MIC with a fixed dosage of 400 mg per day of either gentamicin or tobramycin. Although 400 mg per day provides a high probability of attaining the desired outcome at MIC 0.5 mg/L or less, the likelihood of a successful outcome declines to about 80% at a MIC value of 1.0 mg/L. A MIC value of 2.0 mg/L, which would still be considered susceptible by CLSI guidelines, has a probability of afebrility by day 7 of 53%. Given the possibility of nephrotoxicity and the fact that infections caused by organisms with MIC values greater than 1.0 mg/L have unacceptable probabilities of attaining the desired outcome, even with a 5 mg/kg daily dosage, it is no surprise that clinicians turned away from these agents as new broad-spectrum β-lactam agents became available in the 1980s and 1990s. However, an advanced understanding of the PK and PD of this drug illustrates that they can be administered safely, and with proper dosing, can also provide good clinical outcomes. In this era of resistance, we can turn to these agents once again for the therapy of seriously infected patients.

VANCOMYCIN
Mechanism of Effect

Vancomycin binds to the end of dAla-dAla and interrupts cell wall synthesis. Although a variety of PK and PD monitoring parameters have been suggested for vancomycin, the AUC/MIC ratio appears to be the best predictor of response based on data from animal models and in vitro studies. Collectively, these data suggest that microbiologic success is optimized when the vancomycin AUC/MIC ratio 400 or higher.[39]

Mechanism of Toxicity

Early in its life cycle, vancomycin was associated with significant adverse effects, including infusion-related toxicities, nephrotoxicity, and ototoxicity,[40–42] many of which were largely attributed to impurities in the original formulations. Modern fermentation methods were thought to minimize the onset of these toxicities,

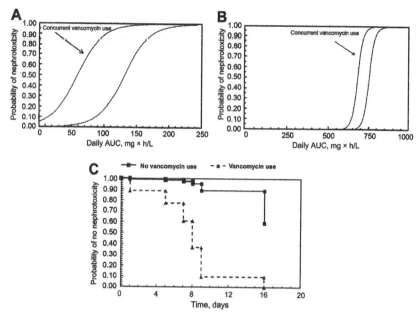

Fig. 7. (*A*) Curve of probability of development of aminoglycoside nephrotoxicity for patients receiving the drug on a twice-daily basis as estimated by multivariate logistic regression analysis. The probability rises as a function of increasing daily exposure to aminoglycoside, as indexed to the AUC. Concurrent vancomycin use provides a marked increase in the probability of nephrotoxicity for equivalent exposure to aminoglycosides, as indexed to the daily AUC. (*B*) Once-daily administration shifts the curves of probability of nephrotoxicity as influenced by daily aminoglycoside AUC to the right. (*Reprint from* Rybak MJ, Abate BJ, Kang SL, et al. Prospective evaluation of the effect of an aminoglycoside dosing regimen on rates of observed nephrotoxicity and ototoxicity. Antimicrob Agents Chemother 1999;43(7):1549–55 [Figure 1]; with permission.) (*C*) Effect of concurrent vancomycin use on the time to the occurrence of nephrotoxicity in patients receiving a twice-daily aminoglycoside regimen. (*Reprint from* Drusano GL, Ambrose PG, Bhavnani SM, et al. Back to the future: using aminoglycosides again and how to dose them optimally. Clin Infect Dis 2007;45(6):753–60 [Figure 2]; with permission.)

particularly nephrotoxicity.[40–42] This notion was supported by early animal model data that demonstrated safety of the "purer" formulations at therapeutic doses.[43]

Although found to be non-nephrotoxic in initial animal model studies, recent animal data suggest that vancomycin is an oxidative stressor in proximal renal tubular cells.[44–49] Additionally, antioxidants and cilastatin have been found to protect against vancomycin-induced kidney damage, further supporting the notion that vancomycin is an oxidative stressor.[47–49] Human data also suggest vancomycin toxicity involves both the proximal tubules and medullary region.[50]

Clinical Correlation for Vancomycin: Balancing Effect and Nephrotoxicity

Although animal and in vitro data suggest the PD target is an AUC/MIC ratio of 400, clinical data are available and remove information is available regarding the relationship between vancomycin exposure and the probability of a good clinical or microbiological outcome. The best data available are from a retrospective evaluation of patients with *Staphylococcus aureus* in a community hospital over

Table 2 Likelihood of attainment of the endpoint of temperature defervescence after a fixed dose of 400 mg per day of either gentamicin or tobramycin as a function of MIC	
MIC Value (mg/L)	Probability of Becoming Afebrile by Day 7
0.25	0.997
0.5	0.948
1.0	0.799
2.0	0.635
4.0	0.635

Abbreviation: MIC, minimum inhibitory concentration.

a 1-year period.[51] Unfortunately, there are a number of limitations to these data. There are only a small number of methicillin-resistant *S aureus* (MRSA) isolates in the database and a number of the patients had combination agent chemotherapy. Nonetheless, a number of different analyses identified exposures between 350 and 400 of AUC/MIC ratio (total drug) as being related to clinical outcome for patients with staphylococcal nosocomial pneumonia. This target plays a major role in the evaluation of vancomycin as a therapeutic agent, particularly with respect to the "MIC-creep" (increase in vancomycin MICs for *S aureus* seen in recent years). With an MIC of 0.5 mg/L, a standard dosage of vancomycin of 1 g every 12 hours provides a reasonable target attainment of 90% with a target of 400 total drug AUC/MIC ratio. When the MIC value increases from 0.5 mg/L to 1.0 or 2.0 mg/L, the target attainment falls to 70% and 22%.[52] These target attainments are clearly suboptimal. This provides the impetus to increase the daily vancomycin dosage to 3 to 4 g per day.

Given the more recent need to increase the dosage to obtain better target attainment rates with increasing MIC values, it was important to examine the consequent nephrotoxicity rates. Lodise and colleagues[53,54] examined this issue in 2 retrospective evaluations. In **Fig. 8**A, the stratified Kaplan-Meier analysis demonstrates that there is a significantly higher rate of nephrotoxicity with higher vancomycin doses. Importantly, there is a linezolid control group included, as linezolid is known to not be associated with nephrotoxicity.[54] In a separate analysis in greater depth, the concentration dependence of vancomycin nephrotoxicity was explored. In **Fig. 8**B, the relationship between vancomycin trough concentration and the probability of nephrotoxicity is displayed. Not surprisingly, there is a major difference in the probability of nephrotoxicity based on residence in the ICU.[53] Given the recommendation for initial trough concentrations of 20 mg/L for serious MRSA infections, one can immediately see that such recommendations will provide a probability of nephrotoxicity of about 35% for patients in the ICU. This allows the immediate inference that if the target of a total drug AUC/MIC ratio is correct, then one cannot attain an appropriate likelihood of a good clinical response without also engendering an unacceptably high likelihood of a nephrotoxic event. This also points out the major importance in identifying a better estimate of the pharmacodynamic target for good clinical response than that currently available. Unfortunately, there is little information available with regard to the protein binding of vancomycin. Previous reports have differed considerably with respect to the amount of free drug.[55] It is, therefore, a high priority to identify the range of protein binding observed clinically for this agent so that the free

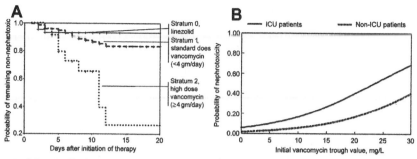

Fig. 8. (*A*) Stratified Kaplan-Meier analysis of time to nephrotoxicity for patients treated with linezolid (stratum 0), those treated with a standard dose of vancomycin (<4 g/d) (stratum 1), and a those treated with a high dose of vancomycin (≥4 g/d) (stratum 2). The overall differences are significant (*P*<.001 by Mantel test). Pairwise analysis demonstrated that strata 0 and 1 are not different. Strata 0 and 2 and strata 1 and 2 are significantly different. For the pairwise analyses, α-decay was performed by Bonferroni adjustment. (*Reprint from* Lodise TP, Lomaestro B, Graves J, et al. Larger vancomycin doses [at least four grams per day] are associated with an increased incidence of nephrotoxicity. Antimicrob Agents Chemother 2008;52(4):1330–36 [Figure 1]; with permission.) (*B*) Graphic representation of the logistic regression–derived nephrotoxicity probability functions. ICU, intensive care unit. (*Reprint from* Lodise TP, Patel N, Lomaestro BM, et al. Relationship between initial vancomycin concentration-time profile and nephrotoxicity among hospitalized patients. Clin Infect Dis 2009;49(4):507–14 [Figure 3]; with permission.)

drug AUC/MIC ratio target can be properly estimated and the true therapeutic window for vancomycin be elucidated for seriously ill patients.

SUMMARY

As patients become sicker and require residence in the intensive care setting, it becomes more and more important to get their antimicrobial chemotherapy right. This requires knowing the organisms and their resistance profile in your specific ICU. It also requires identifying the correct drug or drugs and dosing them according to pharmacodynamic principles, as this will optimize the outcome. Overall optimization of outcome also requires understanding the relationship between exposure and toxicity. Finally, in many instances, particularly in the empiric therapy circumstance, combination therapy becomes a prudent choice. This choice should be optimized for spectrum of activity, maximal cell kill, and ability of the regimen to suppress resistance.

REFERENCES

1. Ibrahim EH, Sherman G, Ward S, et al. The influence of inadequate antimicrobial treatment of bloodstream infections on patient outcomes in the ICU setting. Chest 2000;118:146–55.
2. Kollef MH, Sherman G, Ward S, et al. Inadequate antimicrobial treatment of infections: a risk factor for hospital mortality among critically ill patients. Chest 1999; 115:462–74.
3. Lodise TP Jr, Patel N, Kwa A, et al. Predictors of 30-day mortality among patients with *Pseudomonas aeruginosa* bloodstream infections: impact of delayed appropriate antibiotic selection. Antimicrob Agents Chemother 2007;51:3510–5.
4. Lodise TP, McKinnon PS, Swiderski L, et al. Outcomes analysis of delayed antibiotic treatment for hospital-acquired *Staphylococcus aureus* bacteremia. Clin Infect Dis 2003;36:1418–23.

5. Clinical Laboratory Standards Institute (CLSI). Performance standards for antimicrobial susceptibility testing; twentieth informational supplement. CLSI document M100-S20. Wayne (PA): Clinical and Laboratory Standards Institute; 2010.

6. Clinical and Laboratory Standards Institute/NCCLS Performance standards for antimicrobial disc diffusion tests; Approved standards. CLSI Document M2-M9. 9th edition. Wayne (PA): Clinical and Laboratory Standards Institute; 2006.

7. Craig WA. Pharmacokinetic/pharmacodynamic parameters: rationale for antibacterial dosing of mice and men. Clin Infect Dis 1998;26:1–10 [quiz: 1–2].

8. Drusano GL. Antimicrobial pharmacodynamics: critical interactions of 'bug and drug'. Nat Rev Microbiol 2004;2:289–300.

9. Lodise TP, Lomaestro BM, Drusano GL. Application of antimicrobial pharmacodynamic concepts into clinical practice: focus on beta-lactam antibiotics: insights from the Society of Infectious Diseases Pharmacists. Pharmacotherapy 2006; 26:1320–32.

10. Merrikin DJ, Briant J, Rolinson GN. Effect of protein binding on antibiotic activity in vivo. J Antimicrob Chemother 1983;11:233–8.

11. Bilello JA, Drusano GL. Relevance of plasma protein binding to antiviral activity and clinical efficacy of inhibitors of human immunodeficiency virus protease. J Infect Dis 1996;173:1524–6.

12. Tsuji BT, Bulitta JB, Kelchlin PA, et al. Determining the active fraction of daptomycin against MRSA by evaluating bactericidal activity in the presence of protein and pharmacodynamic (PD) modeling. Poster Presentation at the 49th Interscience Conference on Antimicrobial Agents and Chemotherapy. San Francisco (CA), 2009;A1–1270.

13. Drusano GL, Johnson DE, Rosen M, et al. Pharmacodynamics of a fluoroquinolone antimicrobial agent in a neutropenic rat model of Pseudomonas sepsis. Antimicrob Agents Chemother 1993;37:483–90.

14. Drusano GL, Preston SL, Hardalo C, et al. Use of preclinical data for selection of a phase II/III dose for evernimicin and identification of a preclinical MIC breakpoint. Antimicrob Agents Chemother 2001;45:13–22.

15. Lodise TP Jr, Lomaestro B, Drusano GL. Piperacillin-tazobactam for Pseudomonas aeruginosa infection: clinical implications of an extended-infusion dosing strategy. Clin Infect Dis 2007;44:357–63.

16. Lodise TP Jr, Lomaestro B, Rodvold KA, et al. Pharmacodynamic profiling of piperacillin in the presence of tazobactam in patients through the use of population pharmacokinetic models and Monte Carlo simulation. Antimicrob Agents Chemother 2004;48:4718–24.

17. Lodise TP Jr, Pypstra R, Kahn JB, et al. Probability of target attainment for ceftobiprole as derived from a population pharmacokinetic analysis of 150 subjects. Antimicrob Agents Chemother 2007;51:2378–87.

18. Mouton JW, Schmitt-Hoffmann A, Shapiro S, et al. Use of Monte Carlo simulations to select therapeutic doses and provisional breakpoints of BAL9141. Antimicrob Agents Chemother 2004;48:1713–8.

19. Lodise TP, Sorgel F, Mason B, et al. Penetration of meropenem into epithelial lining fluid of patients with ventilator-associated pneumonia [abstract 1889]. Presented at the 48th Interscience Conference on Antimicrobial Agents and Chemotherapy/46th Annual Meeting of the Infectious Diseases Society of America. Washington, DC, October 2008.

20. Jumbe N, Louie A, Leary R, et al. Application of a mathematical model to prevent in vivo amplification of antibiotic-resistant bacterial populations during therapy. J Clin Invest 2003;112:275–85.

21. Tam VH, Louie A, Fritsche TR, et al. Impact of drug-exposure intensity and duration of therapy on the emergence of *Staphylococcus aureus* resistance to a quinolone antimicrobial. J Infect Dis 2007;195:1818–27.
22. Drusano GL, Liu W, Fregeau C, et al. Differing effects of combination chemotherapy with meropenem and tobramycin on cell kill and suppression of resistance of wild-type *Pseudomonas aeruginosa* PAO1 and its isogenic MexAB efflux pump-overexpressed mutant. Antimicrob Agents Chemother 2009;53:2266–73.
23. Louie A, Grasso C, Bahniuk N, et al. The combination of meropenem and levofloxacin is synergistic with respect to both *Pseudomonas aeruginosa* kill rate and resistance suppression. Antimicrob Agents Chemother 2010;54:2646–54.
24. Gumbo T, Louie A, Deziel MR, et al. Selection of a moxifloxacin dose that suppresses drug resistance in Mycobacterium tuberculosis, by use of an in vitro pharmacodynamic infection model and mathematical modeling. J Infect Dis 2004;190:1642–51.
25. Craig WA, Andes D. Pharmacokinetics and pharmacodynamics of antibiotics in otitis media. Pediatr Infect Dis J 1996;15:255–9.
26. Craig WA. Interrelationship between pharmacokinetics and pharmacodynamics in determining dosage regimens for broad-spectrum cephalosporins. Diagn Microbiol Infect Dis 1995;22:89–96.
27. Drusano GL. How does a patient maximally benefit from anti-infective chemotherapy? Clin Infect Dis 2004;39:1245–6.
28. Kim A, Sutherland CA, Kuti JL, et al. Optimal dosing of piperacillin-tazobactam for the treatment of *Pseudomonas aeruginosa* infections: prolonged or continuous infusion? Pharmacotherapy 2007;27:1490–7.
29. Tam VH, Gamez EA, Weston JS, et al. Outcomes of bacteremia due to *Pseudomonas aeruginosa* with reduced susceptibility to piperacillin-tazobactam: implications on the appropriateness of the resistance breakpoint. Clin Infect Dis 2008;46:862–7.
30. Drusano GL. Prevention of resistance: a goal for dose selection for antimicrobial agents. Clin Infect Dis 2003;36:S42–50.
31. Forrest A, Nix DE, Ballow CH, et al. Pharmacodynamics of intravenous ciprofloxacin in seriously ill patients. Antimicrob Agents Chemother 1993;37:1073–81.
32. Drusano GL, Preston SL, Fowler C, et al. Relationship between fluoroquinolone area under the curve: minimum inhibitory concentration ratio and the probability of eradication of the infecting pathogen, in patients with nosocomial pneumonia. J Infect Dis 2004;189:1590–7.
33. Preston SL, Drusano GL, Berman AL, et al. Pharmacodynamics of levofloxacin: a new paradigm for early clinical trials. JAMA 1998;279:125–9.
34. Uchino S, Kellum JA, Bellomo R, et al. Acute renal failure in critically ill patients: a multinational, multicenter study. JAMA 2005;294:813–8.
35. Mingeot-Leclercq MP, Tulkens PM. Aminoglycosides: nephrotoxicity. Antimicrob Agents Chemother 1999;43:1003–12.
36. Drusano GL, Ambrose PG, Bhavnani SM, et al. Back to the future: using aminoglycosides again and how to dose them optimally. Clin Infect Dis 2007;45:753–60.
37. Rybak MJ, Abate BJ, Kang SL, et al. Prospective evaluation of the effect of an aminoglycoside dosing regimen on rates of observed nephrotoxicity and ototoxicity. Antimicrob Agents Chemother 1999;43:1549–55.
38. Kashuba AD, Nafziger AN, Drusano GL, et al. Optimizing aminoglycoside therapy for nosocomial pneumonia caused by gram-negative bacteria. Antimicrob Agents Chemother 1999;43:623–9.
39. Rybak MJ, Lomaestro BM, Rotschafer JC, et al. Therapeutic monitoring of vancomycin in adults: summary of consensus recommendations from the American

Society of Health-System Pharmacists, the Infectious Diseases Society of America, and the Society of Infectious Diseases Pharmacists. Pharmacotherapy 2009;29: 1275–9.

40. Moellering RC Jr. Vancomycin: a 50-year reassessment. Clin Infect Dis 2006; 42(Suppl 1):S3–4.

41. Rybak MJ. The pharmacokinetic and pharmacodynamic properties of vancomycin. Clin Infect Dis 2006;42(Suppl 1):S35–9.

42. Levine DP. Vancomycin: a history. Clin Infect Dis 2006;42(Suppl 1):S5–12.

43. Aronoff GR, Sloan RS, Dinwiddie CB Jr, et al. Effects of vancomycin on renal function in rats. Antimicrob Agents Chemother 1981;19:306–8.

44. King DW, Smith MA. Proliferative responses observed following vancomycin treatment in renal proximal tubule epithelial cells. Toxicol In Vitro 2004;18: 797–803.

45. Celik I, Cihangiroglu M, Ilhan N, et al. Protective effects of different antioxidants and amrinone on vancomycin-induced nephrotoxicity. Basic Clin Pharmacol Toxicol 2005;97:325–32.

46. Oktem F, Arslan MK, Ozguner F, et al. In vivo evidences suggesting the role of oxidative stress in pathogenesis of vancomycin-induced nephrotoxicity: protection by erdosteine. Toxicology 2005;215:227–33.

47. Cetin H, Olgar S, Oktem F, et al. Novel evidence suggesting an anti-oxidant property for erythropoietin on vancomycin-induced nephrotoxicity in a rat model. Clin Exp Pharmacol Physiol 2007;34:1181–5.

48. Hodoshima N, Nakano Y, Izumi M, et al. Protective effect of inactive ingredients against nephrotoxicity of vancomycin hydrochloride in rats. Drug Metab Pharmacokinet 2004;19:68–75.

49. Toyoguchi T, Takahashi S, Hosoya J, et al. Nephrotoxicity of vancomycin and drug interaction study with cilastatin in rabbits. Antimicrob Agents Chemother 1997;41: 1985–90.

50. Le Moyec L, Racine S, Le Toumelin P, et al. Aminoglycoside and glycopeptide renal toxicity in intensive care patients studied by proton magnetic resonance spectroscopy of urine. Crit Care Med 2002;30:1242–5.

51. Moise-Broder PA, Forrest A, Birmingham MC, et al. Pharmacodynamics of vancomycin and other antimicrobials in patients with Staphylococcus aureus lower respiratory tract infections. Clin Pharmacokinet 2004;43:925–42.

52. Patel N, Grifasi M, Pai M, et al. Vancomycin: we can not get there from here [abstract #193]. Poster Presentation at the 47th Annual Meeting of the Infectious Diseases Society of America. Philadelphia, October 2009.

53. Lodise TP, Patel N, Lomaestro BM, et al. Relationship between initial vancomycin concentration-time profile and nephrotoxicity among hospitalized patients. Clin Infect Dis 2009;49:507–14.

54. Lodise TP, Lomaestro B, Graves J, et al. Larger vancomycin doses (at least four grams per day) are associated with an increased incidence of nephrotoxicity. Antimicrob Agents Chemother 2008;52:1330–6.

55. Berthoin K, Ampe E, Tulkens PM, et al. Correlation between free and total vancomycin serum concentrations in patients treated for gram-positive infections. Int J Antimicrob Agents 2009;34:555–60.

Antimicrobial Pharmacokinetic and Pharmacodynamic Issues in the Critically Ill with Severe Sepsis and Septic Shock

Julie M. Varghese, BPharm (Hons)[a],
Jason A. Roberts, PhD, BPharm (Hons), FSHP[a,b,c],
Jeffrey Lipman, MBBCh, FCICM, MD[a,b],*

KEYWORDS
• Pharmacokinetics • Pharmacodynamics
• Volume of distribution • Clearance • Renal failure
• Renal replacement therapy

Severe sepsis and septic shock are a major challenge for critical care clinicians because of the associated high rates of morbidity and mortality. In the United States, the estimated incidence of severe sepsis is ~3 cases per 1000 population with mortality of 28.6% (215,000 deaths from 750,000 patients diagnosed) per year.[1] Septicemia was listed as the 10th leading cause of death in the United States in 2007.[2]

In critically ill patients with sepsis and septic shock, early and appropriate antimicrobial therapy has been shown to be the predominant factor for reducing mortality.[3,4]

Financial support: National Health and Medical Research Council of Australia (Project Grant 519702; Australian Based Health Professional Research Fellowship 569917).
[a] Burns, Trauma and Critical Care Research Centre, The University of Queensland, Level 7 Block 6, Royal Brisbane & Women's Hospital, Brisbane Queensland 4029, Australia
[b] Department of Intensive Care Medicine, Royal Brisbane and Women's Hospital, Level 3 Ned Hanlon Building, Butterfield Street, Herston, Brisbane 4029, Australia
[c] Department of Pharmacy, Royal Brisbane and Women's Hospital, Level 1 Ned Hanlon Building, Butterfield Street, Herston, Brisbane 4029, Australia
* Corresponding author. Department of Intensive Care Medicine, Royal Brisbane and Women's Hospital, Level 3 Ned Hanlon Building, Butterfield Street, Herston, Brisbane 4029, Australia.
E-mail address: j.lipman@uq.edu.au

Crit Care Clin 27 (2011) 19–34
doi:10.1016/j.ccc.2010.09.006
0749-0704/11/$ – see front matter
criticalcare.theclinics.com

Severe sepsis is defined as sepsis with the failure or dysfunction of more than 1 organ; septic shock is defined as hypotension in the setting of severe sepsis that is unresponsive to fluid resuscitation.[5] The pathophysiologic changes that occur during sepsis, severe sepsis, and septic shock can lead to changes in pharmacokinetic parameters that affect the achievement of pharmacodynamic targets for antimicrobial therapy. This may adversely affect efficacy of antimicrobial therapy in this group of critically ill patients.[6]

This article provides a systematic review of the data on the effect of severe sepsis and septic shock on the pharmacokinetics of antimicrobials and the likely consequences for antimicrobial effect. A rational framework for antimicrobial dosing in these complex patients is also provided.

INTERRELATIONSHIP BETWEEN PHARMACOKINETICS AND PHARMACODYNAMICS

An understanding of pharmacokinetics (PK) and pharmacodynamics (PD) is essential to understand the effect of the many pathophysiologic changes in critically ill patients on antimicrobial concentrations, both in blood and in tissues. Knowledge of PK and PD can be used to personalize dosing to achieve optimized antimicrobial therapy.

PK describes the relationship between the dose administered and the changes in the drug concentration in the body with time. PD, on the other hand, describes the relationship between drug concentration and its pharmacologic effect. **Fig. 1** highlights the relationship between PK and PD. The relevant pharmacokinetic parameters for drug dosing are defined in **Table 1**.

Clearance (CL) and apparent volume of distribution (V_d) can be considered the 2 pharmacokinetic parameters that influence drug dosing most. Half-life ($t_{1/2}$) is related to CL and V_d as represented in the following equation:

$$t_{1/2} = \frac{0.693 \times V_d}{CL} \tag{1}$$

First principles suggest that initial dosing of a drug is determined by V_d, whereas maintenance dosing should be based on clearance. Alterations in CL and V_d of a drug can occur as a result of the pathophysiologic changes during severe sepsis

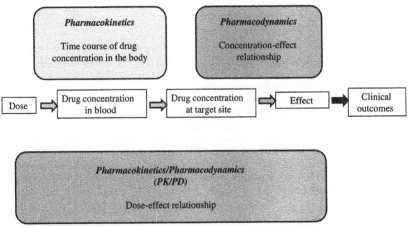

Fig. 1. The relationship between pharmacokinetics (PK) and pharmacodynamics (PD).

Table 1
Relevant PK parameters for drug dosing

PK Parameter	Definition	Description
Clearance (CL)	The volume of blood cleared of drug per unit time	CL measures the irreversible elimination of a drug from the body by excretion and/or metabolism
Volume of distribution (V_d)	Apparent volume of fluid that contains the total drug dose administered at the same concentration as in the plasma	V_d is the parameter that relates the total amount of drug in the body to the plasma concentration
Half-life ($t_{1/2}$)	Time required for the plasma drug concentration to decrease by half	Half-life is dependent on CL and V_d; half-life is increased with a decrease in CL or an increase in V_d
C_{max}	Peak drug concentration during a dosing interval	
C_{min}	Minimum drug concentration during a dosing interval	
AUC_{0-24}	Area under the concentration-time curve from 0 to 24 h	

and septic shock. An understanding of the interrelationship between pathophysiology and PK is of importance to adjust empiric dosing to meet the specific needs of the individual patient to achieve the pharmacodynamic targets associated with maximal antimicrobial efficacy.

Different antimicrobial classes have different PK/PD indices correlated with optimal antimicrobial activity.[7] These are summarized in **Table 2**. Drug dosing regimens should take into consideration the different pharmacodynamic kill characteristics and PK/PD targets for the prescribed antimicrobial, as well as the susceptibility of the organism(s) targeted, to achieve optimal antimicrobial activity.

A general understanding of the physicochemical properties of antimicrobials (eg, degree of hydrophilicity) is useful to further explain the likely pharmacokinetic and pharmacodynamic changes in critically ill patients. **Table 3** provides a summary of the general characteristics of hydrophilic antimicrobials compared with lipophilic agents.

CHANGES IN DISTRIBUTION
Volume of Distribution and Fluid Shifts

The pathogenesis of sepsis is complex and involves the release of endotoxins and exotoxins from pathogens.[8] Endotoxins such as lipopolysaccharides (gram-negative organisms) and lipotechoic acid (gram-positive organisms) are structural components of the bacterial cell wall.[8] Exotoxins are actively secreted toxins mainly produced by gram-positive organisms.[9] These toxins result in the production of various endogenous mediators that can cause endothelial damage and thus increased capillary permeability.[8,10,11] This capillary leak results in fluid shifting from the intravascular space into the interstitial space in a phenomenon described as third spacing. This process serves to increase the V_d for hydrophilic antimicrobials,[12,13] thus resulting in lower plasma and tissue antimicrobial concentrations. Lipophilic drugs, on the other hand, distribute to a greater extent intracellularly and/or into adipose tissue, and

Table 2
PK/PD indices of significance for antimicrobials

Antibiotic Classification	PK/PD Index	Definition of PK/PD Index	Examples of Antibiotics
Time-dependent	T>MIC	Percentage time for which the concentration of a drug remains more than the minimum inhibitory concentration (MIC) during a dosing interval	Beta-lactams Carbapenems Lincosamides
Concentration-dependent	C_{max}/MIC	Ratio of the peak drug concentration to the MIC of the pathogen	Aminoglycosides
Concentration-dependent with time dependence	AUC_{0-24}/MIC	Ratio of the area under the concentration-time curve (AUC) during a 24-h period to the MIC of the pathogen	Fluoroquinolones Glycopeptides Tigecycline

therefore generally have larger V_d to start with and are not greatly influenced by these fluid shifts.

By definition, septic shock is associated with hypotension and initial management is by administration of boluses of intravenous fluids to increase blood pressure. In the presence of increased capillary permeability, administration of large volumes of fluid

Table 3
PK characteristics of antimicrobials based on classification according to hydrophilicity and lipophilicity in general ward patients (General PK) compared with altered PK observed in critically ill patients

	General PK		Altered PK in Critically Ill
Hydrophilic antibiotics	Low	V_d	↑ V_d
	Predominantly renal	CL	↑ or ↓ depending on renal function
	Poor intracellular penetration	Distribution	↓ Interstitial penetration
	Examples: Beta-lactams, carbapenems, aminoglycosides, glycopeptides, linezolid		
Lipophilic antibiotics	High	V_d	Unchanged
	Predominantly hepatic	CL	↑ or ↓ depending on hepatic function
	Good intracellular penetration	Distribution	Unchanged interstitial penetration
	Examples: fluoroquinolones, macrolides, tigecycline, lincosamides		

can lead to an expansion of fluid volume in the interstitial space and an increase in the V_d for hydrophilic antimicrobials. Other possible reasons for edema and fluid retention in critically ill patients may include cardiac failure or renal failure, both of which may also serve to increase V_d of hydrophilic antimicrobials.

Tissue Perfusion, Tissue Penetration, and Target Site Distribution of Antimicrobials

Most infections occur in the interstitial fluid of tissues and may be considered the site of most infections.[14] During septic shock, microvascular perfusion is diminished which, in turn, leads to impaired distribution of drugs to sites of infection, such as soft tissue.

Impaired tissue penetration in patients with severe sepsis and septic shock can be attributed to capillary leakage, tissue edema, and microvascular failure. Several studies have utilized an in vivo sampling technique known as microdialysis in critically ill patients with sepsis and septic shock to measure antimicrobial concentrations in interstitial fluid.[15–18] A study by Joukhadar and colleagues[16] showed that in patients with septic shock, the concentration of piperacillin in interstitial fluid was 5 to 10 times lower than the corresponding plasma concentrations. In this study, interstitial fluid concentrations in healthy volunteers was observed to be 3- to 4-fold higher compared with interstitial fluid concentrations in patients with septic shock. Roberts and colleagues[19] studied piperacillin penetration into interstitial fluid in patients with sepsis and observed subcutaneous tissue concentrations to be 1 to 5 times lower than plasma concentrations. The difference in the level of sickness severity (septic shock vs sepsis) may explain the observed difference in the tissue interstitial fluid concentrations in these studies for piperacillin, where the greater impairment of microvascular perfusion in patients with septic shock is associated with much lower tissue antimicrobial concentrations compared with that observed in patients with sepsis. Higher plasma concentrations may be required to achieve the target concentrations needed in tissues, especially when poor tissue penetration is suspected, such as during septic shock.

Selection and dosing of antimicrobials in patients with severe sepsis and septic shock should consider the potential sites of infection and whether adequate concentrations will be achieved at the focus of infection. For example, in the treatment of bacterial meningitis, penetration of most antimicrobials, including beta-lactams, into the cerebrospinal fluid is limited and high-dose therapy is recommended for this reason.

Protein Binding and Hypoalbuminemia

Albumin, the predominant plasma protein that binds to acidic drugs, is a negative acute phase protein and is often low in critically ill patients. Hypoalbuminemia in critically ill patients with sepsis is mainly caused by increased capillary permeability and leakage into extravascular space,[20] as well as decreased synthesis in the liver. Low plasma albumin levels cause an increase in the unbound (ie, free) fraction of drugs that are usually bound to this protein. Increased unbound concentrations result in increased tissue distribution because it is only the unbound drug that distributes. However, the increased fluid loading that is required in critically ill patients in response to fluid shifts during an acute phase response, means that the interstitial fluid volume in tissues increases. This causes the tissue concentration of antibiotic to remain low, despite the increased amount of drug that has distributed. This effect is particularly significant for highly protein-bound antimicrobials such as ceftriaxone, ertapenem, teicoplanin, and flucloxacillin.[12,21–23] The increased V_d is associated with low plasma concentrations, in which case, larger, or more frequent doses, or modified dosing regimens such as continuous infusion may be required to meet pharmacodynamic targets for these highly protein-bound agents. An initial loading dose may also be required in this situation to account for the increased V_d and ensure adequate drug concentrations are achieved early during antimicrobial therapy.

A recent study examining the PK of flucloxacillin in critically ill patients with hypoalbuminemia observed subtherapeutic unbound plasma levels of flucloxacillin.[23] This highlights the importance of measuring unbound concentrations of highly protein-bound antimicrobials, rather than total concentration alone, as the unbound fraction can change during severe sepsis and septic shock and only the unbound drug confers antimicrobial effect.

CHANGES IN CL
Increased Cardiac Output and Increased CL

The initial hyperdynamic state of sepsis is associated with a high cardiac output and, thus, increased renal blood flow resulting in increased CL of drugs eliminated by glomerular filtration. The administration of fluid as well as the use of inotropes during severe sepsis and septic shock can also lead to an early increase in cardiac output and increased glomerular filtration rate. Hydrophilic antimicrobials are predominantly cleared by the kidneys and increased renal CL results in lower plasma concentrations. Septic shock with renal dysfunction, on the other hand, translates to lower glomerular filtration rates and decreased CL.

Only the unbound or free fraction of a drug can be cleared by the body. Hypoalbuminemia as previously discussed results in an increase in the unbound fraction of highly protein-bound drugs. This translates to an increased renal CL particularly for highly protein-bound hydrophilic antimicrobials.

End-Organ Dysfunction and Decreased CL

Decreased organ perfusion that occurs with sepsis can lead to the development of organ dysfunction including renal and/or hepatic dysfunction. In general, decreased CL and/or metabolism of drugs will result in accumulation of drugs and/or metabolites with the possibility of increased risk of toxicity. It follows that dose reductions need to be considered for these patients, taking into consideration possible alternative mechanisms of CL that may be upregulated in the presence of isolated organ dysfunction.

Renal Replacement Therapy

Sepsis is the most common cause of acute kidney injury and continuous renal replacement therapy (RRT) is often prescribed to remove fluid and wastes from the body. There are different forms of RRT available and different centers use different modes of RRT with different settings. The principles of antimicrobial dosing during continuous renal replacement therapy (CRRT) have recently been reviewed.[24] Multiple factors including the physicochemical properties of the drug, dialysis settings, and patient-related factors can influence the PK of antimicrobials in patients undergoing RRT.[25]

Extended daily dialysis (EDD) is a hybrid form of dialysis that generally runs for 8–12 hours a day and has the combined advantages of intermittent hemodialysis (IHD) and CRRT. This form of dialysis is increasingly being used in some centers and a few recent studies have examined antimicrobial PK in EDD.[26–28] Additional factors that need to be considered include the timing of antimicrobial dosing in relation to EDD treatment and the possible need for supplemental antimicrobial dosing after an EDD session.[29]

Extracorporeal Membrane Oxygenation

Extracorporeal membrane oxygenation (ECMO) may influence antimicrobial kinetics through increasing the V_d for a drug as well as through possible binding of drugs in the ECMO circuit.[30,31] In practice, in the absence of informative data, therapeutic drug monitoring of antimicrobials is recommended where possible in critically ill patients treated with ECMO.

Plasma Exchange

Plasma exchange is a treatment modality that may influence antimicrobial concentrations as a result of extracorporeal removal of drugs.[32] During the procedure, plasma proteins are removed from the body and plasma losses are replaced with donor human albumin. Drugs with a low V_d (<0.3 L/kg) and high protein binding are most likely to be removed during plasma exchange and may require dose adjustments.[33,34] Highly protein-bound drugs such as ceftriaxone and teicoplanin, for example, have been shown to be significantly affected by plasma exchange.[35,36]

CHANGES IN METABOLISM

Decreased hepatic blood flow as a result of sepsis may cause a decrease in drug metabolism.[37] Hepatic metabolism of drugs with a high extraction ratio is primarily dependent on the blood flow. For drugs with a low extraction ratio, metabolism is dependent on the unbound fraction and/or the activity of hepatic enzymes. Clindamycin, for example, has a low extraction ratio and has been shown to have decreased clearance during the hyperdynamic state of sepsis.[38] This antimicrobial is highly bound to alpha$_1$-acid glycoprotein, an acute phase protein that is increased in critical illness. The observed decreased hepatic clearance of clindamycin in sepsis/septic shock is possibly caused by a decrease in enzyme activity or a decrease in fraction unbound considering only the unbound fraction of drug can be cleared hepatically. Decrease in CYP3A4 activity has also been observed in animal models of endotoxin-induced shock.[39]

CHANGES IN ABSORPTION

Critically ill patients with sepsis are not normally administered drugs via the oral route, but if the oral route is used absorption into the systemic circulation is expected to be low. During septic shock, blood flow is directed preferentially to vital organs such as the brain, heart, and lungs. Organs such as the kidney and the gastrointestinal tract become less well perfused. Poor blood perfusion to the peripheries also impairs the systemic absorption of drugs from muscles and subcutaneous tissues. The intravenous route of administration is thus preferred because of the unreliable systemic drug absorption by other routes.

EFFECT OF PK/PD ON SPECIFIC ANTIMICROBIAL CLASSES
Beta-lactams

Beta-lactams are the most commonly prescribed class of antimicrobials and include penicillins and cephalosporins. In general, beta-lactams are hydrophilic in nature and thus predominantly renally cleared with the exception of ceftriaxone and oxacillin, which undergo biliary clearance. Variability exists in terms of protein binding, with high protein binding (~90%) well recognized for ceftriaxone and flucloxacillin.

Beta-lactam antimicrobials have a slow concentration-independent continuous kill characteristic and the time for which the free (or unbound) antimicrobial concentration is maintained above the minimum inhibitory concentration (MIC), $fT_{>MIC}$ is the PK/PD index best correlated to efficacy.[7] A recent study with cefepime and ceftazidime has suggested that a $fT_{>MIC}$ of 100% is associated with better clinical and microbiological cure in serious bacterial infections.[40] Changes in V_d and CL that occur in patients with sepsis can influence the maintenance of adequate $fT_{>MIC}$ for beta-lactams. Some studies of beta-lactams in critically ill patients with sepsis have observed an increased V_d compared with patients who are not critically ill.[12,13] Pharmacokinetic studies of cefepime and cefpirome in critically ill patients with normal serum creatinine levels have shown subtherapeutic plasma levels and high antimicrobial CL with renal elimination linearly related to creatinine clearance.[41] Some patients with normal serum creatinine levels may have large creatinine clearances (more than the generally reported maximum of 120 mL/min) and creatinine clearance was shown to be an independent predictor of antimicrobial clearance.[11] In these patients, measured creatinine clearances may be useful to identify or predict patients who are at risk of underdosing because of increased renal CL. An 8-, 12- or 24-hour creatinine clearance collection[42,43] is the most practical and accurate method to measure renal function in these cases, although a 2-hour creatinine clearance has been shown to be an appropriate substitute.[44]

Pharmacokinetic modeling and dosing simulation indicate that an improved pharmacodynamic profile is achieved with more frequent dosing or extended or continuous infusion (for a fixed total dose) of beta-lactams in critically ill patients.[45–49] This is of particular value for patients with increased renal CL and/or large V_d especially when targeting bacteria with high MICs and subtherapeutic antimicrobial concentrations are likely to result from the pathophysiologic changes that occur during sepsis.[13,19,45,50,51]

Carbapenems

Carbapenems generally have similar kill characteristics to other beta-lactams although the carbapenems do exhibit some postantimicrobial effects (PAE).[7] In vitro data for carbapenems suggest that $fT_{>MIC}$ of at least 40% is required for antibacterial activity. Increased V_d and CL has been observed for carbapenems in critically ill patients.[52,53] Pharmacokinetic studies along with pharmacodynamic modeling indicate that PK/PD targets are better achieved through administration as an extended or continuous infusion.[54–56]

Aminoglycosides

Aminoglycosides have concentration-dependent kill characteristics where a C_{max}/MIC of at least 10 is the PK/PD index related to clinical success.[57] This class also displays a PAE whereby antibacterial activity is prolonged even when drug concentrations decrease to less than the MIC.[58] These PK/PD characteristics support the recommendation for extended interval dosing of aminoglycosides. High trough concentrations of aminoglycosides are related to toxicity with increased risk of toxicity associated with increased drug exposure.

Critically ill patients often display increased V_d for aminoglycosides[59–61] and this translates to decreased C_{max}. Increased sickness severity as measured by the APACHE II score has been shown to be related to higher V_d for aminoglycosides.[62] Weight-based initial dosing of 7 mg/kg for gentamicin and tobramycin, and 20 mg/kg for amikacin is recommended and therapeutic drug monitoring should be performed after the first dose. Once available, the MIC for the pathogen(s) allows further dose adjustments to achieve PK/PD targets.

Glycopeptides

Vancomycin displays moderate protein binding, whereas teicoplanin is highly protein bound.[63] In patients with hypoalbuminemia, increased V_d and CL are possible for teicoplanin because of an increase in the unbound fraction of the drug.[22,64] A teicoplanin loading dose of 6 mg/kg every 12 hours for at least 3 doses followed by once-daily dosing is recommended.[65]

Increased capillary permeability and fluid shifts in the critically ill can lead to increased V_d for vancomycin.[66–68] The optimal PK/PD target for optimal antibacterial activity of vancomycin is not well understood. In vitro and animal studies demonstrate that bacterial killing of vancomycin is time dependent (T>MIC).[69] A neutropenic mouse model demonstrated that area under the curve AUC/MIC ratio is the best predictor of antibacterial activity although a non-neutropenic mouse model demonstrated that C_{max}/MIC was the PK/PD index determining efficacy.[69,70]

In practice, therapeutic drug monitoring of vancomycin in the form of trough concentration monitoring is recommended aiming for C_{min} of between 15 and 20 mg/L to achieve a target AUC/MIC ratio of at least 400 for eradication of *Staphylococcus aureus*.[71] Maintenance doses of up to 30 to 40 mg/kg/d may be required in critically ill patients with increased V_d and/or increased CL to achieve adequate antimicrobial concentrations. Vancomycin can be administered by continuous infusion to improve the PD and to minimize the risk of toxicity associated with the use of large intermittent doses.[72] In patients with renal impairment, dose reduction of glycopeptides is warranted to minimize the risk of toxicity.

Fluoroquinolones

Fluoroquinolones are lipophilic antimicrobials and fluid shifts in critically ill patients have minimal effect on the V_d of this class of antimicrobials.[73] Fluoroquinolones display concentration-dependent kill characteristic with time-dependent effects. In vitro studies have shown that a C_{max}/MIC ratio of 10 is the PK/PD parameter correlated to bacterial eradication.[74] Peak drug concentration may be decreased as a result of fluid shifts in critically ill patients. An AUC/MIC>125 has been shown to be the PK/PD target for ciprofloxacin against gram-negative pathogens for clinical and microbiological cure in critically ill patients.[75]

The results from several pharmacokinetic studies of ciprofloxacin in critically ill patients suggest that a total daily dose of 1200 mg is required in patients with normal renal function to achieve the PK/PD targets that maximize bacterial kill.[76–78] High doses of intravenous ciprofloxacin of up to 1200 mg per day (ie, 600 mg every 12 hours or 400 mg every 8 hours) in patients with normal renal function seem to be safe. Subtherapeutic fluoroquinolone concentrations, on the other hand, have been associated with the emergence of resistance.[79,80] Selection of antimicrobial resistance is associated with suboptimal drug exposure as defined by AUC/MIC<100.[81] The goal for dosing fluoroquinolones is to ensure maximal antimicrobial exposure to maximize achievement of PK/PD target as well as minimize the development of resistance.

Lincosamides

Clindamycin and lincomycin are lipophilic in nature and $fT_{>MIC}$ is the PK/PD index related to efficacy. Unbound drug concentrations should exceed the MIC for at least 40% to 50% of the dosing interval for optimal antimicrobial activity.[82] In critically ill patients with sepsis, hepatic CL of clindamycin has been shown to decrease.[38] Decreased doses are required for clindamycin and lincomycin in patients with hepatic dysfunction. Lincomycin requires dose adjustment in renal impairment.

Linezolid

Linezolid is an oxazolidinone antibacterial that has a weak, reversible, nonselective monoamine oxidase inhibitory activity and the potential for drug interactions should be considered when prescribing this agent. Linezolid is predominantly metabolized in the liver and the metabolites and parent drug are renally cleared.[83] Although hydrophilic in nature, linezolid penetrates well into tissues and has been shown to achieve adequate concentrations in epithelial lining fluid in patients with ventilator-associated pneumonia.[84] The AUC/MIC ratio is the PK/PD index associated with antimicrobial efficacy.[85] Oral bioavailability of linezolid is 100% and a dose of 600 mg every 12 hours is adequate to achieve a pharmacodynamic target of AUC/MIC between 80 and 100 against susceptible organisms with MICs up to 2 to 4 mg/L.[85]

Tigecycline

Tigecycline is a glycycline antimicrobial that has broad spectrum activity including gram-positive, gram-negative, and anaerobic cover.[86] It is lipophilic in nature and has a large V_d indicating extensive distribution into tissues.[87] The AUC/MIC ratio is the PK/PD index that is correlated with efficacy as tigecycline has a long half-life and exhibits a prolonged PAE.[88] The primary route of elimination is biliary excretion.[87] No dosing adjustment is required for tigecycline in renal dysfunction or mild to moderate hepatic dysfunction.

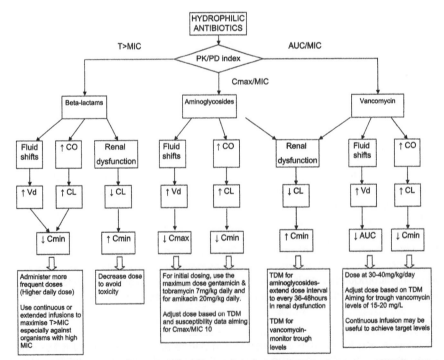

Fig. 2. Flow diagram summarizing the effects of pathophysiologic changes on PK/PD parameters of hydrophilic antibiotics. AUC, area under the curve; C_{max}, maximum drug concentration; C_{min}, minimum drug concentration; CL, clearance; CO, cardiac output; MIC, minimum inhibitory concentration; PK/PD, pharmacokinetic/pharmacodynamic; V_d, volume of distribution.

SUMMARY

In critically ill patients with severe sepsis and septic shock, altered pathophysiology can have a significant influence on pharmacokinetic parameters, particularly V_d and CL, which can then further affect the achievement of pharmacodynamic targets for antimicrobial agents. Failure to achieve pharmacodynamic targets for antimicrobials can result in poor clinical outcomes. Knowledge of the physicochemical properties and PK/PD index associated with maximal activity of an antimicrobial can help clinicians determine if dosage adjustments need to be made. The flow diagrams in **Figs. 2** and **3** summarize the effects of pathophysiologic changes on PK/PD parameters for the different hydrophilic and lipophilic antimicrobials and provide suggested

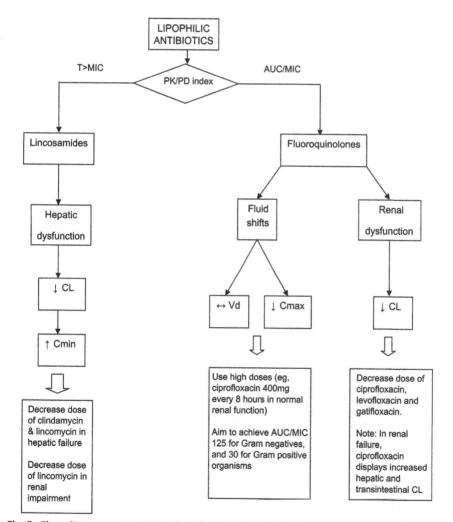

Fig. 3. Flow diagram summarizing the effects of pathophysiologic changes on PK/PD parameters of lipophilic antibiotics. AUC, area under the curve; C_{max}, maximum drug concentration; C_{min}, minimum drug concentration; CL, clearance; CO, cardiac output; MIC, minimum inhibitory concentration; PK/PD, pharmacokinetic/pharmacodynamic; V_d, volume of distribution.

dosing recommendations for the different antimicrobial classes. Hydrophilic time-dependent antimicrobials such as beta-lactams may display decreased C_{min} as a result of large V_d and/or increased CL, whereas hydrophilic concentration-dependent antimicrobials such as the aminoglycosides may display decreased C_{max} as a result of higher V_d in the critically ill patient with sepsis.

Antimicrobial dosing adjustments should take into considerations these potential changes in pharmacokinetic parameters and careful dosage adjustments need to be made particularly in patients with renal and/or hepatic dysfunction. The effect of any extracorporeal treatment modalities on antimicrobial pharmacokinetics also needs to be considered by clinicians. Knowledge of PK/PD properties of antimicrobials can be used to personalize dosing regimens for critically ill patients with sepsis and septic shock not only to maximize antimicrobial activity but also to minimize toxicity and reduce the development of antimicrobial resistance.[89]

REFERENCES

1. Angus DC, Linde-Zwirble WT, Lidicker J, et al. Epidemiology of severe sepsis in the United States: analysis of incidence, outcome, and associated costs of care. Crit Care Med 2001;29(7):1303–10.
2. Xu J, Kochane KD, Murphy SL, et al. Deaths: final data for 2007. National vital statistics report web release. Hyattsville (MD): National Centre for Health Statistics; 2010.
3. Kumar A, Roberts D, Wood KE, et al. Duration of hypotension before initiation of effective antimicrobial therapy is the critical determinant of survival in human septic shock. Crit Care Med 2006;34(6):1589–96.
4. Garnacho-Montero J, Garcia-Garmendia JL, Barrero-Almodovar A, et al. Impact of adequate empirical antimicrobial therapy on the outcome of patients admitted to the intensive care unit with sepsis. Crit Care Med 2003;31(12):2742–51.
5. Bone RC, Balk RA, Cerra FB, et al. Definitions for sepsis and organ failure and guidelines for the use of innovative therapies in sepsis. The ACCP/SCCM Consensus Conference Committee. American College of Chest Physicians/Society of Critical Care Medicine. Chest 1992;101(6):1644–55.
6. Roberts JA, Lipman J. Antibacterial dosing in intensive care: pharmacokinetics, degree of disease and pharmacodynamics of sepsis. Clin Pharmacokinet 2006;45(8):755–73.
7. Craig WA. Pharmacokinetic/pharmacodynamic parameters: rationale for antibacterial dosing of mice and men. Clin Infect Dis 1998;26(1):1–10.
8. Bochud PY, Calandra T. Pathogenesis of sepsis: new concepts and implications for future treatment. BMJ 2003;326:262–6.
9. Opal SM, Cohen J. Clinical gram-positive sepsis: does it fundamentally differ from gram-negative bacterial sepsis? Crit Care Med 1999;27(8):1608–16.
10. Glauser MP, Zanetti G, Baumgartner JD, et al. Septic shock: pathogenesis. Lancet 1991;338(8769):732–6.
11. Bone RC. The pathogenesis of sepsis. Ann Intern Med 1991;115(6):457–69.
12. Joynt GM, Lipman J, Gomersall CD, et al. The pharmacokinetics of once-daily dosing of ceftriaxone in critically ill patients. J Antimicrob Chemother 2001;47(4):421–9.
13. Lipman J, Wallis SC, Rickard CM, et al. Low cefpirome levels during twice daily dosing in critically ill septic patients: pharmacokinetic modelling calls for more frequent dosing. Intensive Care Med 2001;27(2):363–70.

14. Ryan DM. Pharmacokinetics of antimicrobials in natural and experimental superficial compartments in animals and humans. J Antimicrob Chemother 1993; 31(Suppl D):1–16.
15. Buerger C, Plock N, Dehghanyar P, et al. Pharmacokinetics of unbound linezolid in plasma and tissue interstitium of critically ill patients after multiple dosing using microdialysis. Antimicrob Agents Chemother 2006;50(7):2455–63.
16. Joukhadar C, Frossard M, Mayer BX, et al. Impaired target site penetration of beta-lactams may account for therapeutic failure in patients with septic shock. Crit Care Med 2001;29(2):385–91.
17. Joukhadar C, Klein N, Dittrich P, et al. Target site penetration of fosfomycin in critically ill patients. J Antimicrob Chemother 2003;51(5):1247–52.
18. Sauermann R, Delle-Karth G, Marsik C, et al. Pharmacokinetics and pharmacodynamics of cefpirome in subcutaneous adipose tissue of septic patients. Antimicrob Agents Chemother 2005;49(2):650–5.
19. Roberts JA, Roberts MS, Robertson TA, et al. Piperacillin penetration into tissue of critically ill patients with sepsis–bolus versus continuous administration? Crit Care Med 2009;37(3):926–33.
20. Fleck A, Raines G, Hawker F, et al. Increased vascular permeability: a major cause of hypoalbuminaemia in disease and injury. Lancet 1985;1(8432):781–4.
21. Burkhardt O, Kumar V, Katterwe D, et al. Ertapenem in critically ill patients with early-onset ventilator-associated pneumonia: pharmacokinetics with special consideration of free-drug concentration. J Antimicrob Chemother 2007;59(2): 277–84.
22. Pea F, Viale P, Candoni A, et al. Teicoplanin in patients with acute leukaemia and febrile neutropenia: a special population benefiting from higher dosages. Clin Pharmacokinet 2004;43(6):405–15.
23. Ulldemolins M, Roberts JA, Wallis SC, et al. Flucloxacillin dosing in critically ill patients with hypoalbuminaemia: special emphasis on unbound pharmacokinetics. J Antimicrob Chemother 2010;65(8):1771–8.
24. Choi G, Gomersall CD, Tian Q, et al. Principles of antibacterial dosing in continuous renal replacement therapy. Crit Care Med 2009;37(7):2268–82.
25. Pea F, Viale P, Pavan F, et al. Pharmacokinetic considerations for antimicrobial therapy in patients receiving renal replacement therapy. Clin Pharmacokinet 2007;46(12):997–1038.
26. Burkhardt O, Hafer C, Langhoff A, et al. Pharmacokinetics of ertapenem in critically ill patients with acute renal failure undergoing extended daily dialysis. Nephrol Dial Transplant 2009;24(1):267–71.
27. Kielstein JT, Eugbers C, Bode-Boeger SM, et al. Dosing of daptomycin in intensive care unit patients with acute kidney injury undergoing extended dialysis–a pharmacokinetic study. Nephrol Dial Transplant 2010;25(5):1537–41.
28. Swoboda S, Ober MC, Lichtenstern C, et al. Pharmacokinetics of linezolid in septic patients with and without extended dialysis. Eur J Clin Pharmacol 2010; 66(3):291–8.
29. Mushatt DM, Mihm LB, Dreisbach AW, et al. Antimicrobial dosing in slow extended daily dialysis. Clin Infect Dis 2009;49(3):433–7.
30. Mehta NM, Halwick DR, Dodson BL, et al. Potential drug sequestration during extracorporeal membrane oxygenation: results from an ex vivo experiment. Intensive Care Med 2007;33(6):1018–24.
31. Spriet I, Annaert P, Meersseman P, et al. Pharmacokinetics of caspofungin and voriconazole in critically ill patients during extracorporeal membrane oxygenation. J Antimicrob Chemother 2009;63(4):767–70.

32. Kintzel PE, Eastlund T, Calis KA. Extracorporeal removal of antimicrobials during plasmapheresis. J Clin Apher 2003;18(4):194–205.

33. Fauvelle F, Petitjean O, Tod M, et al. Clinical pharmacokinetics during plasma exchange. Therapie 2000;55(2):269–75.

34. Roberts JA, Roberts MS, Robertson TA, et al. A novel way to investigate the effects of plasma exchange on antimicrobial levels: use of microdialysis. Int J Antimicrob Agents 2008;31(3):240–4.

35. Fauvelle F, Lortholary O, Tod M, et al. Pharmacokinetics of ceftriaxone during plasma exchange in polyarteritis nodosa patients. Antimicrob Agents Chemother 1994;38(7):1519–22.

36. Alet P, Lortholary O, Fauvelle F, et al. Pharmacokinetics of teicoplanin during plasma exchange. Clin Microbiol Infect 1999;5(4):213–8.

37. McKindley DS, Hanes S, Boucher BA. Hepatic drug metabolism in critical illness. Pharmacotherapy 1998;18(4):759–78.

38. Mann HJ, Townsend RJ, Fuhs DW, et al. Decreased hepatic clearance of clindamycin in critically ill patients with sepsis. Clin Pharm 1987;6(2):154–9.

39. McKindley DS, Boulet J, Sachdeva K, et al. Endotoxic shock alters the pharmacokinetics of lidocaine and monoethylglycinexylidide. Shock 2002;17(3):199–204.

40. McKinnon PS, Paladino JA, Schentag JJ. Evaluation of area under the inhibitory curve (AUIC) and time above the minimum inhibitory concentration (T>MIC) as predictors of outcome for cefepime and ceftazidime in serious bacterial infections. Int J Antimicrob Agents 2008;31(4):345–51.

41. Lipman J, Wallis SC, Boots RJ. Cefepime versus cefpirome: the importance of creatinine clearance. Anesth Analg 2003;97(4):1149–54.

42. Wells M, Lipman J. Measurements of glomerular filtration in the intensive care unit are only a rough guide to renal function. S Afr J Surg 1997;35(1):20–3.

43. Pong S, Seto W, Abdolell M, et al. 12-hour versus 24-hour creatinine clearance in critically ill pediatric patients. Pediatr Res 2005;58(1):83–8.

44. Herrera-Gutierrez ME, Seller-Perez G, Banderas-Bravo E, et al. Replacement of 24-h creatinine clearance by 2-h creatinine clearance in intensive care unit patients: a single-center study. Intensive Care Med 2007;33(11):1900–6.

45. Lipman J, Wallis SC, Rickard C. Low plasma cefepime levels in critically ill septic patients: pharmacokinetic modeling indicates improved troughs with revised dosing. Antimicrob Agents Chemother 1999;43(10):2559–61.

46. Boselli E, Breilh D, Duflo F, et al. Steady-state plasma and intrapulmonary concentrations of cefepime administered in continuous infusion in critically ill patients with severe nosocomial pneumonia. Crit Care Med 2003;31(8):2102–6.

47. Burgess DS, Hastings RW, Hardin TC. Pharmacokinetics and pharmacodynamics of cefepime administered by intermittent and continuous infusion. Clin Ther 2000;22(1):66–75.

48. Georges B, Conil JM, Cougot P, et al. Cefepime in critically ill patients: continuous infusion versus an intermittent dosing regimen. Int J Clin Pharmacol Ther 2005;43(8):360–9.

49. Roos JF, Bulitta J, Lipman J, et al. Pharmacokinetic-pharmacodynamic rationale for cefepime dosing regimens in intensive care units. J Antimicrob Chemother 2006;58(5):987–93.

50. Roberts JA, Kirkpatrick CM, Roberts MS, et al. Meropenem dosing in critically ill patients with sepsis and without renal dysfunction: intermittent bolus versus continuous administration? Monte Carlo dosing simulations and subcutaneous tissue distribution. J Antimicrob Chemother 2009;64(1):142–50.

51. Roos JF, Lipman J, Kirkpatrick CM. Population pharmacokinetics and pharmaco-dynamics of cefpirome in critically ill patients against Gram-negative bacteria. Intensive Care Med 2007;33(5):781–8.
52. Kitzes-Cohen R, Farin D, Piva G, et al. Pharmacokinetics and pharmacodynamics of meropenem in critically ill patients. Int J Antimicrob Agents 2002;19(2):105–10.
53. Novelli A, Adembri C, Livi P, et al. Pharmacokinetic evaluation of meropenem and imipenem in critically ill patients with sepsis. Clin Pharmacokinet 2005;44(5):539–49.
54. Jaruratanasirikul S, Sriwiriyajan S, Punyo J. Comparison of the pharmacody-namics of meropenem in patients with ventilator-associated pneumonia following administration by 3-hour infusion or bolus injection. Antimicrob Agents Chemo-ther 2005;49(4):1337–9.
55. Li C, Kuti JL, Nightingale CH, et al. Population pharmacokinetic analysis and dosing regimen optimization of meropenem in adult patients. J Clin Pharmacol 2006;46(10):1171–8.
56. Lomaestro BM, Drusano GL. Pharmacodynamic evaluation of extending the administration time of meropenem using a Monte Carlo simulation. Antimicrob Agents Chemother 2005;49(1):461–3.
57. Moore RD, Lietman PS, Smith CR. Clinical response to aminoglycoside therapy: importance of the ratio of peak concentration to minimal inhibitory concentration. J Infect Dis 1987;155:93–9.
58. Vogelman BS, Craig WA. Postantimicrobial effects. J Antimicrob Chemother 1985;15(Suppl A):37–46.
59. Beckhouse MJ, Whyte IM, Byth PL, et al. Altered aminoglycoside pharmacoki-netics in the critically ill. Anaesth Intensive Care 1988;16(4):418–22.
60. Buijk SE, Mouton JW, Gyssens IC, et al. Experience with a once-daily dosing program of aminoglycosides in critically ill patients. Intensive Care Med 2002; 28(7):936–42.
61. Triginer C, Izquierdo I, Fernandez R, et al. Gentamicin volume of distribution in critically ill septic patients. Intensive Care Med 1990;16(5):303–6.
62. Marik PE. Aminoglycoside volume of distribution and illness severity in critically ill septic patients. Anaesth Intensive Care 1993;21(2):172–3.
63. Wilson AP. Clinical pharmacokinetics of teicoplanin. Clin Pharmacokinet 2000; 39(3):167–83.
64. Sanchez A, Lopez-Herce J, Cueto E, et al. Teicoplanin pharmacokinetics in crit-ically ill paediatric patients. J Antimicrob Chemother 1999;44(3):407–9.
65. Pea F, Brollo L, Viale P, et al. Teicoplanin therapeutic drug monitoring in critically ill patients: a retrospective study emphasizing the importance of a loading dose. J Antimicrob Chemother 2003;51(4):971–5.
66. Gous AG, Dance MD, Lipman J, et al. Changes in vancomycin pharmacokinetics in critically ill infants. Anaesth Intensive Care 1995;23(6):678–82.
67. del Mar Fernandez de Gatta Garcia M, Revilla N, Calvo MV, et al. Pharmacoki-netic/pharmacodynamic analysis of vancomycin in ICU patients. Intensive Care Med 2007;33(2):279–85.
68. Llopis-Salvia P, Jimenez-Torres NV. Population pharmacokinetic parameters of vancomycin in critically ill patients. J Clin Pharm Ther 2006;31(5):447–54.
69. MacGowan AP. Pharmacodynamics, pharmacokinetics, and therapeutic drug monitoring of glycopeptides. Ther Drug Monit 1998;20(5):473–7.
70. Rybak MJ. The pharmacokinetic and pharmacodynamic properties of vancomy-cin. Clin Infect Dis 2006;42(S1):S35–9.
71. Rybak MJ, Lomaestro BM, Rotschafer JC, et al. Vancomycin Therapeutic Guide-lines: a summary of consensus recommendations from the infectious diseases

Society of America, the American Society of Health System Pharmacists, and the Society of Infectious Diseases Pharmacists. Clin Infect Dis 2009;49(3):325–7.

72. Pea F, Furlanut M, Negri C, et al. Prospectively validated dosing nomograms for maximizing the pharmacodynamics of vancomycin administered by continuous infusion in critically ill patients. Antimicrob Agents Chemother 2009;53(5):1863–7.

73. Gous A, Lipman J, Scribante J, et al. Fluid shifts have no influence on ciprofloxacin pharmacokinetics in intensive care patients with intra-abdominal sepsis. Int J Antimicrob Agents 2005;26(1):50–5.

74. Blaser J, Stone BB, Groner MC, et al. Comparative study with enoxacin and netilmicin in a pharmacodynamic model to determine importance of ratio of antimicrobial peak concentration to MIC for bactericidal activity and emergence of resistance. Antimicrob Agents Chemother 1987;31(7):1054–60.

75. Forrest A, Nix DE, Ballow CH, et al. Pharmacodynamics of intravenous ciprofloxacin in seriously ill patients. Antimicrob Agents Chemother 1993;37(5):1073–81.

76. Lipman J, Scribante J, Gous AG, et al. Pharmacokinetic profiles of high-dose intravenous ciprofloxacin in severe sepsis. The Baragwanath Ciprofloxacin Study Group. Antimicrob Agents Chemother 1998;42(9):2235–9.

77. Conil JM, Georges B, de Lussy A, et al. Ciprofloxacin use in critically ill patients: pharmacokinetic and pharmacodynamic approaches. Int J Antimicrob Agents 2008;32(6):505–10.

78. van Zanten AR, Polderman KH, van Geijlswijk IM, et al. Ciprofloxacin pharmacokinetics in critically ill patients: a prospective cohort study. J Crit Care 2008;23(3):422–30.

79. Hyatt JM, Schentag JJ. Pharmacodynamic modeling of risk factors for ciprofloxacin resistance in *Pseudomonas aeruginosa*. Infect Control Hosp Epidemiol 2000;21(S1):S9–11.

80. MacGowan A, Rogers C, Bowker K. The use of in vitro pharmacodynamic models of infection to optimize fluoroquinolone dosing regimens. J Antimicrob Chemother 2000;46(2):163–70.

81. Thomas JK, Forrest A, Bhavnani SM, et al. Pharmacodynamic evaluation of factors associated with the development of bacterial resistance in acutely ill patients during therapy. Antimicrob Agents Chemother 1998;42(3):521–7.

82. Craig WA. Does the dose matter? Clin Infect Dis 2001;33(S3):S233–7.

83. Stalker DJ, Jungbluth GL. Clinical pharmacokinetics of linezolid, a novel oxazolidinone antibacterial. Clin Pharmacokinet 2003;42(13):1129–40.

84. Boselli E, Breilh D, Rimmele T, et al. Pharmacokinetics and intrapulmonary concentrations of linezolid administered to critically ill patients with ventilator-associated pneumonia. Crit Care Med 2005;33(7):1529–33.

85. Craig WA. Basic pharmacodynamics of antibacterials with clinical applications to the use of beta-lactams, glycopeptides, and linezolid. Infect Dis Clin North Am 2003;17(3):479–501.

86. Peterson LR. A review of tigecycline – the first glycylcycline. Int J Antimicrob Agents 2008;32(S4):S215–22.

87. Muralidharan G, Micalizzi M, Speth J, et al. Pharmacokinetics of tigecycline after single and multiple doses in healthy subjects. Antimicrob Agents Chemother 2005;49(1):220–9.

88. Meagher AK, Ambrose PG, Grasela TH, et al. Pharmacokinetic/pharmacodynamic profile for tigecycline – a new glycylcycline antimicrobial agent. Diagn Microbiol Infect Dis 2005;52(3):165–71.

89. Roberts JA, Kruger P, Paterson DL, et al. Antimicrobial resistance–what's dosing got to do with it? Crit Care Med 2008;36(5):2433–40.

Appropriateness is Critical

Marta Ulldemolins, PharmD[a,b,c], Xavier Nuvials, MD[a,b],
Mercedes Palomar, MD, PhD[a,b,d], Joan R. Masclans, MD, PhD[a,b],
Jordi Rello, MD, PhD[a,b,c,d],*

KEYWORDS

- Critically ill patient • Susceptibility • Empirical antibiotics
- Pneumonia • Bloodstream infection • Adequate • Optimal

Despite considerable research and clinical effort, management of severe infections in critically ill patients remains an ongoing challenge for physicians. Increased severity of sickness and aggressive medical management, together with reduced susceptibilities of nosocomial pathogens, dramatically increase the complexity of managing severe infections in the intensive care unit (ICU). Critically ill patients are most significantly affected by this issue because it has been estimated than more than 70% are prescribed antibiotics during their ICU stay.[1]

Maximization of antimicrobial efficacy is a priority in the era of multidrug-resistant bacteria given the dearth of new antibiotics in production.[2,3] The dramatic increase in bacterial resistance has led to increased recognition of inappropriate (ie, without in vitro activity against a microorganism) empirical treatment of infections in both community and hospital settings[4,5] that dramatically affects mortality, morbidity,

Financial support: Marta Ulldemolins and Jordi Rello are supported in part by CIBER Enfermedades Respiratorias (CIBERES) and AGAUR 09/SGR/1226; support was also received from FIS 07/90960.

Conflicts of interest: Jordi Rello serves as a consultant for Basilea, Merck & Co, Pfizer Pharmaceuticals, Wyeth, Aerst Pharmaceuticals, Astra-Zeneca, Johnson & Johnson, Novartis, Arpida, Bristol-Myers, Ipsat, and Intercell; has received grant research support from BARD, Pfizer, and Johnson & Johnson; and is on the speakers bureau of Astra-Zeneca, Wyeth, ABLE, Kimberley-Clark, Novartis, Pfizer, and Bayer. Mercedes Palomar serves as a consultant for Johnson & Johnson and is on the speakers bureau of Astra-Zeneca, Wyeth, Pfizer, and Johnson & Johnson. Marta Ulldemolins, Xavier Nuvials, and Joan R. Masclans have no conflicts of interest to disclose.

a Critical Care Department, Vall d'Hebron University Hospital, Passeig de la Vall d'Hebron, 119-129, 08035 Barcelona, Spain

b Vall d'Hebron Research Institute (VHRI), Universitat Autònoma de Barcelona (UAB), Passeig de la Vall d'Hebron, 119–129, 08035 Barcelona, Spain

c Centro de Investigación Biomédica En Red de Enfermedades Respiratorias (CIBERES), Spain

d School of Medicine, Universitat Autònoma de Barcelona, Barcelona, Spain

* Corresponding author. Critical Care Department, Vall d'Hebron University Hospital, Passeig de la Vall d'Hebron, 119-129, 08035 Barcelona, Spain.

E-mail address: jrello.hj23.ics@gencat.cat

Crit Care Clin 27 (2011) 35–51

doi:10.1016/j.ccc.2010.09.007

0749-0704/11/$ – see front matter © 2011 Elsevier Inc. All rights reserved.

and health care resources use. This article addresses the major factors that can lead to inappropriate empirical therapy and describes the effect of inappropriateness on the outcomes of critically ill patients with severe infections. Emerging evidence suggests that in vitro susceptibility is critical but not sufficient for achieving the best outcomes, and other factors have to be carefully considered. Therefore, it is important to revise the meaning of the expression appropriate antibiotic therapy by introducing the concepts of adequate and optimal. Hence, this review also briefly describes the factors that comprise the concepts of appropriate, adequate, and optimal initial antibiotic therapy.

APPROPRIATE, ADEQUATE, AND OPTIMAL ANTIBIOTIC THERAPY

Classically, the in vitro susceptibility of the causal pathogen was considered the reference aspect for antibiotic efficacy in the treatment of severe infections, and defined the concept of appropriate (or concordant) antibiotic therapy.[6] However, this concept is becoming obsolete after the recognition that, although critical, the in vitro susceptibility is not enough for achieving optimal efficacy of antibiotic therapy.[7,8] For example, Rello and colleagues[7] showed that patients with methicillin-resistant Staphylococcus aureus (MRSA) ventilator-associated pneumonia (VAP) prescribed with vancomycin exhibited an excess mortality of 22.7%, which is unacceptable compared with the low mortality of methicillin-sensitive S aureus (MSSA) VAP treated with β-lactams. This finding has led to adjustments in the definition of appropriateness, such as the 1 adopted recently by Vogelaers and colleagues,[9] in which appropriate is defined as "in vitro susceptibility of the causative pathogen and clinical response to the agent administered." In 2000, Kollef[10] proposed a broader definition of adequate antibiotic therapy as "in vitro susceptibility together with proper dosing, proper interval administration, monitoring of drug levels when appropriate, and avoidance of unwanted drug interactions." In 2006, our group proposed that antibiotic therapy could be classified as appropriate, adequate, and optimal on consideration of concrete factors that have a direct effect on achievement of optimal antibiotic efficacy.[11] It follows that appropriate antibiotic therapy would include in vitro susceptibility and early administration, whereas adequate would refer to physicochemistry, and penetration and optimal would consist of pharmacokinetics/pharmacodynamics-driven dosage strategies.[11] The Tarragona strategy was a strategy to manage VAP based on the concepts of appropriate, adequate, and optimal. This paradigm was intended to maximize the likelihood of prescribing the optimal antimicrobial in each case by controlling the factors likely to drive to inappropriateness of therapy.[12] **Fig. 1** represents the components of the antibiotic therapy optimization.

CAUSES OF INAPPROPRIATE ANTIBIOTIC THERAPY

Among many risks for suboptimal outcomes in critically ill patients, inappropriate empirical antibiotic therapy is a modifiable factor that clinicians must always consider. An extensive body of literature has shown that administration of inappropriate (or non-concordant) empirical therapy based on in vitro susceptibilities results in unfavorable clinical outcomes.[13–32] The most common cause of inappropriate empirical antibiotic therapy is infection by a highly resistant pathogen.[33] In the community and in-hospital settings, the incidence of infections resistant pathogens is rising worryingly.[2,33–35] This increases the likelihood of administering inappropriate empirical therapy to patients not expected to be infected by resistant pathogens. In the hospital setting, the occurrence of infections caused by resistant bacteria is determined by the contribution of many factors, whose consideration is required for prediction of likely infective agents

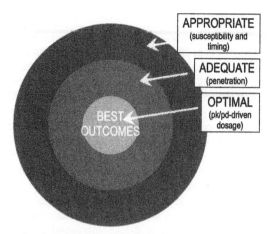

APPROPRIATE
(susceptibility and timing)

ADEQUATE
(penetration)

OPTIMAL
(pk/pd-driven dosage)

BEST OUTCOMES

Fig. 1. The components of appropriate, adequate, and optimal antibiotic therapy.

in order to avoid inappropriate empirical therapies. The most relevant of these are described later.

Prior Antibiotic Exposure

The administration of previous antibiotic therapy has an important effect on the ecology of patient's microflora, which can ultimately lead to infection with resistant strains of high-risk pathogens.[36] In 1993, Rello and colleagues[9] showed that the cause of VAP was significantly different in critically ill patients who received previous antibiotic therapy compared with patients who did not receive previous antibiotics. Previous antibiotic therapy resulted in a much higher incidence of infections caused by high-risk pathogens such as *Pseudomonas aeruginosa*[37,38] or MRSA,[39] with important increases in the mortality (up to 9 times higher).[37] Other groups have confirmed this observation.[40–43] If the previous antibiotics were broad-spectrum antibiotics, an independent association with high-risk pathogens has also been found.[40] Knowledge about previous prescription of antimicrobial agents is paramount. This knowledge determines likely antibiotic resistances and guides therapy for present and further infectious episodes.

Prolonged Length of Stay in the Hospital and Previous Hospitalization

Prolonged length of stay (LOS) in the hospital and previous hospitalization also increase the likelihood of being colonized by resistant bacteria, which are likely to be the causal agents of subsequent severe infections.[40,44–47] Chen and colleagues[46] showed that patients who came from the community but had been recently discharged from the hospital had a higher risk of being infected by antimicrobial-resistant bacteria. In their study, previous carriage of antimicrobial-resistant bacteria in the past 360 days and previous stay in the ICU in the past 180 days were independent risk factors for antimicrobial-resistant bacteremia. Similarly, Bonten and colleagues[47] studied the risk factors for being colonized and infected by vancomycin-resistant enterococci (VRE) in a cohort of critically ill patients and found that prolonged LOS in the hospital before the ICU increased the risk of colonization on ICU admission (odds ratio [OR] 4.65 when in-hospital LOS>3 days).

Presence of Invasive Devices

Endotracheal intubation, intravascular catheterization, and urinary catheterization in critically ill patients also increase the predisposition to acquiring infections by resistant bacteria. Richards and colleagues[48] analyzed the data from a large ICU surveillance program and found that 87% of primary bloodstream infections were associated with central lines, 86% of nosocomial pneumonia was associated with mechanical ventilation, and 95% of urinary tract infections were associated with urinary catheters. The most common causal pathogens of these infections were coagulase-negative staphylococci with intravascular catheters, *P aeruginosa* and *Acinetobacter* spp with endotracheal intubation and fungal infections by *Candida* spp with urinary catheters. Regarding respiratory infections, prolonged mechanical ventilation is also associated with a higher incidence of resistant pathogens In VAP. Trouillet and colleagues[40] performed a study to determine risk factors for VAP caused by high-risk pathogens in critically ill patients and found that mechanical ventilation for more than 7 days was associated with a 6-fold increased probability of high-risk microorganisms.

Local Susceptibilities

Knowledge on local susceptibilities is paramount for avoiding the choice of inappropriate empirical therapy. There is extensive evidence in the literature that supports the belief that the spectrum of nosocomial pathogens likely to cause severe infections differs among different sites and even among different departments of the same institution.[49–51] A study by Rello and colleagues[49] focused on the variations in the cause of VAP in critically ill patients from 4 different settings and reported significant variations in the incidence of high-risk pathogens, which particularly affected the number of pneumonias caused by MRSA, *P aeruginosa* and *Acinetobacter* spp among sites. These results have been confirmed with hospital-acquired pneumonia (HAP) and VAP by other studies.[50,52,53] A large European study described significant differences in the prevalence and antibiotic sensitivity patterns of the causal agents for nosocomial pneumonia in 27 ICUs from 9 European countries.[50] For instance, Turkey and Greece had a high prevalence of *Acinetobacter* species in HAP/VAP episodes, whereas *P aeruginosa* was commonly found in Italy and Portugal and Enterobacteriaceae species were common in Germany and Belgium. These data suggest that, instead of following general recommendations, antimicrobial prescribing practices for nosocomial infections should be based on up-to-date information of the pattern of multiresistant isolates from each institution. Although the 1996 American Thoracic Society guidelines for the management of nosocomial pneumonia failed to recognize local susceptibilities as a key factor for reducing the rate of inappropriate prescription,[54] this recommendation was incorporated in the most recent edition of these guidelines as one of the most important factors to guide physicians' antimicrobial selection.[44]

Admission Category and Underlying Diseases

Admission category also determines the likely causal pathogens of an infection and should be considered when choosing empirical antimicrobials. For example, in VAP, causal agents in patients with trauma differ significantly from patients without trauma. MSSA is the predominant pathogen in comatose multiple-trauma patients,[55] and nasal MSSA colonization at time of severe injury may increase the risk of MSSA pneumonia. The results of a large European study on HAP and VAP suggest that admission category drove physicians' choice, because trauma patients received more non–anti-*Pseudomonas* spp cephalosporins, whereas surgical patients were prescribed more aminoglycosides.[56] Underlying diseases also have a causal role by predisposing the patient to be infected by specific organisms. For example, patients with chronic obstructive pulmonary disease are at increased risk for *Haemophilus influenzae*, *Moraxella catarrhalis*, or *Streptococcus pneumoniae* infections, and cystic fibrosis increases the risk of *P aeruginosa* and *S aureus* infections.[44]

Colonization Pressure by Resistant Pathogens

It has been suggested that in ICUs, where antibiotic pressure is very high, increased colonization rates by high-risk pathogens may affect cross-acquisition of these microorganisms, probably because of an increased chance of physical contact between health care workers and patients colonized with resistant bacteria making any lapses in compliance of the infection control measures more likely to result in pathogen spread. The number of patients already colonized (colonization pressure) by resistant pathogens may be an important factor in increasing the probabilities of cross-colonization and cross-infection to other patients. This effect was shown by Bonten and colleagues[57] with VRE. This group found that colonization pressure was the most important variable affecting VRE acquisition, and that the median time for a noncolonized patient to acquire VRE was significantly decreased with higher colonization pressures.[57] Therefore, high colonization pressures by resistant pathogens in the ICU could be also a marker of suspicion for resistant pathogens to be found in nosocomial infections and to be targeted by empirical therapy.

EFFECTS OF INAPPROPRIATENESS ON DIFFERENT KINDS OF INFECTION

Provision of appropriate empirical antimicrobials greatly affects morbidity and mortality in hospitalized patients. A large multicenter international study evaluated the effect of appropriateness on mortality and hospital LOS in a large cohort of hospitalized patients with severe infections, both community acquired and hospital acquired. Notably, inappropriate initial antibiotic treatment was prescribed to more than one-third of the patients, with similar proportions in the 3 investigational sites.[31] All-cause 30-day mortalities were significantly higher in patients with inappropriate antibiotics (20.1% vs 11.8%, $P = .001$), and hospital LOS was increased by more than 2 days in the inappropriate treatment group ($P = .024$). Similarly, Kumar and colleagues[32] recently published a study of 5715 patients in ICUs with septic shock, showing that mortality was higher when empirical antibiotic therapy was inappropriate (52.0%) than when appropriate (10.3%). Inappropriateness was confirmed to be independently associated with mortality by multivariate logistic regression (OR, 8.99; 95% CI, 6.60–12.23; $P<.0001$). Moreover, inappropriateness was significantly associated with the isolated microorganism, fungal species being the microorganisms that were most frequently treated inappropriately (56.4% of the cases),[32] followed by gram-positive organisms (22.2%).

Regarding other concrete clinical scenarios, the effect of inappropriateness on outcomes has also been shown in a variety of infectious causes, detailed later.

Nosocomial Pneumonia

Pneumonia is the most frequent nosocomial infection described in critically ill patients. Rates of pneumonia are considerably higher among patients in the ICU than in wards, and the risk for developing pneumonia is higher in intubated patients receiving mechanical ventilation.[58] However, despite extensive research and clinical experience with this disease, controversy regarding optimal management still exists. Because of the unacceptably high mortality and morbidity of this complication,[59] maximization of the effectiveness of the therapeutic arsenal is mandatory. Patients with a diagnosis of nosocomial pneumonia who receive appropriate antibiotic therapy are more than twice as likely to survive.[13,14] The effects of inappropriate antibiotic therapy on patient outcomes and resources use are well described in the literature. **Fig. 2** summarizes the results of some of the most relevant studies in VAP.

Rello and colleagues[14] found that, in patients with VAP, both crude and attributable mortalities decreased significantly in patients who received appropriate empirical antibiotics (63.0% vs 41.5% for crude and 37.0% vs 15.4% for attributable mortality). Luna and colleagues[29] assessed the appropriateness of therapy based on the results of bronchoalveolar lavage (BAL) cultures in critically ill patients with nosocomial pneumonia, and reported similar findings (91.2% vs 37.5% mortality in inappropriate vs appropriate therapy). Other studies have confirmed these results with VAP and HAP.[18,19,27,28] Regarding LOS in the ICU, Dupont and colleagues[19] showed that inappropriateness resulted in more ICU days (12 ± 11 days vs 20 ± 24 days, P = .01). A recent meta-analysis on the effect of inappropriate antibiotic therapy on mortality in patients with VAP has been published.[60] The investigators pooled the results of 10 clinical studies on patients with VAP and found that, both when using an unadjusted and an adjusted model, the odds ratio for death increased greatly when inappropriate therapy was prescribed (OR, 2.34; 95% CI, 1.51–3.63 for unadjusted data, and OR, 3.03; 95% CI, 1.12–8.19 for adjusted data). In these studies, most of the episodes of inappropriate treatment were caused by bacterial resistance to the empirically administered antibiotics rather than the presence of atypical pathogens.[14,18] High-risk pathogens such as *P aeruginosa*, *Acinetobacter* spp, and MRSA are common in VAP and HAP[50] and should be targeted when risk factors are present to minimize the chances of inappropriateness and bad outcomes.

The Infectious Diseases Society of North America, the American College of Chest Physicians, the Society of Critical Care Medicine, and the American Thoracic Society have recently published a position paper with recommendations for the design of

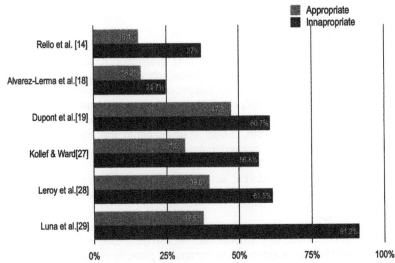

Fig. 2. The mortality in appropriate versus appropriate empirical antibiotic treatment of VAP.

further clinical trials for HAP and VAP.[61] The investigators emphasize that clinical trials for HAP and VAP usually exclude patients with infections caused by organisms resistant to standard comparator drugs from enrollment. These patients would be more likely to receive inappropriate empirical therapy with the comparator drug. Therefore, new antibacterial drugs will probably not be tested in the scenarios that would benefit most from the new treatment and achieve superior efficacy compared with the gold standard. However, extreme gram-negative drug resistance (XDR) has created a situation in which superiority trials can be performed, because the investigational drug can show clinical benefit compared with the standard therapy because of the lack of an approved alternative to which the pathogen is susceptible. These kinds of studies are desirable and should be supported to advance clinical therapy and to improve treatment of HAP and VAP.

Bloodstream Infections

Bloodstream infections (BSI) are among the most serious complications found in critically ill patients, with high associated mortality, morbidity, and health care expenses.[62] The Center of Disease Control's National Nosocomial Infections Surveillance System has reported that BSI account for up to 20% of the nosocomial infections in critically ill patients,[48] with approximately 80% of those related to the use of invasive devices such as intravascular catheters.[62] The spectrum of causal agents that frequently cause BSI in the ICU is broad, and mainly comprises staphylococci and gram-negative bacteria with coagulase-negative staphylococci by far the most frequent single pathogen.[63,64] However, the incidence of infections caused by high-risk gram-negative bacilli, gram-positive cocci, and nonbacterial pathogens has been rising during the 3 past decades, even in the community setting,[65] with high rates of *Enterococcus* spp, MRSA, *P aeruginosa*, and *Candida* spp[64] that may increase the likelihood of provision of inappropriate empirical antibiotic therapy. Moreover, certain clinical scenarios increase the likelihood that specific pathogens will need to be covered. For instance, immunocompromised patients, patients who have received red blood cell transfusions, patients who have undergone abdominal surgery, who are receiving total parenteral nutrition, are colonized by yeasts, or with femoral catheters are more likely to have BSI by *Candida* spp,[66] and patients with femoral or jugular lines, with severe sepsis, or with septic shock are more likely to be infected by gram-negative bacteria.[54]

Many studies have focused on the effect of inappropriateness on outcomes of BSI in critically ill patients,[21–26,30] and have shown that patients who receive inappropriate empirical antibiotics are at more than a 2-fold risk of dying. **Fig. 3**[60] summarizes the findings of some of the studies focused on mortality in BSI depending on appropriateness of empirical treatment.

Valles and colleagues[30] studied the prognosis of community-acquired BSI in a cohort of critically ill patients from 30 Spanish ICUs and reported that the factor with the greatest effect on mortality was administration of inappropriate empirical antibiotic therapy (mortality 69.4% vs 37% in inappropriate vs appropriate, OR for mortality with inappropriate empirical antibiotic 3.23, 95% CI 1.52–6.82), especially when vasopressors were required. Similar findings were reported when studying hospital-acquired BSI. Leibovici and colleagues[25] studied the evolution of nosocomial bacteremia in 3413 patients and found that the fatality rate in patients given appropriate treatment was 20%, whereas in patients given inappropriate treatment it was 34% ($P = .0001$, OR 2.1, 95% CI 1.8–2.4). They also reported significant differences in LOS in the hospital between groups. The hospital LOS for patients who survived was 9 days (range 0–117 days) for patients who received appropriate empirical

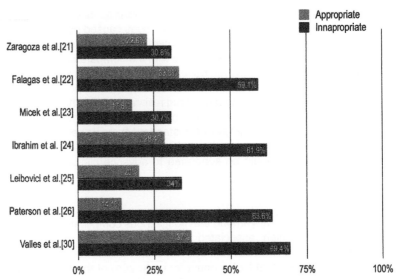

Fig. 3. The mortality in appropriate versus appropriate empirical antibiotic treatment of bloodstream infections.

antibiotics, and 11 days (range 0–209 days) for patients given inappropriate antibiotics (P = .0001). For patients who died, the median hospital LOS was 5 days (range 0–120 days) for those given appropriate antibiotic treatment, and 4 days (range 1–83 days) for those given inappropriate treatment (P = .03).[25] Schramm and colleagues[67] performed a retrospective cohort analysis of the influence of appropriate therapy on outcomes of sterile-site infections by hospital-acquired MRSA and community-acquired MRSA (CA-MRSA). They reported statistically higher hospital mortality in patients receiving inappropriate initial antimicrobial treatment within 24 hours of a positive culture than for those receiving appropriate initial treatment (26.1% vs 16.6%; P = .015). The investigators recommended initial empirical antimicrobial treatment regimens targeting MRSA in patients at risk for this infection or in a high-incidence area.[67] Kumar and colleagues[32] reported that appropriate therapy in primary bloodstream infections without an obvious clinical source in patients with septic shock was associated with a 17.6-fold better survival than inappropriate initial therapy (47.5% vs 2.7%, respectively). A recent meta-analysis pooled the data from 22 clinical studies and showed an adjusted OR for mortality of 2.28 (95% CI 1.43–3.65) when empirical antibiotics were inappropriate.[60]

Severe Skin and Soft Tissue Infections

Skin and soft tissue infections (SSTI) can result in critical illness and require ICU admission. _S aureus_ and group A streptococci are the most common causal agents of SSTI, followed by other bacteria such as _Clostridium_ spp.[68] Antibiotics are a crucial element in the management of SSTI. The selection of the appropriate antibiotic is driven by many factors, especially after the increase in the rate of infections caused by CA-MRSA.[69,70] In the United States, CA-MRSA has been reported to be the causal pathogen of 59% of the SSTI that arrive at emergency departments.[70]

Inappropriate empirical antibiotic therapy has significantly effects in the resolution of SSTI. Chuck and colleagues[71] designed an algorithm for the empirical treatment of severe SSTI in the emergency department, where they prompted physicians to use antibiotics active against CA-MRSA for complicated infections. When they analyzed outcome data regarding appropriateness of treatment, they reported that patients who underwent surgical drainage and received appropriate antibiotics had much better clinical cures (100%) compared with those who only underwent drainage but received inappropriate empirical therapy (33%).[71] Ruhe and colleagues[72] retrospectively studied the resolution of noncomplicated SSTI in 492 adult patients with CA-MRSA and found that 95% of patients with appropriate antibiotic, versus 87% with inappropriate antibiotic, resolved satisfactorily from the infection ($P = .01$). Multivariate analysis showed failure to initiate appropriate antibiotics within 48 hours as the only factor determining treatment failure (OR 2.80, 95% CI 1.26–6.22).

Meningitis

Bacterial meningitis is caused by severe infections that require prompt administration of effective antibiotics. Community-acquired bacterial meningitis has a high rate of an unfavorable outcome in adults (34%), with the most common causal pathogens being *Streptococcus pneumoniae*, *Neisseria meningitides*, and *Listeria monocytogenes*.[73] Pneumococcal meningitis leads to higher death rates and more unfavorable outcomes than meningococcal pneumonia.[73] Because of the increase in the incidence of strains of *S pneumoniae* resistant to penicillin in many countries such as the United States,[74] an increased risk of inappropriateness of empirical treatment has been identified. Accordingly, high mortalities have been observed in meningitis episodes caused by penicillin-resistant pneumococcal strains. A multi-center study of 156 consecutive adults hospitalized for pneumococcal meningitis shown that 38% of the identified strains were nonsusceptible to penicillin G. The multivariate analysis identified isolation of a nonsusceptible pneumococcus strain as one of the factors that most increased the OR for death (OR 6.83, 95% CI 2.94–20.8, $P<.0004$), together with delays of more than 3 hours in the administration of antibiotics (OR 14.12, 95% CI 3.93–50.9; $P<.0004$).[75] Other studies have focused on the effect of inappropriateness on outcomes of severe meningitis caused by other pathogens, with compelling results.[76–78] Lu and colleagues[76] studied the prognostic factors of gram-negative meningitis in 77 patients and found that 100% of patients who received inappropriate therapy died because of the infectious episode, compared with 38% mortality with appropriate therapy. Inappropriate empirical antibiotics resulted in an independent predictor of higher mortality in the logistic regression model.[76] The same group reported similar results with *Klebsiella* spp meningitis in adults during a 13-year period (100% death in inappropriate vs 24.4% in appropriate antibiotics).[78]

ADEQUATE ANTIBIOTIC THERAPY

The terms antimicrobial and antibiotic include many compounds that considerably differ in physicochemistry. Chemically, the distribution coefficient between water and lipids classifies a molecule as hydrophilic or lipophilic. This property determines the tissues to which drug molecules will preferentially distribute. Hydrophilic drugs will distribute mainly in the intravascular and extracellular body water, whereas lipophilic antibiotics can cross barriers and distribute intracellularly and into the lipid tissues.[79] This characteristic determines the amount of drug that will be able to reach certain organs, which is directly proportional to the pharmacologic effect. For example, to reach tissues and organ systems such as the lung, the central nervous system, or the bone marrow, many physiologic barriers must be crossed. These barriers may reduce the rate and extent of antibiotic distribution, and concentrations achieved at the target site may be suboptimal. The glycopeptide vancomycin is an example of an antimicrobial that can exhibit suboptimal penetration into key target organs. Vancomycin is highly hydrophilic and has been shown to penetrate poorly into lung tissue and pulmonary epithelial lining fluid (ELF) (5:1 blood/tissue and 6:1 blood/ELF ratio).[80,81] Another case is ceftriaxone, which achieves concentrations in the central nervous system that are between 1.5% and2.5% of the plasma concentrations as a consequence of its hydrophilicity and its high level of protein binding.[82] Hence, it is important to take into account the target organ system or tissue where the infection is located, and select antimicrobials likely to achieve therapeutic concentrations at the target site.

OPTIMAL ANTIBIOTIC THERAPY

Optimal antibiotic therapy includes the consideration of factors beyond susceptibility, minimum inhibitory concentration (MIC) of the bacteria, and tissue concentrations of the drug. Selection of the optimal dosage is complex because specific drug and patient characteristics must be considered individually and in aggregate. First, the pharmacokinetic/pharmacodynamic behavior of each antimicrobial and the particular physiology of critically ill patients must be taken into account.[83] Different antimicrobials exhibit different bacterial killing characteristics associated with certain pharmacodynamic indices. Antibiotics whose mechanism of action is though the inhibition of nucleic acid or protein synthesis have a postantibiotic effect (PAE), with inhibition of bacterial growth even when concentrations are lower than the MIC.[84] For this reason, administration of high doses of these drugs once or twice daily is generally preferred to multiple and frequent dosing (concentration-dependent killing). In contrast, antibiotics that inhibit the bacterial wall synthesis, such as β-lactams, kill bacteria more slowly and do not have a clinically significant PAE. Accordingly, such drugs must maintain a concentration at the infection site that is greater than the MIC of the pathogen for a certain period of time to achieve optimal effectiveness (time-dependent killing).[84] Therefore, dosage regimens must be adjusted to these specific pharmacodynamic properties to optimize bacterial killing.

In addition, critically ill patients exhibit several physiologic alterations that may affect antimicrobial pharmacokinetics and result in underdosing. The clinical management of hypotension or septic shock is likely to include fluid resuscitation and inotropes, leading to early increased renal blood flow and augmented renal clearances,[85,86] which translates into faster elimination of hydrophilic drugs. In this circumstance, higher-than-standard daily doses of the antimicrobial may be required. Also, because of capillary leakage and hypoalbuminemia, among other causes,[87,88] the volume of distribution of many hydrophilic antimicrobials is likely to increase greatly.[89–91] Consequently, increased loading doses could be necessary to achieve therapeutic concentrations on the first day of therapy.

RECOMMENDATIONS

As detailed earlier, inappropriate empirical therapy is a modifiable determinant of poor outcomes that clinicians must address aggressively. Broad-spectrum antibiotics, in monotherapy or in combination where appropriate, should be prescribed empirically when high-risk pathogens are suspected. Likely pathogens should be targeted depending on risk factors described previously. Local susceptibility surveillance data should be updated regularly to keep clinicians aware of local resistance patterns.

Once culture results are available, reassessment of the prescribed antimicrobial regimen with potential de-escalation to narrower-spectrum drugs is recommended to reduce the antibiotic selection pressure and decrease the development of antibiotic resistance.[92,93] Development of acute-care antimicrobial bundles could improve the rate of appropriate prescription of antibiotics at the bedside, and may be the next major step in the process of optimization of infection management.[94] A care bundle for the management of VAP has recently been proposed by our group. The components of this bundle are summarized in **Box 1**.[95] This review emphasizes the importance of administering early and broad-spectrum antimicrobials with consideration of risk factors and local susceptibilities in order to avoid inappropriateness of therapy. Afterward, de-escalation based on culture results and shortening of the duration of therapy where possible are strongly recommended.[95] Further advances in the creation and validation of management care bundles for severe infections in the ICU are required. Moreover, therapeutic drug monitoring (TDM) of peak and/or trough concentrations would be helpful in the optimization of antibiotic therapy. Knowledge of trough concentration values allows clinicians to assess whether dosing leads to concentration/time profiles for optimal therapy, and to make appropriate adjustments as needed to reach therapeutic values. Drugs such as glycopeptides and aminoglycosides are regularly monitored in the clinical setting; however, the application of TDM principles to β-lactams (the most prescribed class of antibiotics) would be desirable because of the great variations in the pharmacokinetics of these drugs in critically ill patients.[96] A recently published paper prospectively used TDM for evaluating whether β-lactam dosing led to optimal levels in patients in ICUs. This study showed that 50.4% of patients were underdosed at the first TDM sample, requiring dose increases.[97] More prospective work on the potential and usefulness of using TDM as a strategy for optimizing antibiotic dosing of β-lactams in patients in ICUs is highly recommendable.

Box 1
The domains of the care bundle for the management of VAP in the ICU

VAP management care

Bundle VAP diagnosis

Early chest radiograph with interpretation by an expert within 1 hour

Immediate reporting of the Gram stain findings and cells from the respiratory secretions analysis

VAP treatment

Immediate administration of broad-spectrum antibiotics following microbiological sampling

Empirical therapy based on assessment of assessment local surveillance data and risk factors for resistant bacteria

De-escalation of antibiotics in responding patients once culture results are available

Assessment of response to treatment within 72 hours

Short therapy duration (8 days) if patient is on an appropriate regimen and not infected by a multidrug-resistant pathogen

Adapted from Rello J, Chastre J, Cornaglia G, et al. European care bundle for the management of ventilator-associated pneumonia. J Crit Care 2010. [Epub ahead of print].

SUMMARY

The pathophysiology of severe infections and the complexity of nosocomial pathogens make the optimization of the antimicrobial management of severe infections extremely difficult. In critically ill patients with severe infections, inappropriate empirical treatment is often associated with the presence of microorganisms resistant to the usual antibiotics. Such resistant organisms are increasingly being found in both community-acquired and nosocomial infections. Previous receipt of antibiotics, prolonged LOS in the hospital, admission category, local susceptibilities, colonization pressure, and presence of invasive devices increase the likelihood of being infected by resistant pathogens. Administration of inappropriate empirical antibiotics significantly worsens outcomes and increases health care expenses in many severe infections such as nosocomial pneumonia, meningitis, SSTI, and bloodstream infections. These and other serious infections require appropriate empirical antimicrobial therapy, ideally with an agent that covers both gram-positive and gram-negative pathogens. Clinicians should include local antimicrobial resistance pattern data (antibiograms) and known risk factors for high-risk pathogens in their decision making regarding empirical therapy in order to improve quality of care and outcomes. Moreover, emerging evidence suggests that appropriate empirical therapy is critical but not sufficient to achieve the best patient outcomes. Consideration of issues beyond in vitro susceptibility, such as antimicrobial physicochemistry, tissue penetration, and pharmacokinetic/pharmacodynamic-driven dosing is required for the optimization of antimicrobial use in the ICU. Further clinical research on this area is strongly recommended.

REFERENCES

1. Vincent JL, Rello J, Marshall J, et al. International study of the prevalence and outcomes of infection in intensive care units. JAMA 2009;302(21):2323–9.
2. Paterson DL, Doi Y. A step closer to extreme drug resistance (XDR) in gram-negative bacilli. Clin Infect Dis 2007;45(9):1179–81.
3. Pharmaceutical Research and Manufactures of America. Available at: http://www.phrma.org/newmedicines/. Accessed November 16, 2009.
4. Rello J, Valles J. Mortality as an outcome in hospital-acquired pneumonia. Infect Control Hosp Epidemiol 1998;19(10):795–7.
5. Deleo FR, Otto M, Kreiswirth BN, et al. Community-associated methicillin-resistant *Staphylococcus aureus*. Lancet 2010;375(9725):1557–68.
6. Pea F, Viale P. The antimicrobial therapy puzzle: could pharmacokinetic-pharmacodynamic relationships be helpful in addressing the issue of appropriate pneumonia treatment in critically ill patients? Clin Infect Dis 2006;42(12):1764–71.
7. Rello J, Sole-Violan J, Sa-Borges M, et al. Pneumonia caused by oxacillin-resistant *Staphylococcus aureus* treated with glycopeptides. Crit Care Med 2005; 33(9):1983–7.
8. Stein GE, Wells EM. The importance of tissue penetration in achieving successful antimicrobial treatment of nosocomial pneumonia and complicated skin and soft-tissue infections caused by methicillin-resistant *Staphylococcus aureus*: vancomycin and linezolid. Curr Med Res Opin 2010;26(3):571–88.
9. Vogelaers D, De Bels D, Foret F, et al. Patterns of antimicrobial therapy in severe nosocomial infections: empiric choices, proportion of appropriate therapy, and adaptation rates–a multicentre, observational survey in critically ill patients. Int J Antimicrob Agents 2010;35(4):375–81.

10. Kollef MH. Inadequate antimicrobial treatment: an important determinant of outcome for hospitalized patients. Clin Infect Dis 2000;31(Suppl 4):S131–8.
11. Rello J, Mallol J. Optimal therapy for methicillin-resistant *Staphylococcus aureus* pneumonia: what is the best dosing regimen? Chest 2006;130(4):938–40.
12. Sandiumenge A, Diaz E, Bodi M, et al. Therapy of ventilator-associated pneumonia. A patient-based approach based on the ten rules of "The Tarragona Strategy". Intensive Care Med 2003;29(6):876–83.
13. Celis R, Torres A, Gatell JM, et al. Nosocomial pneumonia. A multivariate analysis of risk and prognosis. Chest 1988;93(2):318–24.
14. Rello J, Gallego M, Mariscal D, et al. The value of routine microbial investigation in ventilator-associated pneumonia. Am J Respir Crit Care Med 1997;156(1):196–200.
15. Garnacho-Montero J, Garcia-Garmendia JL, Barrero-Almodovar A, et al. Impact of adequate empirical antibiotic therapy on the outcome of patients admitted to the intensive care unit with sepsis. Crit Care Med 2003;31(12):2742–51.
16. Garnacho-Montero J, Ortiz-Leyba C, Herrera-Melero I, et al. Mortality and morbidity attributable to inadequate empirical antimicrobial therapy in patients admitted to the ICU with sepsis: a matched cohort study. J Antimicrob Chemother 2008;61(2):436–41.
17. Kollef MH, Sherman G, Ward S, et al. Inadequate antimicrobial treatment of infections: a risk factor for hospital mortality among critically ill patients. Chest 1999; 115(2):462–74.
18. Alvarez-Lerma F. Modification of empiric antibiotic treatment in patients with pneumonia acquired in the intensive care unit. ICU-Acquired pneumonia study group. Intensive Care Med 1996;22(5):387–94.
19. Dupont H, Mentec H, Sollet JP, et al. Impact of appropriateness of initial antibiotic therapy on the outcome of ventilator-associated pneumonia. Intensive Care Med 2001;27(2):355–62.
20. Magnotti LJ, Schroeppel TJ, Fabian TC, et al. Reduction in inadequate empiric antibiotic therapy for ventilator-associated pneumonia: impact of a unit-specific treatment pathway. Am Surg 2008;74(6):516–22.
21. Zaragoza R, Artero A, Camarena JJ, et al. The influence of inadequate empirical antimicrobial treatment on patients with bloodstream infections in an intensive care unit. Clin Microbiol Infect 2003;9(5):412–8.
22. Falagas ME, Kasiakou SK, Rafailidis PI, et al. Comparison of mortality of patients with *Acinetobacter baumannii* bacteraemia receiving appropriate and inappropriate empirical therapy. J Antimicrob Chemother 2006;57(6):1251–4.
23. Micek ST, Lloyd AE, Ritchie DJ, et al. *Pseudomonas aeruginosa* bloodstream infection: importance of appropriate initial antimicrobial treatment. Antimicrob Agents Chemother 2005;49(4):1306–11.
24. Ibrahim EH, Sherman G, Ward S, et al. The influence of inadequate antimicrobial treatment of bloodstream infections on patient outcomes in the ICU setting. Chest 2000;118(1):146–55.
25. Leibovici L, Shraga I, Drucker M, et al. The benefit of appropriate empirical antibiotic treatment in patients with bloodstream infection. J Intern Med 1998;244(5): 379–86.
26. Paterson DL, Ko WC, Von Gottberg A, et al. Antibiotic therapy for *Klebsiella pneumoniae* bacteremia: implications of production of extended-spectrum beta-lactamases. Clin Infect Dis 2004;39(1):31–7.
27. Kollef MH, Ward S. The influence of mini-BAL cultures on patient outcomes: implications for the antibiotic management of ventilator-associated pneumonia. Chest 1998;113(2):412–20.

28. Leroy O, Meybeck A, d'Escrivan T, et al. Impact of adequacy of initial antimicrobial therapy on the prognosis of patients with ventilator-associated pneumonia. Intensive Care Med 2003;29(12):2170–3.

29. Luna CM, Vujacich P, Niederman MS, et al. Impact of BAL data on the therapy and outcome of ventilator-associated pneumonia. Chest 1997;111(3):676–85.

30. Valles J, Rello J, Ochagavia A, et al. Community-acquired bloodstream infection in critically ill adult patients: impact of shock and inappropriate antibiotic therapy on survival. Chest 2003;123(5):1615–24.

31. Fraser A, Paul M, Almanasreh N, et al. Benefit of appropriate empirical antibiotic treatment: thirty-day mortality and duration of hospital stay. Am J Med 2006; 119(11):970–6.

32. Kumar A, Ellis P, Arabi Y, et al. Initiation of inappropriate antimicrobial therapy results in a fivefold reduction of survival in human septic shock. Chest 2009; 136(5):1237–48.

33. Kollef MH. Optimizing antibiotic therapy in the intensive care unit setting. Crit Care 2001;5(4):189–95.

34. Johnson PN, Rapp RP, Nelson CT, et al. Characterization of community-acquired *Staphylococcus aureus* infections in children. Ann Pharmacother 2007;41(9): 1361–7.

35. Ho PL, Cheng VC, Chu CM. Antibiotic resistance in community-acquired pneumonia caused by *Streptococcus pneumoniae*, methicillin-resistant *Staphylococcus aureus*, and *Acinetobacter baumannii*. Chest 2009;136(4):1119–27.

36. Flaherty JP, Weinstein RA. Infection control and pneumonia prophylaxis strategies in the intensive care unit. Semin Respir Infect 1990;5(3):191–203.

37. Rello J, Ausina V, Ricart M, et al. Impact of previous antimicrobial therapy on the etiology and outcome of ventilator-associated pneumonia. Chest 1993;104(4): 1230–5.

38. Rello J, Ausina V, Ricart M, et al. Risk factors for infection by *Pseudomonas aeruginosa* in patients with ventilator-associated pneumonia. Intensive Care Med 1994;20(3):193–8.

39. Rello J, Torres A, Ricart M, et al. Ventilator-associated pneumonia by *Staphylococcus aureus*. Comparison of methicillin-resistant and methicillin-sensitive episodes. Am J Respir Crit Care Med 1994;150(6 Pt 1):1545–9.

40. Trouillet JL, Chastre J, Vuagnat A, et al. Ventilator-associated pneumonia caused by potentially drug-resistant bacteria. Am J Respir Crit Care Med 1998;157(2): 531–9.

41. Fagon JY, Chastre J, Domart Y, et al. Nosocomial pneumonia in patients receiving continuous mechanical ventilation. Prospective analysis of 52 episodes with use of a protected specimen brush and quantitative culture techniques. Am Rev Respir Dis 1989;139(4):877–84.

42. Husni RN, Goldstein LS, Arroliga AC, et al. Risk factors for an outbreak of multidrug-resistant *Acinetobacter* nosocomial pneumonia among intubated patients. Chest 1999;115(5):1378–82.

43. Edmond MB, Ober JF, Weinbaum DL, et al. Vancomycin-resistant *Enterococcus faecium* bacteremia: risk factors for infection. Clin Infect Dis 1995;20(5):1126–33.

44. American Thoracic Society/Infectious Diseases Society of America. Guidelines for the management of adults with hospital-acquired, ventilator-associated, and healthcare-associated pneumonia. Am J Respir Crit Care Med 2005;171(4): 388–416.

45. Tacconelli E, Cataldo MA, De Pascale G, et al. Prediction models to identify hospitalized patients at risk of being colonized or infected with multidrug-resistant

Acinetobacter baumannii calcoaceticus complex. J Antimicrob Chemother 2008; 62(5):1130–7.

46. Chen SY, Wu GH, Chang SC, et al. Bacteremia in previously hospitalized patients: prolonged effect from previous hospitalization and risk factors for antimicrobial-resistant bacterial infections. Ann Emerg Med 2008;51(5):639–46.

47. Bonten MJ, Slaughter S, Hayden MK, et al. External sources of vancomycin-resistant enterococci for intensive care units. Crit Care Med 1998;26(12):2001–4.

48. Richards MJ, Edwards JR, Culver DH, et al. Nosocomial infections in medical intensive care units in the United States. National Nosocomial Infections Surveillance System. Crit Care Med 1999;27(5):887–92.

49. Rello J, Sa-Borges M, Correa H, et al. Variations in etiology of ventilator-associated pneumonia across four treatment sites: implications for antimicrobial prescribing practices. Am J Respir Crit Care Med 1999;160(2):608–13.

50. Koulenti D, Lisboa T, Brun-Buisson C, et al. Spectrum of practice in the diagnosis of nosocomial pneumonia in patients requiring mechanical ventilation in European intensive care units. Crit Care Med 2009;37(8):2360–8.

51. Dancer SJ, Coyne M, Robertson C, et al. Antibiotic use is associated with resistance of environmental organisms in a teaching hospital. J Hosp Infect 2006; 62(2):200–6.

52. Valles J, Mesalles E, Mariscal D, et al. A 7-year study of severe hospital-acquired pneumonia requiring ICU admission. Intensive Care Med 2003; 29(11):1981–8.

53. Hansen S, Schwab F, Behnke M, et al. National influences on catheter-associated bloodstream infection rates: practices among national surveillance networks participating in the European HELICS project. J Hosp Infect 2009; 71(1):66–73.

54. Hospital-acquired pneumonia in adults. Diagnosis, assessment of severity, initial antimicrobial therapy, and preventive strategies. A consensus statement, American Thoracic Society, November 1995. Am J Respir Crit Care Med 1996; 153(5):1711–25.

55. Agbaht K, Lisboa T, Pobo A, et al. Management of ventilator-associated pneumonia in a multidisciplinary intensive care unit: does trauma make a difference? Intensive Care Med 2007;33(8):1387–95.

56. Rello J, Ulldemolins M, Lisboa T, et al. Determinants of choice and prescription patterns in empiric antibiotic Therapy for HAP/VAP. Eur Respir J 2010. [Epub ahead of print].

57. Bonten MJ, Slaughter S, Ambergen AW, et al. The role of "colonization pressure" in the spread of vancomycin-resistant enterococci: an important infection control variable. Arch Intern Med 1998;158(10):1127–32.

58. Kollef MH. Epidemiology and risk factors for nosocomial pneumonia. Emphasis on prevention. Clin Chest Med 1999;20(3):653–70.

59. McEachern R, Campbell GD Jr. Hospital-acquired pneumonia: epidemiology, etiology, and treatment. Infect Dis Clin North Am 1998;12(3):761–79.

60. Kuti EL, Patel AA, Coleman CI. Impact of inappropriate antibiotic therapy on mortality in patients with ventilator-associated pneumonia and blood stream infection: a meta-analysis. J Crit Care 2008;23(1):91–100.

61. Spellberg B, Talbot G. Recommended design features of future clinical trials of antibacterial agents for hospital-acquired bacterial pneumonia and ventilator-associated bacterial pneumonia. Clin Infect Dis 2010;51(Suppl 1):S150–70.

62. Spengler RF, Greenough WB 3rd. Hospital costs and mortality attributed to nosocomial bacteremias. JAMA 1978;240(22):2455–8.

63. Rello J, Ricart M, Mirelis B, et al. Nosocomial bacteremia in a medical-surgical intensive care unit: epidemiologic characteristics and factors influencing mortality in 111 episodes. Intensive Care Med 1994;20(2):94–8.
64. Valles J, Leon C, Alvarez-Lerma F. Nosocomial bacteremia in critically ill patients: a multicenter study evaluating epidemiology and prognosis. Spanish Collaborative Group for Infections in Intensive Care Units of Sociedad Espanola de Medicina Intensiva y Unidades Coronarias (SEMIUC). Clin Infect Dis 1997;24(3):387–95.
65. Steinberg JP, Clark CC, Hackman BO. Nosocomial and community-acquired Staphylococcus aureus bacteremias from 1980 to 1993: impact of intravascular devices and methicillin resistance. Clin Infect Dis 1996;23(2):255–9.
66. Chow JK, Golan Y, Ruthazer R, et al. Risk factors for albicans and non-albicans candidemia in the intensive care unit. Crit Care Med 2008;36(7):1993–8.
67. Schramm GE, Johnson JA, Doherty JA, et al. Methicillin-resistant Staphylococcus aureus sterile-site infection: the importance of appropriate initial antimicrobial treatment. Crit Care Med 2006;34(8):2069–74.
68. Brook I. Microbiology and management of soft tissue and muscle infections. Int J Surg 2008;6(4):328–38.
69. Crum NF, Lee RU, Thornton SA, et al. Fifteen-year study of the changing epidemiology of methicillin-resistant Staphylococcus aureus. Am J Med 2006;119(11): 943–51.
70. Moran GJ, Krishnadasan A, Gorwitz RJ, et al. Methicillin-resistant S. aureus infections among patients in the emergency department. N Engl J Med 2006;355(7): 666–74.
71. Chuck EA, Frazee BW, Lambert L, et al. The benefit of empiric treatment for methicillin-resistant Staphylococcus aureus. J Emerg Med 2010;38(5):567–71.
72. Ruhe JJ, Smith N, Bradsher RW, et al. Community-onset methicillin-resistant Staphylococcus aureus skin and soft-tissue infections: impact of antimicrobial therapy on outcome. Clin Infect Dis 2007;44(6):777–84.
73. van de Beek D, de Gans J, Spanjaard L, et al. Clinical features and prognostic factors in adults with bacterial meningitis. N Engl J Med 2004; 351(18):1849–59.
74. Whitney CG, Farley MM, Hadler J, et al. Increasing prevalence of multidrug-resistant Streptococcus pneumoniae in the United States. N Engl J Med 2000;343(26): 1917–24.
75. Auburtin M, Wolff M, Charpentier J, et al. Detrimental role of delayed antibiotic administration and penicillin-nonsusceptible strains in adult intensive care unit patients with pneumococcal meningitis: the PNEUMOREA prospective multicenter study. Crit Care Med 2006;34(11):2758–65.
76. Lu CH, Chang WN, Chuang YC, et al. The prognostic factors of adult gram-negative bacillary meningitis. J Hosp Infect 1998;40(1):27–34.
77. Geyik MF, Kokoglu OF, Hosoglu S, et al. Acute bacterial meningitis as a complication of otitis media and related mortality factors. Yonsei Med J 2002;43(5):573–8.
78. Lu CH, Chang WN, Chang HW. Klebsiella meningitis in adults: clinical features, prognostic factors and therapeutic outcomes. J Clin Neurosci 2002;9(5):533–8.
79. Rowland M, Tozer TN. Clinical pharmacokinetics. Concepts and applications. 3rd edition. Philadelphia: Lippincott Williams & Wilkins; 1995.
80. Cruciani M, Gatti G, Lazzarini L, et al. Penetration of vancomycin into human lung tissue. J Antimicrob Chemother 1996;38(5):865–9.
81. Lamer C, de Beco V, Soler P, et al. Analysis of vancomycin entry into pulmonary lining fluid by bronchoalveolar lavage in critically ill patients. Antimicrob Agents Chemother 1993;37(2):281–6.

82. Chandrasekar PH, Rolston KV, Smith BR, et al. Diffusion of ceftriaxone into the cerebrospinal fluid of adults. J Antimicrob Chemother 1984;14(1):127–30.
83. Burgess DS. Curbing resistance development: maximizing the utility of available agents. J Manag Care Pharm 2009;15(Suppl 5):S5–9.
84. Craig WA. Post-antibiotic effects in experimental infection models: relationship to in-vitro phenomena and to treatment of infections in man. J Antimicrob Chemother 1993;31(Suppl D):149–58.
85. Fuster-Lluch O, Geronimo-Pardo M, Peyro-Garcia R, et al. Glomerular hyperfiltration and albuminuria in critically ill patients. Anaesth Intensive Care 2008;36(5): 674–80.
86. Udy AA, Roberts JA, Boots RJ, et al. Augmented renal clearance: implications for antibacterial dosing in the critically ill. Clin Pharmacokinet 2010;49(1):1–16.
87. Fleck A, Raines G, Hawker F, et al. Increased vascular permeability: a major cause of hypoalbuminaemia in disease and injury. Lancet 1985;1(8432):781–4.
88. Ulldemolins M, Roberts JA, Rello J, et al. The effects of hypoalbuminemia on optimizing antibiotic dosing in critically ill patients. Clin Pharmacokinet, in press.
89. Roberts JA, Roberts MS, Robertson TA, et al. Piperacillin penetration into tissue of critically ill patients with sepsis–bolus versus continuous administration? Crit Care Med 2009;37(3):926–33.
90. Ulldemolins M, Roberts J, Wallis S, et al. Flucloxacillin dosing in critically ill patients with hypoalbuminemia - special emphasis on unbound pharmacokinetics. J Antimicrob Chemother 2010;65(8):1771–8.
91. Marik PE. Aminoglycoside volume of distribution and illness severity in critically ill septic patients. Anaesth Intensive Care 1993;21(2):172–3.
92. Kollef M. Appropriate empirical antibacterial therapy for nosocomial infections: getting it right the first time. Drugs 2003;63(20):2157–68.
93. Rello J, Vidaur L, Sandiumenge A, et al. De-escalation therapy in ventilator-associated pneumonia. Crit Care Med 2004;32(11):2183–90.
94. Cooke FJ, Holmes AH. The missing care bundle: antibiotic prescribing in hospitals. Int J Antimicrob Agents 2007;30(1):25–9.
95. Rello J, Chastre J, Cornaglia G, et al. European care bundle for the management of ventilator-associated pneumonia. J Crit Care 2010. [Epub ahead of print].
96. Roberts JA, Lipman J. Pharmacokinetic issues for antibiotics in the critically ill patient. Crit Care Med 2009;37(3):840–51.
97. Roberts JA, Ulldemolins M, Roberts MS, et al. Therapeutic drug monitoring of beta-lactams in critically ill patients: proof of concept. Int J Antimicrob Agents 2010;36(4):332–9.

Antimicrobial Therapy for Life-threatening Infections: Speed is Life

Duane J. Funk, MD, FRCP(C)[a], Anand Kumar, MD[b,c],*

KEYWORDS

• Antimicrobial therapy • Septic shock
• Early therapy • Survival

> *This thing all things devours:*
> *Birds, beasts, trees, flowers;*
> *Gnaws iron, bites steel*
> *Grinds hard stones to meal;*
> *Slays king, ruins town,*
> *And beats High Mountain down.*

The answer to this riddle, from JRR Tolkien's *The Hobbit* is time. In the context of acute illness, time is always a critical issue. Physicians routinely attempt to reverse or slow the temporal progression of illness to improve the lives of patients. Those of us who practice critical care have also tried to use time to our advantage. The trauma surgeons amongst us were the first to develop the concept of the golden hour that was critical to the survival of those with traumatic and hemorrhagic shock.[1] This concept subsequently expanded to cardiogenic and obstructive shock with the use of thrombolytics for myocardial infarction[2] and more recently, obstructive shock caused by massive pulmonary embolism.[3]

In recent decades, the importance of rapid initiation of appropriate antimicrobial therapy for life-threatening infection has become apparent. In the late 1970s and early 1980s, pediatricians, emergentologists, and infectious diseases physicians began to recognize the critical importance of rapid antimicrobial therapy for pediatric meningitis. This knowledge has translated into internationally accepted guidelines that mandate initiation of appropriate antimicrobial therapy as quickly as possible after

---

[a] Department of Anesthesia, Section of Critical Care Medicine, 2nd Floor Harry Medovy House, University of Manitoba, Winnipeg, Manitoba R3E 1X2, Canada
[b] Section of Infectious Diseases, Section of Critical Care Medicine, Health Sciences Centre, University of Manitoba, JJ399d, 700 William Street, Winnipeg, Manitoba R3A-1R9, Canada
[c] Robert Wood Johnson Medical School, University of Medicine and Dentistry, New Jersey, NJ, USA
* Corresponding author. Robert Wood Johnson Medical School, University of Medicine and Dentistry, New Jersey, NJ.
E-mail address: akumar61@yahoo.com

Crit Care Clin 27 (2011) 53–76
doi:10.1016/j.ccc.2010.09.008
0749-0704/11/$ – see front matter © 2011 Elsevier Inc. All rights reserved.

recognition of potential bacterial meningitis (preferably within an hour or less).[4] During the 1990s, the importance of rapid initiation of appropriate antimicrobials for community-acquired pneumonia (CAP) became appreciated[5] and was eventually integrated into Joint Commission on Accreditation of Health care Organizations (JHACO) guidelines. In the last decade, the critical importance of time to effective antimicrobial therapy in the context of bacteremia/candidemia and particularly septic shock has come to the forefront.[6,7] International guidelines for sepsis and septic shock management have, throughout the decade, included a recommendation for rapid (<1 hour) initiation of antimicrobial therapy.[8]

Nonetheless, there remains controversy about this issue in the broader context. Some of these concerns have to do with the retrospective methodology of studies that have yielded evidence of a relationship between outcome and antimicrobial delay.[9] Much of the work supporting this relationship is confounded by other therapeutic factors. Biologic plausibility may also be an issue for mild disease.[10] Fortunately, interventional studies that support the proposition that early initiation of appropriate antimicrobial therapy is the key factor in determining survival from severe infections have recently been published. This article describes the concept of early appropriate therapy, and reviews the evidence behind the early administration of antimicrobials as a key determinant in survival from septic shock, bacteremia/candidemia, pneumonia, and meningitis.

WHAT CONSTITUTES EARLY AND APPROPRIATE ANTIMICROBIAL THERAPY?

The concept of what constitutes early appropriate therapy is discussed further in another article in this issue. However, when describing appropriate therapy, many factors must be taken into account. Most of the current studies on appropriate therapy have defined this as the selection of an antimicrobial that has in vitro activity against the organism that was isolated from the index culture. Other studies have defined appropriate as consistent with current practice guidelines for the particular site of infection (ie, ventilator-acquired pneumonia [VAP]).

When defining appropriate therapy, the use of culture results should be the gold standard, as the antibiograms of organisms at different institutions or even on different wards within a given institution show great variability.[11,12] This definition, although microbiologically sound, ignores the unique pharmacokinetics and pharmacodynamics of antimicrobials, particularly in the critically ill. Elements that may affect appropriateness include route of administration, dose and dosing schedule (ie, optimization of pharmacokinetic indices in view of alterations in absorption, volume of distribution, and drug elimination kinetics in the critically ill), penetration and cidality of the antimicrobial agent, and the use of combination therapy in some contexts (eg, *Pseudomonas* infection).

Clinicians assessing the extensive literature on the benefit of initiation of appropriate antimicrobial therapy for life-threatening infections should be aware that the term appropriate therapy intrinsically includes a time element. That provision of microbiologically inappropriate antimicrobials simply represents a marker of delayed delivery of appropriate therapy (assuming the patient lives long enough) should be obvious. When defined as the use of an antimicrobial without activity for the causative pathogen, inappropriate therapy is fundamentally equivalent to no therapy at all. Therefore, almost all studies that have favored appropriate rather than inappropriate initial antimicrobial therapy for serious infections can be interpreted to be favoring early rather than delayed antimicrobial therapy.

The rest of this article deals with the specific infections where data have shown that time to appropriate therapy is a key factor in survival. Limitations of the current literature are also highlighted.

ANIMAL DATA

Few experimental animal studies have examined the effect of delays of antimicrobial therapy on outcome in systemic infections such as sepsis. Knudsen and colleagues[13] and Fridmodt-Moller and Thomsen[14] have demonstrated a critical effect of timing of antimicrobial therapy relative to intraperitoneal inoculation of S. pneumoniae into mice. The degree of bacterial propagation and survival was shown to be highly dependent on antimicrobial timing with 100% mortality if penicillin was initiated at 24 hours after inoculation. Similarly, Greisman and colleagues[15] have shown that sequential delays in aminoglycoside therapy after intraperitoneal or intravenous inoculation of enteric organisms (Escherichia coli, Proteus mirabilis, and Klebsiella pneumoniae) results in progressive increases in mortality from 0% to 90% to 100%. Kumar and colleagues[16] have examined the relationship between peritonitis induction using implantation of an E coli–containing fibrin/α-cellulose clot encased in a gelatin capsule, the onset of hypotension, and outcome in mice. A critical inflection point with respect to survival occurred between 12 and 15 hours after sepsis induction, the point at which physiologically relevant hypotension was manifested. Antibiotic therapy before 12 hours yielded less than 15% mortality but after 15 hours there was more than 80% mortality. Heart rate diverged by 6 hours after sepsis induction, whereas cardiac output and stroke volume divergence did not occur until 18 to 24 hours after sepsis induction. Antibiotic administration 12 hours or longer after E coli capsule implant was associated with persistence of increased circulating lactate, tumor necrosis factor α (TNF)α, and interleukin-6 levels.

This study pointed out the potential importance of rapidity of effective antimicrobial therapy on risk of death once hypotension is present. In healthy animals, only a modest increase in mortality occurs with delayed therapy before the hypotension of early septic shock. However, once such hypotension is present, mortality risk increases rapidly and death eventually becomes inevitable irrespective of any intervention, a process of irreversible shock that had previously been described only for hemorrhagic shock.[17,18] These data suggest that sustained hypotension in septic shock is associated with irreversible injury leading to inevitable deterioration and death many hours after the initial injury. This study provides a biologic rationale for a linkage between delays in initiation of effective antimicrobial therapy and outcome of septic shock in humans.

HUMAN STUDIES
Inflammatory Markers and Organ Failure

Several studies have examined the role of delays in initiation of effective antimicrobial therapy and persistence of inflammatory markers and/or development of organ failure. Calbo and colleagues[19] showed that patients with pneumococcal pneumonia with a longer time of evolution presented with higher levels of proinflammatory cytokines (TNFα) and a higher expression of acute phase proteins (including C-reactive protein and fibrinogen). This study parallels the finding in the mouse study by Kumar and colleagues[16] with respect to persistence of increased TNFα in untreated sepsis.

Bagshaw and colleagues[20] have also demonstrated in a multivariate analysis of more than 4500 patients with septic shock that delays in initiation of appropriate antimicrobial therapy are associated with increased risk and severity of renal injury.

Similarly, Iscimen and colleagues[21] have shown using multivariate analysis that the risk of acute lung injury in patients with septic shock is positively related to increasing delays in initiation of appropriate antimicrobial therapy. Garnacho-Montero and colleagues[22] have demonstrated a relationship between antimicrobial delay and increase in the Sequential Organ Failure Assessment (SOFA) score in patients with sepsis. Thus, any finding of increased mortality with delays in initiation of antimicrobial therapy for serious infections in humans is supported by congruent inflammatory injury and organ dysfunction data.

Mortality Studies

Sepsis and septic shock

The most life-threatening infectious disease that intensivists confront is septic shock. With a mortality of 30% to 40%, the early recognition and treatment of this disease is key to improving survival. If early antimicrobial therapy has an effect on mortality, this is the disease where the largest effect should be realized. Numerous studies have looked at time to antimicrobial therapy in septic shock, and virtually all have found a reduction in mortality when antimicrobials were given in a timely fashion.

Kumar and colleagues have provided the most direct data on the question of the specific effect of early appropriate antimicrobial therapy on survival in septic shock. Parallel to our earlier experimental mouse study, we retrospectively looked at the duration of hypotension before initiation of effective antimicrobial therapy in 2731 adult patients with septic shock.[6] The delay to initial administration of effective antimicrobial therapy was shown to be the single strongest predictor of survival.

Initiation of effective antimicrobial therapy within the first hour after onset of septic shock–related hypotension was associated with 79.9% survival to hospital discharge (**Fig. 1**). For every additional hour to effective antimicrobial initiation in the first 6 hours

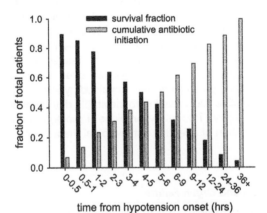

time from hypotension onset (hrs)

Fig. 1. Cumulative initiation of effective antimicrobial therapy and survival in septic shock. In a large retrospective study of septic shock, Kumar and colleagues demonstrated that median time to effective/appropriate antimicrobial therapy was 6 hours and that for every hour delay more than the first 6 hours, the projected mortality increased by 7.6%/h. X axis represents time (hours) after first documentation of septic shock–associated hypotension. Black bars represent the fraction of patients surviving to hospital discharge and the gray bars represent the cumulative fraction of patients having received effective antimicrobials at any given time point. (*From* Kumar A, Roberts D, Wood KE, et al. Duration of hypotension before initiation of effective antimicrobial therapy is the critical determinant of survival in human septic shock. Crit Care Med 2006;34:1589–96; with permission.)

after onset of hypotension, survival dropped an average of 7.6%. With effective antimicrobial initiation between the first and second hour after onset of hypotension, survival had already dropped to 70.5%. With effective antimicrobial therapy delay of 5 to 6 hours after hypotension onset, survival was just 42.0% and 25.4% by 9 to 12 hours. The adjusted odds ratio of death was already significantly increased by the second hour after onset of hypotension and the ratio continued to climb with longer delays (**Fig. 2**).

Substantial delays before initiation of effective therapy have been shown in several studies of serious infections.[5,23–25] In septic shock, the median time to delivery of effective antimicrobial therapy after initial onset of recurrent/persistent hypotension was 6 hours.[6] Only 14.5% of all patients who had not received effective antimicrobials before shock received them within the first hour of documentation of onset of recurrent or persistent hypotension (see **Fig. 1**). Only 51.4% had received them by 6 hours after onset of hypotension. Even 12 hours after the first occurrence of recurrent or sustained hypotension, 29.8% of patients had not received effective antimicrobial therapy. The effect was sustained across a broad group of organisms including gram-negatives, gram-positives, and *Candida* species.

After adjustment for various comorbidities (including the number of presenting organ failures), therapeutic variables (use of mechanical ventilation, drotrecogin-alpha and low-dose steroids) and severity of illness (APACHE II score [Acute Physiology and Chronic Health Evaluation]), the delay in initiation of antimicrobial therapy remained the strongest correlate of outcome. Although often referred to as linear, a graphic representation of the relationship between antimicrobial delay relative to onset of hypotension and outcome in human septic shock suggests a logarithmic decay of survival probability (**Fig. 3**).

The strong relationship between delays in antimicrobial therapy and outcome in septic shock (and less so, sepsis) have been confirmed by several other groups. In these studies, time to effective antimicrobial therapy has been assessed in the context of rapidity of vasopressor initiation,[26] polymorphisms of inflammatory genes,[22] or time

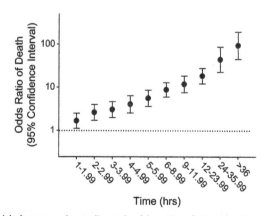

Time (hrs)

Fig. 2. Mortality risk (expressed as adjusted odds ratio of death) with increasing delays in initiation of effective antimicrobial therapy. Bars represent 95% CI. An increased risk of death is already present by the second hour after hypotension onset (compared with the first hour after hypotension onset). The risk of death continues to increase up to more than 36 hours after hypotension onset. (*From* Kumar A, Roberts D, Wood KE, et al. Duration of hypotension before initiation of effective antimicrobial therapy is the critical determinant of survival in human septic shock. Crit Care Med 2006;34:1589–96; with permission.)

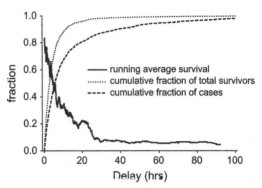

Fig. 3. The running average of the fraction of 250 patients with septic shock surviving to hospital discharge from fast to slowest antimicrobial initiation time after documentation of hypotension (n = 5715). Decay of survival probability seems to represent a logarithmic function. Approximately 90% of survivors of septic shock received appropriate antimicrobial therapy within 12 hours of documentation of hypotension.

to qualification for early goal-directed therapy.[27] Benefit has even been shown in patients with cancer with septic shock, a group with exceptionally high mortality (>65%).[28] In a study on candidemic septic shock, multivariate analysis demonstrated that a delay in antimicrobial administration of greater than 15 hours after initial positive blood cultures resulted in a significant increase in mortality.[29]

With respect to invasive *Candida* infections, Hsu and colleagues[30] have recently also shown that administration of an echinocandin within 72 hours of initial positive culture is associated with a higher response rate, improved time to clinical stability, and decreased length of stay (LOS). Similarly, Hood and colleagues[31] have shown that early initiation (<4 hours after presentation) of antimicrobial therapy for about 24,000 cases of complicated urinary tract infections requiring hospital admission (most of whom likely had sepsis) was associated with decreased hospital LOS.

Using the 2008 Surviving Sepsis guidelines recommendations as a guide, many hospitals have implemented a bundled approach to the treatment of septic shock.[32] Several studies have shown an improvement in outcome of sepsis/septic shock when such bundles are used.[33–39] However, Barochia and colleagues[40] have shown that the only consistent element of therapy that bundle implementation affected in studies to date was time to antimicrobial and appropriateness of initial antimicrobial therapy.

Efforts have been made to specifically delineate the role of each individual part of the bundle on the overall reduction in mortality. In a prospective study of 316 patients with severe sepsis/septic shock in Brazil, the individual parts of the Surviving Sepsis bundle were evaluated to determine their role in mortality reduction.[41] The administration of antimicrobials within 120 minutes of the diagnosis and the collection of blood cultures were the only interventions that seemed to affect mortality (odds ratio [OR] for early antimicrobials = 0.44, 95% confidence interval [CI] 0.23–0.87, $P<.009$). In this study, appropriate early antimicrobials were delivered to patients 71.7% of the time.

Similar data were generated in a study from Finland in which the effect of different bundle elements including central mixed venous oxygen saturation was assessed in multivariate analysis in 92 patients with septic shock presenting from the community.[42] About one-third of patients achieved 4 or more of the bundle elements. Among the bundle elements, only administration of antimicrobials within 3 hours of admission was associated with improved outcome, even when APACHE II score was added to the model. In another prospective observational study from Spain, 2796 patients with severe sepsis/septic shock were evaluated for the role of each of the bundle elements in the Surviving Sepsis campaign on mortality.[43] Again, early antimicrobials were 1 of only 2 interventions that significantly reduced mortality, the other being the administration of drotrecogin-alpha in the case of multiorgan failure from sepsis. In this study, 85% of patients received an antimicrobial within 6 hours of the diagnosis of sepsis.

Gurnani and colleagues[44] examined the outcomes of 118 patients in a single center after the implementation of a sepsis bundle. Bundle implementation (with associated improvements in antimicrobial delay and early fluid resuscitation volumes) was associated with decreased pressor days, ventilator days, and intensive care unit (ICU) LOS as well as 28-day (but not in-hospital) mortality. The time interval from documentation of shock to empiric antimicrobial therapy (less than or more than 4.5 hours), but not fluid variables, was independently associated with outcome.

Several studies have failed to find a significant association between antimicrobial timing and mortality in sepsis or septic shock. One prospective Spanish study (comparing 396 patients after bundle intervention with 84 historical controls) found that the only individual intervention associated with a reduced mortality in regression analysis was the achievement of a central mixed venous oxygen saturation of 70% or more.[37] However, in this study, there was no significant improvement in either the administration of broad-spectrum antimicrobials or central mixed venous oxygen saturation in the intervention group and the historical controls (49% vs 57.3% for antimicrobial administration, $P = .168$). Compliance with the antimicrobial delivery aspect of the bundle was significantly lower than in other studies that have reported a benefit. It is possible that the lack of a beneficial effect of antimicrobials in this study was not seen because of the lack of improvement in this part of the bundle, and the low rate of appropriate antimicrobials overall. In addition, the analysis suggested an unusually strong degree of covariation among bundle elements rendering statistical differentiation of the effect of individual bundle elements difficult.

A similar negative result for early antimicrobial administration was seen in a Portuguese community-acquired sepsis bundle study involving more than 4000 patients.[34] In this study, only collection of blood cultures was associated with improved outcome. In another study of 182 patients with surgical sepsis, only the use of activated protein C was associated with improved outcome.[45] A major problem with all these studies may be the difficulty of defining the baseline point from the point of view of timing of therapies. However, in all these studies, mortality at least trended in favor of earlier antimicrobial therapy.

Given the ethical challenges in study design, just 1 randomized study of early antimicrobial initiation in septic shock has been documented in the literature.[46] In this Australian study, 198 patients with septic shock requiring transport in a rural environment were randomized to broad-spectrum prehospital antimicrobials or standard care (antimicrobials on arrival at hospital). All patients received standard fluid resuscitation in the field. The (3.4 ± 2.6)-hour relative delay to initial antimicrobial administration after emergency department admission in the control group was significantly greater than in patients receiving prehospital antimicrobials ($P = .02$). The 28-day mortality was significantly reduced to 42.4% in the intervention group compared with 56.7% in the control group ($P = .049$, OR = 0.56; 95% CI = 0.32–1.00). Length of hospital stay was similarly reduced in patients randomized to prehospital antimicrobial therapy.

In most of the studies looking at time and appropriateness of antimicrobial therapy, anywhere from 20% to 40% of patients received inappropriate treatment. It is therefore critically important to consider how to improve on the institution of broad-spectrum antimicrobial therapy based on the presumed source of sepsis, antibiogram at the particular institution (or even within the ICU), and risk factors for resistant organisms. The current weight of evidence supports the early institution of appropriate antimicrobial therapy in patients with septic shock and perhaps less strongly, sepsis. Obstacles to delivering optimal antimicrobial therapy including delayed diagnosis of a serious infection and poor selection of antimicrobials must be overcome to reduce mortality.

Bacteremia/fungemia

In one of the first studies to suggest that a delay in delivery of timely antimicrobials to patients with bacteremia adversely affected outcome, Bodey and colleagues[47] retrospectively reviewed 410 cases of Pseudomonas bacteremia in 1985. They discovered that a delay in appropriate antimicrobials of 1 to 2 days resulted in a decrease in the cure rate from 74% to 46%. However, this study did not address mortality. Similar, but more recent work showed that patients (n = 100) who were bacteremic with Pseudomonas and received their antimicrobials more than 52 hours after the blood culture was drawn had more than double the mortality of patients who received their antimicrobials before this time period (44 vs 19%, $P = .008$).[48] In a multivariate analysis, delayed therapy was independently associated with a 4.1-fold increase in 30-day mortality (95% CI 1.2–13.9, $P = .03$).

Kang and colleagues[49] also demonstrated increased mortality with delays of more than 24 hours from the time blood cultures were drawn in 136 patients with Pseudomonas bacteremia. A trend toward progressive mortality with increasing delays was also seen. Notably, 85% of the patients had septic shock. Significant subsets of patients in all 3 studies had delays in delivery of more than 1 to 2 days. Similar data have been developed for multidrug resistant Klebsiella bloodstream infection where a delay of more than 72 hours to appropriate antibiotic therapy was associated with an increased mortality risk in adjusted analysis.[50]

At first glance, these lengthy times to appropriate therapy for Pseudomonas and other gram-negative bacteremia seem disturbing, considering the disease has a mortality of 18% to 61%.[48,49] However, it is not surprising that these delays occur, as Pseudomonas and other gram-negatives found in the ICU are often resistant to several antimicrobials. So, unless clinicians are specifically suspicious of Pseudomonas or another resistant gram-negative, therapy may often be initially inappropriate and will not be altered to an active agent until the results of cultures and sensitivity are available, usually after several days.

Typical risk factors for Pseudomonas infection, including immunocompromised state, need for hemodialysis, ICU admission, and residence in a nursing home should alert the clinician to begin treatment with antipseudomonal therapy.[51,52] Similar delays in treatment are seen with Staphylococcus aureus bacteremia. This organism can be methicillin resistant in more than 50% of cases. Unless clinicians are suspicious that a patient is at risk for methicillin-resistant Staphylococcus aureus, inappropriate therapy may be initially prescribed pending preliminary sensitivity results. Lodise and colleagues[53] looked at the effect of antimicrobial delay on mortality in Staphylococcus aureus bacteremia. Using regression analysis, they determined that the break point for mortality increase in Staphylococcus aureus bacteremia was 44.75 hours, similar to that seen with Pseudomonas bacteremia. In this study, delayed antimicrobial therapy for Staphylococcus aureus was found to confer a 3.8-fold increase in hospital mortality. Other studies have yielded similar results with Staphylococcus aureus bacteremia.[54] Bacteremic pneumococcal pneumonia has also been shown to be sensitive to delays in appropriate antimicrobial therapy. Garnacho-Montero and colleagues[55] showed that a delay of more than 4 hours from admission to start of adequate antimicrobial treatment (adjusted hazard ratio [aHR] 2.62, 95% CI 1.06–6.45; P = .037) and severe sepsis or septic shock (aHR 5.06, 95% CI 1.63–15.71; P = .005) were independently associated with in-hospital mortality.

Candidemia is another infection where substantial delays in initiation of appropriate antimicrobial therapy may occur. Fernandez and colleagues[56] showed a median delay of 43.3 and 98.1 hours in the initiation of appropriate antimicrobial therapy for *Candida albicans* and *Candida glabrata* infections respectively (from the time the index culture was drawn). Such delays are often related to the lack of recognition of the possibility of a *Candida* infection (which precludes appropriate empiric therapy initiation) and pro-longed turnaround time for the culture results from the microbiology laboratory given the slow growth rate of the organism.[57] The effect of this delay in initiation of antifungal therapy on mortality has been studied extensively in the last few years.

Blot and colleagues[58] had shown as early as 2002 that a delay of antifungal therapy of more than 48 hours after the index blood culture was associated with an increased mortality of 78% from 44%. Later, Morrell and colleagues[59] demonstrated that in a multivariate regression analysis only APACHE II score and administration of anti-fungal therapy greater than 12 hours after blood cultures were drawn was associated with an increase in mortality of patients with *Candida* blood stream infections (CBSI) (**Fig. 4**). The risk of death was nearly doubled when therapy for CBSI was delayed for greater than 12 hours. The specific antifungal agents used were not defined, and approximately 25% of patients had septic shock. Garey and colleagues[7] have also examined this issue in 230 patients with candidemia treated with fluconazole from 4 American medical centers. They found that hospital mortality was significantly linked to delay in fluconazole initiation (after the first positive blood culture). In regression analysis, this delay and APACHE II score were independently associated with outcome.

There have been studies of bacteremia that have failed to show decreased survival with increased delays in appropriate antimicrobial therapy. Lin and colleagues[60] examined more than 1500 episodes of monomicrobial bacteremia. They found that

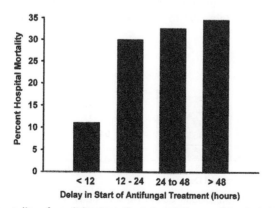

Fig. 4. Hospital mortality of candidemic patients in relation to delay in initiating antifungal therapy after index positive blood culture. Mortality risk climbs with increasing delays. (*From* Morrell M, Fraser VJ, Kollef MH. Delaying the empiric treatment of *Candida* bloodstream infection until positive blood culture results are obtained: a potential risk factor for hospital mortality. Antimicrob Agents Chemother 2005;49:3640–5; with permission.)

in the presence of neutropenia (absolute neutrophil count <100 cells/μL), a delay in effective antimicrobial therapy beyond 24 hours after draw of a positive blood culture was associated with an increased risk of death. In their adjusted analysis, neutropenia and a delay in antimicrobials were associated with an adjusted OR of risk of death of 18 (95% CI 2.84–114.5, P<.01). However, a delay-dependent mortality risk was not seen in non-neutropenic patients. Only 9.5% of patients in this study had septic shock. Similarly, Carona and colleagues[61] have also suggested a lack of relationship between delays of antimicrobial therapy and outcome in bacteremic ICU cases (of whom more than one-third had septic shock).

In summary, the discovery of bacteremia or candidemia in an acutely ill patient is always of major concern to the clinician. Delayed antimicrobial therapy results in an increase in mortality, however the adverse effect of antimicrobial delays is more limited than for septic shock and longer periods are required to manifest an adverse effect. Nonetheless, rapid initiation of appropriate empiric therapy in patients suspected of bacteremia or candidemia is clearly warranted.

Pneumonia

Timely administration of antimicrobials has been recognized as a key element in the survival of patients with CAP. The time to antimicrobial delivery for patients presenting to the emergency department (ED) with pneumonia is a quality measure for Joint Commission on Accreditation of Healthcare Organizations (JCAHO). Current JCAHO recommendations are that patients receive antimicrobials within 6 hours of presentation to hospital with evidence of CAP.[62] This suggestion was based on retrospective cohort analyses by Meehan and colleagues[5] and Houck and colleagues.[23]

In the first key paper on this subject, Meehan and colleagues[5] used the Medicare quality indicator system, a data collection system that tracks the care of hospitalized Medicare patients, to look at 14,069 patients older than 65 years presenting to the emergency room with pneumonia. The study found that antimicrobial administration within 8 hours of presenting to hospital was associated with a lower 30-day mortality (OR = 0.85, 95% CI 0.75–0.96). The odds ratio of death, however, increased gradually with longer delays (**Fig. 5**). The study was not designed to answer the question of whether or not the antimicrobials prescribed were appropriate.

Houck and colleagues,[23] using a similar approach, queried the Center for Medicare and Medicaid services database to look at time to antimicrobial administration in

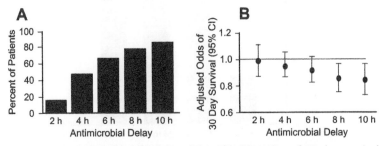

Fig. 5. Distribution of antimicrobial delays (*A*) and odds ratios of 30-day survival (*B*) in patients more than age 65 years presenting to the ER with community-acquired pneumonia. Approximately 25% of patients did not receive antimicrobial therapy after 8 hours in the ER; mortality in this group was significantly increased. (*From* Meehan TP, Fine MJ, Krumholz HM, et al. Quality of care, process, and outcomes in elderly patients with pneumonia. JAMA 1997;278:2080–4; with permission.)

13,771 hospitalized patients older than 65 years of age with CAP. Again, the database was not able to make the determination of appropriate therapy, but there was a reduction of in-hospital mortality of patients who received antimicrobials within 4 hours of emergency room (ER) admission (6.8% vs 7.4%, adjusted OR = 0.85, 95% CI 0.74–0.98). After adjustment for admission severity of illness, decreased 30-day mortality was found for elderly patients with CAP in whom antibiotics were administered within 4 hours (or within 2 hour for immunocompromised patients) in a large pre- and post-intervention study by Kahn and colleagues.[63]

Battleman and colleagues[64] used a slightly different approach by randomly selecting 100 patients with CAP from each of 7 institutions. In logistic regression, each of 3 primary quality parameters was shown to be associated with reduced length of hospital stay: (1) initial antimicrobial treatment in the ED (OR = 0.31; 95% CI 0.19–0.48); (2) appropriate antimicrobial selection (OR = 0.55; 95% CI 0.35–0.88); and (3) antimicrobial door-to-needle time (OR = 1.75 per 8 hours; 95% CI 1.34–2.29).

Other studies have confirmed these findings for general CAP,[65] bacteremic pneumococcal CAP,[55] Legionella pneumonia,[66,67] ICU pneumonia,[68] and ventilator-acquired pneumonia.[69] In addition, several studies that have assessed the effect of CAP guidelines (that include recommendations on rapid antimicrobial administration) have noted an improvement in mortality with implementation.[63,70,71] However, none of these studies specifically examined the role of improvements in time to antimicrobials in relation to outcome.

Not all studies confirm the existence of antimicrobial delay–dependent adverse effects. In a recent article by Cheng and colleagues,[72] the time to antimicrobial administration was not associated with survival. This study was much smaller than those preciously mentioned (501 patients), and the median time to antimicrobial administration was only 2.7 hours. Ninety-one percent of patients received antimicrobials within the JCAHO proscribed 8 hours. This was in contrast to the studies Meehan and colleagues[5] and Houck and colleagues[23] where antimicrobial administration was within 8 hours 75.5% and 85.8% of the time, respectively. The criticisms of the study by Cheng and colleagues[72] were that median time to antimicrobial administration was already low, and most patients received antimicrobials within the appropriate time frame. Furthermore, patients who were at the greatest risk of death (pneumonia severity index of IV or V) received their antimicrobials earlier than those who were less ill. These factors confound the time/mortality association.

At least 2 other studies have similarly failed to demonstrate evidence of a benefit of early antimicrobial therapy in CAP.[73,74] In the study of more than 1000 patients with CAP in 38 American medical centers by Dedier and colleagues,[73] achievement of process-of-care markers including time to antimicrobials of less than 8 hours was not associated with outcome (time to clinical stability, LOS, and inpatient mortality). However, there seemed to be marked confounding in the study with more severely ill patients consistently receiving earlier antimicrobial therapy. With respect to the study by Silber and colleagues,[74] the patient population assessed was limited to those with mild to moderate CAP. Based on the studies of septic shock discussed earlier, the benefit of early antimicrobial therapy seems to be greatest in the most severely ill and may be lacking in those with only modest disease.

The assessment of oxygenation status in these patients also plays a role in their survival. Blot and colleagues[75] looked at the delay in oxygen assessment in patients with pneumonia and found that a delay of greater than 1 hour was associated with a longer median time to antimicrobial administration (6 vs 3 hours). If this oxygen assessment was delayed even further (to >3 hours), the result was an increased risk of death (OR = 2.24, 95% CI 1.17–4.30). The lack of recognition of severity of illness (based on an oxygenation defect) in these patients with CAP probably results in the delay in antimicrobials. Patients with an atypical presentation of their pneumonia (ie, afebrile, or not hypoxic), or with an altered mental state were at higher risk of not receiving their antimicrobials in a timely fashion.[65]

Meningitis

Acute bacterial meningitis is an infectious disease emergency with mortality and morbidity of 25% and 60%, respectively.[76,77] The data for the early administration of antimicrobials in bacterial meningitis are at least as extensive as with CAP, and are no less compelling. But as with pneumonia, the data are not entirely definitive because no prospective randomized studies have been performed and likely never will be.

Many retrospective studies have shown a relationship between delays in antimicrobial therapy and outcome of bacterial meningitis. However, others have failed to demonstrate such a relationship. The positive studies are notable for indexing delays to clinical/physiologic markers such as altered level of consciousness (LOC) and other clinical manifestations (similar to the indexing to hypotension in Kumar and colleagues[6,16] study of septic shock). This approach seems to yield the most consistently positive results.

For example, Lepur and Barsic[78] examined 268 adult patients with community-acquired bacterial meningitis in Croatia. Among patients with a poor clinical outcome, the start of appropriate antimicrobial treatment in relation to the onset of first symptoms and particularly to the onset of consciousness disturbance was significantly delayed ($P = .018$ and $P<.001$, respectively) compared with the favorable group. Earlier adequate antimicrobial treatment related to the onset of overt altered LOC was independently associated with favorable outcome (OR = 11.19; 95% CI 4.37–32.57; $P<.001$). This effect was incremental with longer delays associated with worse outcome. No relationship was found between time from hospital presentation to antimicrobial administration and outcome. Another notable element of this study is the long durations of time involved. Mean time to antimicrobial administration from hospital arrival was 1.21 ± 0.9 SD days.

Aronin and colleagues[79] have similarly found an association between antimicrobial delays and outcome when the patient's condition had progressed to the highest stage of clinical severity. Many investigators have demonstrated that severity of neurologic presentation and/or time of antimicrobial administration is closely linked to outcome.[77,80,81]

Others have focused on door-to-needle time. Miner and colleagues[82] retrospectively looked at their database of 171 cases of bacterial meningitis. Of the patients who presented to the hospital with meningitis, 76% of them received their antimicrobials in the ED, with a mean time to administration of 68 ± 13 minutes. The remaining 24% of patients received their antimicrobials after being admitted to the hospital, with a median time to antimicrobials of 6 ± 9 hours. The mortality of the patients who received their antimicrobials earlier in the ED was 7.9%, whereas the group who received their antimicrobials as inpatients had a mortality of 29% ($P = .003$).

Similarly, Auburtin and colleagues[83] sought to prospectively identify factors associated with mortality and morbidity in adults admitted to ICUs with pneumococcal meningitis. Among 156 patients, 3 variables were independently associated with 3-month mortality: Simplified Acute Physiology Score II (OR = 1.12; 95% CI 1.072–1.153; $P = .002$); isolation of a nonsusceptible strain (OR = 6.83; 95% CI 2.94–20.8; $P<.0001$), and an interval of more than 3 hours between hospital admission and administration of antimicrobials (OR = 14.12; 95% CI 3.93–50.9; $P<.0001$).

In the most recent study, Koster-Rasmussen and colleagues[84] studied all 186 patients presenting with bacterial meningitis in eastern Denmark in a 2-year period. Delay of antibiotic therapy (door-to-needle time) was independently associated with unfavorable outcome (OR = 1.09/h, CI 1.01–1.19) among the 125 adult cases (**Fig. 6**). In the group of 109 adults receiving adequate antibiotic therapy within 12 hours, the association between antibiotic delay and unfavorable outcome was an astonishing 30% per hour delay (OR = 1.30/h, CI 1.080–1.57). Although the median time to appropriate antimicrobial therapy among adults was 2 hours, almost 20% were delayed beyond 12 hours. Mortality outcomes paralleled unfavorable results.

In another study by Proulx and colleagues[25], a delay in antimicrobial administration of greater than 6 hours (door-to-needle time) among 123 cases of adult bacterial meningitis was associated with an 8.4 times increased risk of death (95% CI 1.7–40.9) in regression analysis. This effect of treatment delay on mortality was incremental. Increasing the length of time to antimicrobial administration increased the risk of death, with a delay of greater than 8 to 10 hours resulting in mortality of 75%.

Two other interesting findings from this study deserve mention. First, the failure to administer antimicrobials before transfer from another institution was associated with a 21.8-fold increase in the risk of death. This study took place at a referral facility, and the need for diagnostic computed tomography (CT) scanning of the head was the most common reason for transfer. The time delay in transferring the patients engendered the antimicrobial delay. The other surprising finding from the study was the diagnostic sequence for meningitis. In this relatively recent study (2005), less than 40% of physicians used a decision pathway that involved the administration of antimicrobials before other interventions such as diagnostic lumbar puncture (LP) or CT scan of the head. Twenty-two percent of physicians in the study performed a CT scan, and then an LP before administering antimicrobials. In studies of the CT findings in bacterial meningitis, less than 2.7% to 5% of patients showed evidence of significant mass effect; almost all of these patients exhibited clinical findings of the abnormality.[85,86] Concerns about precipitating transtentorial herniation with an LP, although valid, are still not an excuse to delay antimicrobial administration.

Several other studies have demonstrated that antimicrobial delays in acute bacterial meningitis are associated with poor outcomes, particularly for meningococcal

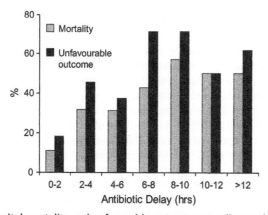

Fig. 6. Rate of hospital mortality and unfavorable outcome according to the treatment delay in time interval in acute bacterial meningitis. (*Data from* Koster-Rasmussen R, Korshin A, Meyer CN. Antibiotic treatment delay and outcome in acute bacterial meningitis. J Infect 2008;57:449–54.)

meningitis; studies have suggested that administration of drug by family practitioners in the community may improve outcomes.[76,87–91] Others have questioned these results.[77,92,93]

Some clinicians argue that delivery of antimicrobials before a diagnostic LP results in sterilization of the cerebrospinal fluid (CSF) and thus the inability to identify a causative organism. Although this is potentially the case, antimicrobials do not alter the CSF biochemistry and cytology sufficiently to alter the diagnostic yield. Furthermore, a causative diagnosis may be made from the CSF Gram stain or antigen tests. The minimization of door-to-needle time in this deadly disease should take precedence over all other diagnostic tests, based on these studies.

Most patients with meningitis present to clinicians who have limited experience in diagnosing and treating this disease. The prototypical clinical presentation of fever, altered LOC, and nuchal rigidity is not always present, making the diagnosis challenging. Clinicians should have a low threshold of instituting antimicrobials in patients who are at risk of this disease, even before the results of CSF analysis are available.

Limitations of Human Data

The question of whether delays in antimicrobial therapy for acute life-threatening infection including meningitis, pneumonia, bacteremia, invasive candidiasis, sepsis, and septic shock have a significant effect on outcome is a critical one. Given the difficulties in developing an ethical trial design, prospective randomized data may be almost impossible to generate. As a consequence, an answer has to be inferred from appropriate experimental animal models, retrospective or prospective cohort analyses, and before-after interventions. However, these approaches have significant limitations, which may explain some of the divergent results seen in studies.

First, confounding is a major issue. Patients who present with a more obvious or more severe presentation may receive earlier assessment and antimicrobial therapy. These patients may also have more intact or robust immune systems which could explain the better outcomes in this group. Alternately, it is possible that less ill patients with a higher probability of survival may receive faster antimicrobials because their clinical condition is more easily and rapidly assessed. Divergent results in different trials could be accounted for, in part, by variations in the nonrandom distribution of patients to early or delayed therapy. For example, some studies have shown that sicker patients often get earlier therapy, whereas those with atypical presentations are significantly delayed.[65,94,95] Confounding seems inconsistent between studies making comparisons difficult.

Second, variations in study results may occur as a consequence of the quality of the data collected. Administrative database studies[5,23] necessarily use data that have not been assessed for the individual patient. Such databases are known to have high error/miscoding rates relative to study designs in which data are collected by trained abstractors. In addition, these studies can necessarily only examine standard data collection elements such as when the first dose of antimicrobial was given (irrespective of whether it was appropriate or not). This can be a substantial issue because 20% to 40% of initial antimicrobials may be inappropriate in some circumstances.[96,97]

A third cause of inconsistency in results can be the use of different points for indexing of when antimicrobials are started. This is an obvious issue with administrative databases because, typically, only the arrival time to hospital and time of antimicrobial dispensing from the pharmacy are recorded routinely. The study by Leper and Barsic[78] was notable in demonstrating a significant relationship between the onset of altered LOC and antimicrobial administration. This study failed to demonstrate a relationship between ER admission time and antimicrobial administration with respect to clinical outcome of patients with bacterial meningitis. The studies reviewed in this article suggest that outcomes may be more closely linked to the time between occurrence of important pathophysiologic responses (hypotension for septic shock, altered LOC for meningitis) and antimicrobial administration than administrative events (hospital or ER admission) and antimicrobial administration.

Fourth, the studies examined within each clinical syndrome indicate substantial variations in the degree and pace of illness. The studies of meningitis and bacteremia/sepsis/septic shock seem to suggest that the ability to show a statistical relationship between antimicrobial delays and outcome may be substantially contingent on the degree of illness being studied. Radetsky and colleagues[98] have suggested that any connection between a delay in the treatment of bacterial meningitis and outcome depends on the presenting clinical pattern. With an early presentation and modest clinical illness, relatively short delays (even on the order of days) may not substantially affect survival or be associated with severe sequelae. On the other hand, late presentations with fulminant illness may show no substantial response to any antimicrobial therapy. Only clinically overt presentations where a risk of irreversible injury is imminent may demonstrate sensitivity to delays in administration of antimicrobial therapy. A similar phenomenon may exist with bacteremia/sepsis/septic shock. Bacteremia or candidemia without sepsis-induced organ failure is a relatively mild disease with a low mortality risk (compared with septic shock with the same organisms). In such situations, relatively short delays in antimicrobial therapy are unlikely to yield evidence of adverse outcomes. Accordingly, the studies that do show an effect of antimicrobial delays show break points in the range of days rather than hours.[48,53,59,99] In contrast, several studies show that hours (or less) make a difference with septic shock.[6,27,28] For this reason, mild to moderate CAP should not be expected to demonstrate evidence of sensitivity to modest variations in antimicrobial delays.[74]

As a statistical issue, the intrastudy range of values of antimicrobial delivery delays may be an important source of variation in study results. If the range of delays is similar (whether very short or very long), then it would not be possible in logistic regression to show any effect of such delays. The studies by Lepur and Barsic[78] on meningitis and by Kumar and colleagues[6] on septic shock showed a very broad range of delays from minutes to days. In contrast, some other studies showed very short antimicrobial delays, which may make it much harder to demonstrate an effect without extremely large datasets.

With respect to non-necrotizing pneumonia without septic shock and bacteremia/fungemia, it is not clear that a solid pathophysiologic rationale to support sensitivity of mortality to antimicrobial delay exists. The authors believe that to exhibit such sensitivity, the condition under study must pose a risk of irreversible and irreplaceable organ injury. Septic shock and meningitis fit that criteria, the former because multiple, simultaneous organ failure can rarely be reversed even with maximal support. However, non-necrotizing pneumonia, bacteremia, and sepsis without shock do not. One possibility to be considered is that it is the subset of patients with septic shock or who develop septic shock that drive antimicrobial delay sensitivity in these groups.

Antimicrobial Delays

Health care professionals do not intentionally delay administration of antimicrobials in patients recognized to have life-threatening infection. The occurrence of delays is a consequence of difficulties in the prompt assessment of these patients and deficiencies in recognizing them as being at high risk of death and increased LOS with a delay in antimicrobial administration. Barriers to timely antimicrobial administration are consistently present across all serious infections.

Identified barriers to timely administration of antimicrobials for CAP have been described in the literature.[100] These barriers include a lack of education of physicians, a lack of appreciation of the severity of pneumonia in the elderly, and increased work intensity in busy EDs.[94,101] A major cause of delays is transfer of the patient to wards before antimicrobials are given. Atypical presentations with a lack of fever and toxicity or an altered mental state can also prevent prompt recognition and treatment.[65,94] Similarly, atypical nonclassic meningitis presentations without fever and severely altered mental status may not be recognized, engendering significant delays.[94,95] Provision of diagnostic procedures (CT and LP) and administrative delays related to transfer to general wards or other facilities are also associated with significant delays.[25,95,102,103] Staffing issues relative to patient demand can also clearly play a significant role.[101,104] With respect to sepsis, septic shock, and bacteremia, a similar list of potential causes (and recommended solutions) for delay can be generated (**Box 1**).[105]

Box 1
Causes of delay of effective antimicrobial therapy and a potential approach to reduce them

Causes of delays in administration of antimicrobials in severe infection and septic shock

1. Failure to recognize infection in a timely way

2. Failure to recognize that hypotension represents septic shock

3. Effect of inappropriate antimicrobial initiation (delays administration of appropriate antimicrobials

4. Failure to appreciate risk of resistant organisms in certain scenarios (eg, immunocompromised versus immunosuppressed; antecedent antimicrobial use) leading to inappropriate initial antimicrobials

5. Wait for blood cultures from intravenous technicians before giving antibiotic

6. Requirement for 2 nurses to check for potential drug sensitivity before dosing of antimicrobials

7. Transfer from ER before ordered antibiotics given

8. Failure to use stat orders

9. Failure to recognize that administration of inappropriate antimicrobials is equivalent to absent antimicrobial therapy when responding to clinical failure (ie, should not delay appropriate antimicrobials because inappropriate drugs recently given)

10. No specified order with multiple drug regimens so that key drug (usually most expensive and hardest to access) may be given last

11. Administrative/logistic delays (nursing/pharmacy/ward clerk)

Potential approaches to minimize delays in initiation of empiric antimicrobial therapy

1. The presence of hypotension in a patient with known or suspected infection should be considered to be septic shock in the absence of a definitive alternate explanation

2. No transfer from ER before ordered antibiotics given

3. All initial orders for any intravenous antibiotic automatically stat

4. Syndrome-based, algorithm-driven guidelines similar to meningitis and neutropenic sepsis with designated broad-spectrum antimicrobial regimen at each center

5. Antimicrobial order to include sequence and time limit (eg, within 30 minutes of order)

6. First intravenous dose of most broad-spectrum agents (ie, β-lactam/carbapenems) push by physician

7. Health care worker and support staff education; a team approach

Available data suggest that it is not difficult to reduce antimicrobial delivery delays especially when delays are substantial to begin with. Natsch and colleagues[106] developed a program of guidelines and education to facilitate timely antibiotic administration in the ER. The program consisted of guidelines on handling patients with serious infections and on ordering immediate treatment, guidelines on obtaining culture samples, lectures to medical and nursing staff, improvement of availability of antibiotics in the ED, and removal of financial restraints on stocking and ordering of antibiotics. The investigators were able to decrease median door-to-needle time from 5.0 hours to 3.2 hours ($P = .04$). Similarly, Rollins and colleagues[107] reduced average time to antimicrobial therapy from 6.8 to 3.6 hours at 1 institution within 6 months of the introduction of an ER preadmission procedure, an antibiotic treatment protocol, and a sputum collection protocol.

Even when door-to-needle times are low, appropriate strategies can reduce delays even further. Tuijn and colleagues[108] were able to take approximately 30 minutes off a 3-hour time primarily by emphasizing the need to administer antimicrobials in the ER before patients were transferred to the wards. Our own data show that much greater delays occur on inpatient wards than the ER.

Vogtlander and colleagues[109] have shown that although the time from writing the order to antimicrobial administration was 2.7 hours, this time could be reduced by 1 hour ($P = .003$) with simple administrative maneuvers and staff training.

The most reliable approach to decreasing the time to antimicrobial administration for acute life-threatening infections is to take a systems-based approach in which all members of the health care team are stakeholders in this process.[110] This allows for the early recognition of serious infectious disease and the rapid institution of therapy. This involves nurses to perform a rapid and focused assessment of these patients, physicians to accurately diagnose the disease, and a pharmacy and transport system that delivers the appropriate antimicrobials to the patients in as short a time as possible. When this systems-based approach is undertaken, improvements in the time to antimicrobial administration can be realized. Such improvements should translate into a significant cost benefit particularly for high-risk patients.[107,111]

SUMMARY

For decades, health care workers faced the challenge of how to adequately treat life-threatening infections. To a great extent, the primary focus on improving outcomes has centered on improvement in resuscitation, deployment of antimicrobials of increasing potency, and development of novel adjunctive therapies. However, a critical appraisal of available studies conclusively shows that the early recognition of life-threatening infection and rapid initiation of appropriate antimicrobial therapy is the critical element in reducing mortality. The challenge that hospitals now face is how best to implement systems to facilitate this goal. The processes to accomplish this goal has already been demonstrated in various aspects of medical care including provision of rapid surgical therapy after trauma and rapid interventions to open blocked coronary arteries in acute myocardial infarction. The fundamental requirement is the involvement all members of the health care team, including physicians, nurses, and pharmacists.

An important slogan used in the training of health care workers with respect to revascularization of arteries in acute myocardial infarction and obstructive stroke has been "Time is tissue." If that is so, then an appropriate rule for life-threatening infections, particularly septic shock is "Speed is life."

REFERENCES

1. Blow O, Magliore L, Claridge JA, et al. The golden hour and the silver day: detection and correction of occult hypoperfusion within 24 hours improves outcome from major trauma. J Trauma 1999;47:964–9.
2. Boersma E, Maas AC, Deckers JW, et al. Early thrombolytic treatment in acute myocardial infarction: reappraisal of the golden hour. Lancet 1996;348:771–5.
3. Wood KE. Major pulmonary embolism: review of a pathophysiologic approach to the golden hour of hemodynamically significant pulmonary embolism. Chest 2002;121:877–905.
4. Tunkel AR, Hartman BJ, Kaplan SL, et al. Practice guidelines for the management of bacterial meningitis. Clin Infect Dis 2004;39:1267–84.
5. Meehan IP, Fine MJ, Krumholz HM, et al. Quality of care, process, and outcomes in elderly patients with pneumonia. JAMA 1997;278:2080–4.
6. Kumar A, Roberts D, Wood KE, et al. Duration of hypotension before initiation of effective antimicrobial therapy is the critical determinant of survival in human septic shock. Crit Care Med 2006;34:1589–96.
7. Garey KW, Rege M, Pai MP, et al. Time to initiation of fluconazole therapy impacts mortality in patients with candidemia: a multi-institutional study. Clin Infect Dis 2006;43:25–31.
8. Dellinger RP, Carlet JM, Masur H, et al. Surviving Sepsis campaign guidelines for management of severe sepsis and septic shock. Crit Care Med 2004;32: 858–73.
9. Pines JM, Isserman JA, Hinfey PB. The measurement of time to first antibiotic dose for pneumonia in the emergency department: a white paper and position statement prepared for the American Academy of Emergency Medicine. J Emerg Med 2009;37:335–40.
10. Cheng AC, Buising KL. Time to first antibiotic dose in community-acquired pneumonia: time for a change: response to letter. Ann Emerg Med 2009;54: 312–3.
11. Green DL. Selection of an empiric antibiotic regimen for hospital-acquired pneumonia using a unit and culture-type specific antibiogram. J Intensive Care Med 2005;20:296–301.
12. Kaufman D, Haas CE, Edinger R, et al. Antibiotic susceptibility in the surgical intensive care unit compared with the hospital-wide antibiogram. Arch Surg 1998;133:1041–5.
13. Knudsen JD, Frimodt-Moller N, Espersen F. Pharmacodynamics of penicillin are unaffected by bacterial growth phases of *Streptococcus pneumoniae* in the mouse peritonitis model. J Antimicrob Chemother 1998;41:451–9.
14. Frimodt-Moller N, Thomsen VF. The pneumococcus and the mouse protection test: inoculum, dosage and timing. Acta Pathol Microbiol Immunol Scand B Microbiology 1986;94:33–7.
15. Greisman SE, DuBuy JB, Woodward CL. Experimental gram-negative bacterial sepsis: prevention of mortality not preventable by antibiotics alone. Infect Immun 1979;25:538–57.
16. Kumar A, Haery C, Paladugu B, et al. The duration of hypotension before the initiation of antibiotic treatment is a critical determinant of survival in a murine model of *Escherichia coli* septic shock: association with serum lactate and inflammatory cytokine levels. J Infect Dis 2006;193:251–8.
17. Wiggers CJ, Ingraham RC, Dillie J. Hemorrhagic-hypotension shock in locally anesthetized dogs. Am J Phys 1945;143:126–33.

18. Wiggers CJ. Experimental haemorrhage shock. In: Physiology of shock. 1st edition. New York: Harvard University Press (The Commonwealth Fund), 1950. p. 121–43.
19. Calbo E, Alsina M, Rodriguez-Carballeira M, et al. The impact of time on the systemic inflammatory response in pneumococcal pneumonia. Eur Respir J 2010;35:614–8.
20. Bagshaw SM, Lapinsky S, Dial S, et al. Acute kidney injury in septic shock: clinical outcomes and impact of duration of hypotension prior to initiation of antimicrobial therapy. Intensive Care Med 2009;35:871–81.
21. Iscimen R, Cartin-Ceba R, Yilmaz M, et al. Risk factors for the development of acute lung injury in patients with septic shock: an observational cohort study. Crit Care Med 2008;36:1518–22.
22. Garnacho-Montero J, Aldabo-Pallas T, Garnacho-Montero C, et al. Timing of adequate antibiotic therapy is a greater determinant of outcome than are TNF and IL-10 polymorphisms in patients with sepsis. Crit Care 2006;10:R111.
23. Houck PM, Bratzler DW, Nsa W, et al. Timing of antibiotic administration and outcomes for Medicare patients hospitalized with community-acquired pneumonia. Arch Intern Med 2004;164:637–44.
24. Natsch S, Kullberg BJ, Van der Meer JW, et al. Delay in administering the first dose of antibiotics in patients admitted to hospital with serious infections. Eur J Clin Microbiol Infect Dis 1998;17:681–4.
25. Proulx N, Frechette D, Toye B, et al. Delays in the administration of antibiotics are associated with mortality from adult acute bacterial meningitis. QJM 2005; 98:291–8.
26. Subramanian S, Yilmaz M, Rehman A, et al. Liberal vs. conservative vasopressor use to maintain mean arterial blood pressure during resuscitation of septic shock: an observational study. Intensive Care Med 2008;34:157–62.
27. Gaieski DF, Pines JM, Band RA, et al. Impact of time to antibiotics on survival in patients with severe sepsis or septic shock in whom early goal-directed therapy was initiated in the emergency department. Crit Care Med 2010;38:1045–53.
28. Larche J, Azoulay E, Fieux F, et al. Improved survival of critically ill cancer patients with septic shock. Intensive Care Med 2003;29:1688–95.
29. Patel GP, Simon D, Scheetz M, et al. The effect of time to antifungal therapy on mortality in candidemia associated septic shock. Am J Ther 2009;16:508–11.
30. Hsu DI, Nguyen M, Nguyen L, et al. A multicentre study to evaluate the impact of timing of caspofungin administration on outcomes of invasive candidiasis in non-immunocompromised adult patients. J Antimicrob Chemother 2010;65: 1765–70.
31. Hood HM, Allman RM, Burgess PA, et al. Effects of timely antibiotic administration and culture acquisition on the treatment of urinary tract infection. Am J Med Qual 1998;13:195–202.
32. Dellinger RP, Levy MM, Carlet JM, et al. Surviving Sepsis campaign: international guidelines for management of severe sepsis and septic shock: 2008. Crit Care Med 2008;36:296–327 [erratum appears in Crit Care Med 2008; 36(4):1394–6].
33. Nguyen HB, Corbett SW, Steele R, et al. Implementation of a bundle of quality indicators for the early management of severe sepsis and septic shock is associated with decreased mortality. Crit Care Med 2007;35:1105–12.
34. Cardoso T, Carneiro A, Ribeiro O, et al. Reducing mortality in severe sepsis with the implementation of a core 6-hour bundle: results from the Portuguese community-acquired sepsis study (SACiUCI study). Crit Care 2010;14:R83.

35. Thiel SW, Asghar MF, Micek ST, et al. Hospital-wide impact of a standardized order set for the management of bacteremic severe sepsis. Crit Care Med 2009;37(3):819–24.
36. Lefrant JY, Muller L, Raillard A, et al. Reduction of the severe sepsis or septic shock associated mortality by reinforcement of the recommendations bundle: a multicenter study. Ann Fr Anesth Reanim 2010;29:621–8.
37. Castellanos-Ortega A, Suberviola B, García-Astudillo LA, et al. Impact of the Surviving Sepsis campaign protocols on hospital length of stay and mortality in septic shock patients: results of a three-year follow-up quasi-experimental study. Crit Care Med 2010;38:1036–43.
38. Ferrer R, Artigas A, Levy MM, et al. Improvement in process of care and outcome after a multicenter severe sepsis educational program in Spain. JAMA 2008;299:2294–303.
39. Kortgen A, Niederprüm P, Bauer M. Implementation of an evidence-based "standard operating procedure" and outcome in septic shock. Crit Care Med 2006;34:943–9.
40. Barochia AV, Cui X, Vitberg D, et al. Bundled care for septic shock: an analysis of clinical trials. Crit Care Med 2010;38:668–78.
41. de Sousa AG, Junior CJF, Santos GPD, et al. The impact of each action in the Surviving Sepsis campaign measures on hospital mortality of patients with severe sepsis/septic shock. Einstein 2008;6:323–7.
42. Varpula M, Karlsson S, Parviainen I, Finnsepsis Study Group, et al. Community-acquired septic shock: early management and outcome in a nationwide study in Finland. Acta Anaesthesiol Scand 2007;51:1320–6.
43. Ferrer R, Artigas A, Suarez D, et al. Effectiveness of treatments for severe sepsis: a prospective, multicenter, observational study. Am J Respir Crit Care Med 2009;180:861–6.
44. Gurnani PK, Patel GP, Crank CW, et al. Impact of the implementation of a sepsis protocol for the management of fluid-refractory septic shock: a single-center, before-and-after study. Clin Ther 2010;32:1285–93.
45. Pestana D, Espinosa E, Sangnesa-Molina JR, et al. Compliance with a sepsis bundle and its effect on intensive care unit mortality in surgical septic shock patients. J Trauma 2010. [Epub ahead of print].
46. Chamberlain D. Prehospital administered intravenous antimicrobial protocol for septic shock: a prospective randomized clinical trial [abstract]. Crit Care 2009; 13(Suppl 1):P317.
47. Bodey GP, Jadeja L, Elting L. Pseudomonas bacteremia. Retrospective analysis of 410 episodes. Arch Intern Med 1985;145:1621–9.
48. Lodise TP, Patel N, Kwa A, et al. Predictors of 30-day mortality among patients with Pseudomonas aeruginosa bloodstream infections: impact of delayed appropriate antibiotic selection. Antimicrob Agents Chemother 2007;51: 3510–5.
49. Kang CI, Kim SH, Kim HB, et al. Pseudomonas aeruginosa bacteremia: risk factors for mortality and influence of delayed receipt of effective antimicrobial therapy on clinical outcome. Clin Infect Dis 2003;37:745–51.
50. Anderson DJ, Engemann JJ, Harrell LJ, et al. Predictors of mortality in patients with bloodstream infection due to ceftazidime-resistant Klebsiella pneumoniae. Antimicrob Agents Chemother 2006;50:1715–20.
51. Cheong HS, Kang CI, Wi YM, et al. Clinical significance and predictors of community-onset Pseudomonas aeruginosa bacteremia. Am J Med 2008; 121(8):709–14.

52. Kang CI, Kim SH, Park WB, et al. Risk factors for antimicrobial resistance and influence of resistance on mortality in patients with bloodstream infection caused by *Pseudomonas aeruginosa*. Microb Drug Resist 2005;11:68–74.

53. Lodise TP, McKinnon PS, Swiderski L, et al. Outcomes analysis of delayed antibiotic treatment for hospital-acquired *Staphylococcus aureus* bacteremia. Clin Infect Dis 2003;36:1418–23.

54. Khatib R, Saeed S, Sharma M, et al. Impact of initial antibiotic choice and delayed appropriate treatment on the outcome of *Staphylococcus aureus* bacteremia. Eur J Clin Microbiol Infect Dis 2006;25:181–5.

55. Garnacho-Montero J, Garcia-Cabrera E, Diaz-Martin A, et al. Determinants of outcome in patients with bacteraemic pneumococcal pneumonia: importance of early adequate treatment. Scand J Infect Dis 2010;42:185–92.

56. Fernandez J, Erstad BL, Petty W, et al. Time to positive culture and identification for *Candida* blood stream infections. Diagn Microbiol Infect Dis 2009;64:402–7.

57. Taur Y, Cohen N, Dubnow S, et al. Effect of antifungal therapy timing on mortality in cancer patients with candidemia. Antimicrob Agents Chemother 2010;54:184–90.

58. Blot SI, Vandewoude KH, Hoste EA, et al. Effects of nosocomial candidemia on outcomes of critically ill patients. Am J Med 2002;113:480–5.

59. Morrell M, Fraser VJ, Kollef MH. Delaying the empiric treatment of *Candida* bloodstream infection until positive blood culture results are obtained: a potential risk factor for hospital mortality. Antimicrob Agents Chemother 2005;49:3640–5.

60. Lin MY, Weinstein RA, Hota B. Delay of active antimicrobial therapy and mortality among patients with bacteremia: impact of severe neutropenia. Antimicrob Agents Chemother 2008;52:3188–94.

61. Corona A, Bertolini G, Lipman J, et al. Antibiotic use and impact on outcome from bacteraemic critical illness: the Bacteraemia Study in Intensive Care (BASIC). J Antimicrob Chemother 2010;65:1276–85.

62. Mitka M. JCAHO tweaks emergency departments' pneumonia treatment standards. JAMA 2007;297:1758.

63. Kahn KL, Rogers WH, Rubenstein LV, et al. Measuring quality of care with explicit process criteria before and after implementation of the DRG-based prospective payment system. JAMA 1990;264:1969–73.

64. Battleman DS, Callahan M, Thaler HT. Rapid antibiotic delivery and appropriate antibiotic selection reduce length of hospital stay of patients with community-acquired pneumonia: link between quality of care and resource utilization. Arch Intern Med 2002;162:682–8.

65. Waterer GW, Kessler LA, Wunderink RG. Delayed administration of antibiotics and atypical presentation in community-acquired pneumonia. Chest 2006;130: 11–5.

66. Gacouin A, Le Tulzo Y, Lavoue S, et al. Severe pneumonia due to *Legionella pneumophila*: prognostic factors, impact of delayed appropriate antimicrobial therapy. Intensive Care Med 2002;28:686–91.

67. Heath CH, Grove DI, Looke DFM. Delay in appropriate therapy of *Legionella* pneumonia associated with increased mortality. Eur J Clin Microbiol Infect Dis 1996;15:286–90.

68. Mathevon T, Souweine B, Traore O, et al. ICU-acquired nosocomial infection: impact of delay of adequate antibiotic treatment. Scand J Infect Dis 2002; 34(11):831–5.

69. Iregui M, Ward S, Sherman G, et al. Clinical importance of delays in the initiation of appropriate antibiotic treatment for ventilator-associated pneumonia. Chest 2002;122:262–8.

70. Dean NC, Bateman KA, Donnelly SM, et al. Improved clinical outcomes with utilization of a community-acquired pneumonia guideline. Chest 2006;130:794–9.
71. McGarvey RN, Harper JJ. Pneumonia mortality reduction and quality improvement in a community hospital. QRB Qual Rev Bull 1993;19:124–30.
72. Cheng AC, Buising KL. Delayed administration of antibiotics and mortality in patients with community-acquired pneumonia. Ann Emerg Med 2009;53:618–24.
73. Dedier J, Singer DE, Chang Y, et al. Processes of care, illness severity, and outcomes in the management of community-acquired pneumonia at academic hospitals. Arch Intern Med 2001;161:2099–104.
74. Silber SH, Garrett C, Singh R, et al. Early administration of antibiotics does not shorten time to clinical stability in patients with moderate-to-severe community-acquired pneumonia. Chest 2003;124:1790–004.
75. Blot SI, Rodriguez A, Solé-Violán J, et al. Effects of delayed oxygenation assessment on time to antibiotic delivery and mortality in patients with severe community-acquired pneumonia. Crit Care Med 2007;35:2509–14.
76. Hussein AS, Shafran SD. Acute bacterial meningitis in adults: a 12-year review. Medicine 2000;79:360–8.
77. Quagliarello VJ, Scheld WM. Treatment of bacterial meningitis. N Engl J Med 1997;336:708–16.
78. Lepur D, Barsic B. Community-acquired bacterial meningitis in adults: antibiotic timing in disease course and outcome. Infection 2007;35:225–31.
79. Aronin SI, Peduzzi P, Quagliarello VJ. Community-acquired bacterial meningitis: risk stratification for adverse clinical outcome and effect of antibiotic timing. Ann Intern Med 1998;129:862–9.
80. Lu CH, Huang CR, Chang WN, et al. Community-acquired bacterial meningitis in adults: the epidemiology, timing of appropriate antimicrobial therapy, and prognostic factors. Clin Neurol Neurosurg 2002;104:352–8.
81. van de BD, de Gans J, Spanjaard L, et al. Clinical features and prognostic factors in adults with bacterial meningitis. N Engl J Med 2004;351(18):1849–59.
82. Miner JR, Heegaard W, Mapes A, et al. Presentation, time to antibiotics, and mortality of patients with bacterial meningitis at an urban county medical center. J Emerg Med 2001;21:387–92.
83. Auburtin M, Wolff M, Charpentier J, et al. Detrimental role of delayed antibiotic administration and penicillin-nonsusceptible strains in adult intensive care unit patients with pneumococcal meningitis: the PNEUMOREA prospective multicenter study. Crit Care Med 2006;34:2758–65.
84. Koster-Rasmussen R, Korshin A, Meyer CN. Antibiotic treatment delay and outcome in acute bacterial meningitis. J Infect 2008;57:449–54.
85. Hasbun R, Abrahams J, Jekel J, et al. Computed tomography of the head before lumbar puncture in adults with suspected meningitis. N Engl J Med 2001;345:1727–33.
86. Gopal AK, Whitehouse JD, Simel DL, et al. Cranial computed tomography before lumbar puncture: a prospective clinical evaluation. Arch Intern Med 1999;159:2681–5.
87. Strang JR, Pugh EJ. Meningococcal infections: reducing the case fatality rate by giving penicillin before admission to hospital. Br Med J 1992;305:141–3.
88. Cartwright K, Reilly S, White D, et al. Early treatment with parenteral penicillin in meningococcal disease. Br Med J 1992;305:143–7.
89. Barquet N, Domingo P, Cayla JA, et al. Meningococcal disease in a large urban population (Barcelona, 1987–1992): predictors of dismal prognosis. Barcelona Meningococcal Disease Surveillance Group. Arch Intern Med 1999;159:2329–40.

90. Lala HM, Mills GD, Barratt K, et al. Meningococcal disease deaths and the frequency of antibiotic administration delays. J Infect 2007;54:551–7.
91. Bonsu BK, Harper MB. Fever interval before diagnosis, prior antibiotic treatment, and clinical outcome for young children with bacterial meningitis. Clin Infect Dis 2001;32:566–72.
92. Sorensen HT, Nielsen GL, Schonheyder HC, et al. Outcome of pre-hospital antibiotic treatment of meningococcal disease. J Clin Epidemiol 1998;51:717–21.
93. Norgard B, Sorensen HT, Jensen ES, et al. Pre-hospital parenteral antibiotic treatment of meningococcal disease and case fatality: a Danish population-based cohort study. J Infect 2002;45:144–51.
94. Pines JM, Morton MJ, Datner EM, et al. Systematic delays in antibiotic administration in the emergency department for adult patients admitted with pneumonia. Acad Emerg Med 2006;13:939–45.
95. Talan DA, Zibulewsky J. Relationship of clinical presentation to time to antibiotics for the emergency department management of suspected bacterial meningitis. Ann Emerg Med 1993;22(11):1733–8.
96. Kumar A, Ellis P, Arabi Y, et al. Initiation of inappropriate antimicrobial therapy results in a five-fold reduction of survival in human septic shock. Chest 2009;136:1237–48.
97. Kollef MH, Sherman G, Ward S, et al. Inadequate antimicrobial treatment of infections: a risk factor for hospital mortality among critically ill patients. Chest 1999;115:462–74.
98. Radetsky M, Feigin RD, Kaplan SL, et al. Duration of symptoms and outcome in bacterial meningitis: an analysis of causation and the implications of a delay in diagnosis. Pediatr Infect Dis J 1992;11:694–701.
99. Garey KW, Pai MP, Suda KJ, et al. Inadequacy of fluconazole dosing in patients with candidemia based on Infectious Diseases Society of America (IDSA) guidelines. Pharmacoepidemiol Drug Saf 2007;16:919–27.
100. Barlow G, Nathwani D, Myers E, et al. Identifying barriers to the rapid administration of appropriate antibiotics in community-acquired pneumonia. J Antimicrob Chemother 2007;61:442–51.
101. Pines JM, Localio AR, Hollander JE, et al. The impact of emergency department crowding measures on time to antibiotics for patients with community-acquired pneumonia. Ann Emerg Med 2007;50:510–6.
102. Talan DA, Guterman JJ, Overturf GD, et al. Analysis of emergency department management of suspected bacterial meningitis. Ann Emerg Med 1989;18(8):856–62.
103. Pines JM. Timing of antibiotics for acute, severe infections. Emerg Med Clin North Am 2008;26:245–57.
104. Houck PM, Bratzler DW. Administration of first hospital antibiotics for community-acquired pneumonia: does timeliness affect outcomes? Curr Opin Infect Dis 2005;18:151–6.
105. Kumar A. Early antimicrobial therapy in severe sepsis and septic shock. Curr Infect Dis Rep 2010;12:336–44.
106. Natsch S, Kullberg BJ, Meis JF, et al. Earlier initiation of antibiotic treatment for severe infections after interventions to improve the organization and specific guidelines in the emergency department. Arch Intern Med 2000;160:1317–20.
107. Rollins D, Thomasson C, Sperry B. Improving antibiotic delivery time to pneumonia patients: continuous quality improvement in action. J Nurs Care Qual 1994;8(2):22–31.

108. van Tuijn CF, Luitse JS, van der Valk M, et al. Reduction of the door-to-needle time for administration of antibiotics in patients with a severe infection: a tailored intervention project. Quicker, faster, better? Neth J Med 2010;68:123–7.

109. Vogtlander NP, Van Kasteren ME, Natsch S, et al. Improving the process of antibiotic therapy in daily practice: interventions to optimize timing, dosage adjustment to renal function, and switch therapy. Arch Intern Med 2004;164(11): 1206–12.

110. Funk D, Sebat F, Kumar A. A systems approach to the early recognition and rapid administration of best practice therapy in sepsis and septic shock. Curr Opin Crit Care 2009;15:301.

111. Barlow G, Nathwani D, Williams F, et al. Reducing door-to-antibiotic time in community-acquired pneumonia: controlled before-and-after evaluation and cost-effectiveness analysis. Thorax 2007;62:67–74.

Pharmacodynamic Approaches to Optimizing Beta-Lactam Therapy

Jared L. Crandon, PharmD, BCPS[a],
David P. Nicolau, PharmD, FCCP, FIDSA[a,b],*

KEYWORDS

• Beta-lactam • Pharmacodynamics • Prolonged infusion
• Continuous infusion

As a class, beta-lactam antibiotics have been a mainstay of therapy since the inception of penicillin approximately 60 years ago. Today, clinical practice guidelines for nearly all infection sites recommend the use of beta lactams, often as first-line therapy.[1–3] Given their popularity and favorable safety profile, it is no wonder that there has been considerable interest in developing strategies to most effectively use beta-lactam therapy. Dating back to those first days of penicillin, it was noted that there was an observed benefit to prolonging the infusion time or dosing more frequently.[4,5] Since that time, considerable research has been performed to help understand and justify these dosing strategies. This article discusses the pharmacology behind these dosing strategies and presents some of the contemporary literature describing the perceived and observed clinical benefits.

BETA-LACTAM PHARMACODYNAMICS

The potency of antimicrobials is determined in vitro by the lowest antibiotic concentration required to inhibit visual growth of the test organism (minimum inhibitory concentration [MIC]) and the interpretation of these values is straight forward; the lower the MIC the more potent the compound. How this in vitro potency translates to in vivo efficacy is exceedingly more complex and is described using pharmacodynamics. Simply put, the pharmacodynamics of antimicrobials describes the relationship between the shape of the concentration-time curve and the efficacy of the compound as a function of the MIC. The 3 recognized pharmacodynamic parameters are the ratio of the area under the free drug concentration-time profile and the MIC ($fAUC/MIC$), the ratio of the

[a] Center for Anti-Infective Research and Development, Hartford Hospital, 80 Seymour Street, Hartford, CT 06102, USA
[b] Division of Infectious Diseases, Hartford Hospital, 80 Seymour Street, Hartford, CT 06102, USA
* Corresponding author. Center for Anti-Infective Research and Development, Hartford Hospital, 80 Seymour Street, Hartford, CT 06102.
E-mail address: dnicola@harthosp.org

Crit Care Clin 27 (2011) 77–93
doi:10.1016/j.ccc.2010.11.004
0749-0704/11/$ – see front matter © 2011 Elsevier Inc. All rights reserved.

criticalcare.theclinics.com

maximal free drug concentration and the MIC (fC_{max}/MIC), and the percentage of the dosing interval that free drug concentrations remain above the MIC ($fT>MIC$).[6] For each class of antimicrobials, one or more of these pharmacodynamic relationships are indefinable as predictive of in vivo efficacy. For the beta lactams, a clear relationship has been noted between $fT>MIC$ and antimicrobial activity using in vitro and in vivo models of infection, as well as clinical data. As such, optimization of beta-lactam therapy rests solely on the ability to maximize the $fT>MIC$.

In designing dosing regimens aimed at optimizing beta-lactam therapy, it is important to understand what targets ($fT>MIC$) are required to maximize antibacterial activity. Generally speaking, these data are derived from animal models of infection and differ slightly between classes of beta lactams. From these animal-based studies, it is recognized that the $fT>MIC$ required for stasis (ie, no bacterial growth or killing) is 20% for carbapenems, 30% for penicillins, and 40% for cephalosporins against gram-negative organisms. Similarly, maximal efficacy, often denoted as an approximate 2-log decrease in colony forming units, requires a $fT>MIC$ of 40% for carbapenems, 50% for penicillins, and 50% to 70% for cephalosporins.[7,8]

In clinical practice, the efficacy of a given compound is dependent on several variables often not well represented or inherently controlled for within animal models or in vitro studies. Examples of these variables include patient comorbid conditions (ie, peripheral vascular disease, renal function, obesity, and so forth), severity of illness, site of infection, host immune status, and nondrug interventions (ie, surgical intervention, intravenous line removal, and so forth). Despite these potential confounders, clinical studies evaluating $fT>MIC$ targets for beta lactams have found values remarkably similar to animal models. Two studies recently conducted by the authors' group evaluating microbiological response to meropenem[9] and cefepime[10] in hospitalized subjects, the authors noted that $fT>MIC$ of 54% and 66% were required for predictable response, respectively. Similarly, a study evaluating several antibiotics for the treatment of otitis media in children found a $fT>MIC$ of 40% to 50% was required to achieve cure rates of 80% to 85% for penicillins[11] and another study evaluating middle ear fluid concentrations of cefprozil found that the poor clinical outcomes associated with MICs greater than 1 μg/mL coincided with a lack of pharmacodynamic target attainment in the middle ear fluid.[12] Given the deficiency of clinical pharmacodynamic studies and the known correlation between clinical and animal-derived data, most investigators and clinicians rely on animal-derived targets to guide therapeutic decisions.

OPTIMAL DOSING STRATEGIES

When considering the outcome of treating patients for infection there are 3 factors involved: the patient, the pathogen, and the drug.[13] Within this triad, the only modifiable factor is the drug itself, allowing manipulation of both antibiotic selection and dosing regimen. With respect to the dosing regimen, there are 3 ways to alter the shape of the concentration time profile: changes to dose, dosing interval, and infusion time (**Fig. 1**). Of these methods, alterations to dose offer the least benefit in changing $fT>MIC$, the parameter of interest for beta lactams. For example, at an MIC of 32 μg/mL, increasing the dose of piperacillin-tazobactam from 3.375 g (30-minute infusion) to 4.5 g (30-minute infusion) in the median patient as derived from a recent population kinetic model[14] results in a minimal increase in $fT>MIC$ (see **Fig. 1A, B**). However, decreasing the dosing interval (see **Fig. 1C**) or increasing the length of infusion (see **Fig. 1D**) can have considerable impacts on $fT>MIC$, thereby optimizing therapy. These differences are even more profound when one considers the variability around these pharmacokinetic parameters through mathematics.[14,15] It should be noted that

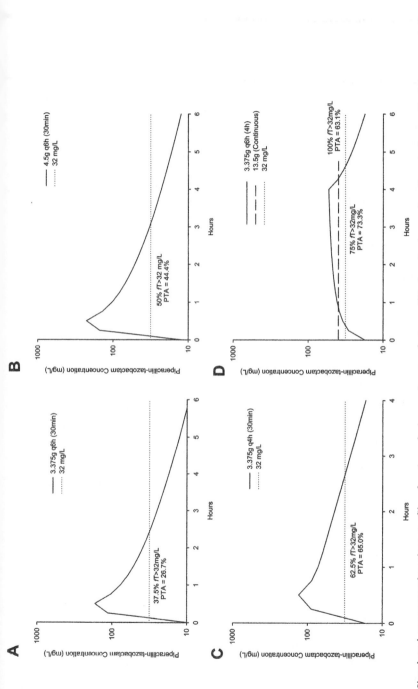

Fig. 1. (*A–D*) Simulated concentration-time profile of various dosing regimens of piperacillin-tazobactam using the median patient in a population pharmacokinetic model to determine *f*T>32 mg/L and incorporating variability to calculate the probability of target attainment (PTA) at 32 mg/L. (*Pharmacokinetic data from* Lodise TP Jr, Lomaestro B, Rodvold KA, et al. Pharmacodynamic profiling of piperacillin in the presence of tazobactam in patients through the use of population pharmacokinetic models and Monte Carlo simulation. Antimicrob Agents Chemother 2004;48:4718–24.)

Fig. 1 represent the median patient in the pharmacokinetic model and thus 50% of patients given these doses will have $fT>MIC$ less than indicated.

MONTE CARLO SIMULATION

Before the age of computers, comparisons between dosing regimens required the administration of an antibiotic to volunteers or patients at the various doses followed by analysis and comparison of the individual concentration-time profiles. In the present day, pharmacokinetic data of even a single dose coupled with Monte Carlo simulation allows these sorts of comparative analyses in only a few strokes of the keyboard. For pharmacokinetic purposes, Monte Carlo simulation is simply a semirandom number generator that incorporates the distributions of variability around pharmacokinetic parameters in a population to simulate drug concentration-time profiles for a large number of conjured individuals. For beta lactams, these simulated pharmacokinetic profiles can then be used to determine the probability that a given dosing regimen will achieve a target $fT>MIC$ across a range of MICs likely to be observed in the clinic, referred to as probability of target attainment (PTA). The importance of applying variability around pharmacokinetics parameters is emphasized in **Fig. 1**. Namely, although the $fT>32$ µg/mL for the simulated median patient was well above pharmacodynamic targets for several doses, none of the doses resulted in optimal ($\geq$90%) PTAs at that MIC.

Fig. 2A shows the results of a Monte Carlo analysis simulating patients with normal renal function (creatinine clearance of 50 to 120 mL/min) using a cefepime population pharmacokinetic model derived in patients with ventilator-associated pneumonia (VAP).[16] The PTA curves shown in this figure represent the likelihood that a given cefepime regimen will achieve a $fT>MIC$ greater than or equal to 50% across the range of MICs. At an MIC of 8 µg/mL, only the 2 g every 8 hours (3-hour infusion) regimen resulted in an optimal PTA (93.8%). In comparison, a 2 g every 8 hour regimen given as a standard 30-minute infusion achieved a PTA of only 85.8%. This finding again highlights the usefulness of prolonging the infusion time. In a clinical scenario where the MIC of the infecting pathogen is known, these data can aid in appropriate dose selection.

These data can also be applied to a distribution of isolate MICs to evaluate the likelihood that a given dosing regimen will achieve adequate PTAs against the bacteria residing in the clinical population; the sum of the resulting fractions is referred to as the cumulative fraction of response (CFR). The authors recently conducted an example of this type of analysis using MIC data for *Pseudomonas aeruginosa* and *Acinetobacter baumannii* isolates collected from 56 hospitals in the United States as part of the 2008 Tracking Resistance in the United States Today (TRUST-12) surveillance program.[17] It was noted that prolonged infusions of all beta lactams resulted in increased CFRs relative to standard infusions, thus increasing the likelihood that the chosen regimen will provide adequate coverage clinically. The degree at which prolonging the infusion impacted the CFR was dependent on the MIC distribution of the isolates. For 2 g every 8 hours of cefepime, the increases in PTA garnered by prolonging the infusion time to 3 hours (see **Fig. 2**A) resulted in an increase from 60.9% to 64.0% for *A baumannii* and an increase from 90.1% to 93.2% for *P aeruginosa*.[16,17] In the case of *A baumannii*, the MIC distribution is shifted to the right (ie, high MICs), thus modulating the dosing regimen does little to improve exposures. Conversely for *P aeruginosa*, the 30-minute infusion of cefepime already maximized exposures, thus prolonging the infusion adds little apparent advantage. Taken collectively, it can be concluded that to appreciated dose optimization, one must understand the MIC distribution for the pathogen of interest. In most instances, this would require additional information from the microbiology department as a simple interpretive report (ie, susceptible, intermediate, or resistant) is clearly

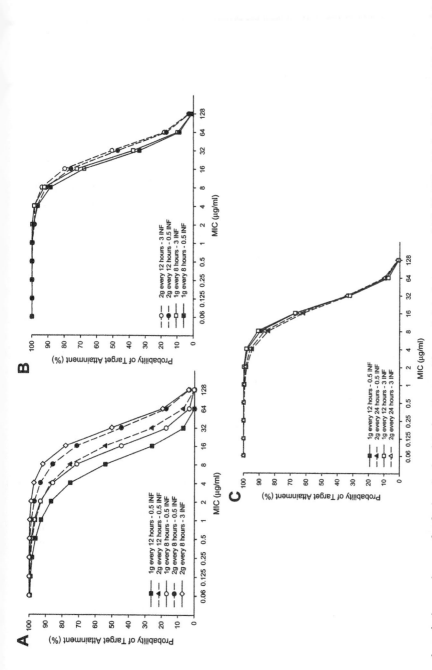

Fig. 2. PTA for various dosing regimens of cefepime in simulated patients with creatinine clearances of (*A*) 50–120 mL/min, (*B*) 30–49 mL/min, anc (*C*) 10–29 mL/min. (*From* Nicasio AM, Ariano RE, Zelenitsky SA, et al. Population pharmacokinetics of high-dose, prolonged-infusion cefepime in adult crit-ically ill patients with ventilator-associated pneumonia. Antimicrob Agents Chemother 2009;53:1476–81; with permission.)

lacking. Moreover, recent data suggest that the MIC reported by many of the automated susceptibility systems used in clinical laboratories may differ from the gold standard broth microdilution method, necessitating the use of another more reliable method (ie, broth microdilution, E test, and so forth).[18,19]

USING MONTE CARLO TO GUIDE CLINICAL PRACTICE

Undoubtedly, the ability to apply Monte Carlo simulation to a large population of isolates provides important insight into the pharmacodynamics of a particular dosing strategy. However, when these data are generated from a local distribution of isolates, they can offer a direct correlate to patient care within a given hospital or better a specific area within a hospital. Such an analysis was recently conducted at the authors' hospital (Hartford Hospital, Hartford, CT, USA) while developing a clinical pathway for the treatment of VAP.[20] In this study, the authors collected respiratory isolates from subjects within each of the intensive care units (ICU) and evaluated the potencies of the most commonly used antimicrobial agents. Because *P aeruginosa* accounted for a large proportion of respiratory infections and exhibited high rates of resistance in the authors' institution, doses were chosen to target this pathogen. Using Monte Carlo simulation, the authors evaluated the CFR of various beta-lactam regimens against the distribution of *P aeruginosa* in each of the ICUs. For the beta-lactam portion of the authors' 3-drug regimen for VAP,[1] they found that for subjects with normal renal function, cefepime 2 g every 8 hours (3-hour prolonged infusion) resulted in the highest CFRs in the neurotrauma and surgical ICUs and meropenem 2 g every 8 hours (3-hour prolonged infusion) had the highest probably of target attainments in the medical ICU. Based on these findings, a clinical dosing pathway was added to the authors' computerized physician order entry system to ensure that orders placed for patients within the respective units would result in therapy most likely to optimize pharmacodynamics against the isolates found in a given unit. A similar approach was taken at the Albany Medical Center Hospital (Albany, NY, USA) to optimize dosing of piperacillin-tazobactam against *P aeruginosa*.[21] Unlike the previous study centered on optimizing therapy against resistant pathogens, this analysis was designed to optimize piperacillin-tazobactam therapy against isolates defined as susceptible by the Clinical Laboratory Standards Institute. With the aid of Monte Carlo simulation, the investigators concluded that piperacillin-tazobactam 3.375 g every 8 hours (4-hours prolonged infusion) provided a significantly better probability of achieving pharmacodynamic targets relative to standard 30-minute infusions given every 4 or 6 hours. Based on these findings, all subjects treated with piperacillin-tazobactam in their hospital were given the pharmacodynamically optimized regimen.[21]

OPTIMIZING PHARMACODYNAMICS IN ANIMAL MODELS

There is a wealth of in vivo information available evaluating the efficacy of beta lactams dosed in such a way as to optimize the pharmacodynamic properties. The overwhelming majority of these studies were preformed by decreasing the time between consecutive doses and comparing those with an increased time between doses. Although these studies are important to help solidify the notion that $fT>MIC$ is the pharmacodynamic parameter of interest for beta lactams, they offer little in direct application to clinical practice. There are, however, an increasing number of studies in the more recent literature that help to construct the bridge between animal models and clinical practice. These studies are designed with dosing regimens simulating human pharmacokinetic profiles in mice and offer a unique insight into how a potential modification in dosing impacts in vivo efficacy. A recent set of studies performed by the authors' group compared the efficacy of various human-simulated regimens of doripenem against *P aeruginosa* in a murine thigh infection model. The first evaluated the changes in bacterial density observed for a 500 mg every 8 hours (1-hour infusion) regimen to that of a pharmacodynamically optimized 500 mg every 8 hours (4-hour infusion) dose against isolates with a range of doripenem MICs.[22] Both regimens resulted in bactericidal activity against isolates with MICs less than or equal to 2 μg/mL. However, at and MIC of 4 μg/mL, the 4-hour infusion regimen (*f*T>MIC 52.5%) resulted in statistically better efficacy than the 1-hour infusion (*f*T>MIC 30%) against 2 of 4 isolates tested. A follow-up study evaluated the effectiveness of 1- and 2-g regimens of doripenem given as 4-hour infusions against isolates with increased MICs (range: 2 to 32 μg/mL).[23] In line with predictions from Monte Carlo simulation,[24,25] 1- and 2-g doses resulted in predictable efficacy against isolates with MICs less than or equal to 8 μg/mL and less than or equal to 16 μg/mL, respectively.

Given the experimental difficulty in administering continuous infusions to animals, there is little literature available evaluating the comparative efficacy of intermittent and continuous infusions of beta lactams in animal models of infection. In a series of studies conducted in the mid to late 1980s using a rat model, Roosendaal and colleagues sought to evaluate the effects of continuous infusion ceftazidime for the treatment of *Klebsiella pneumoniae* lung infection.[26–30] In one example, using mortality as an endpoint for efficacy, the investigators compared the total daily dose required to keep 50% of animals alive for 16 days after 4 days of ceftazidime treatment (50% protective dose [PD_{50}]) when given either as a continuous infusion or intermittently (every 8 hours).[26] Depending on the incubation time, they found the PD_{50} of the continuous infusion to be 8% to 25% of that required for intermittent infusions, highlighting the concept that efficacy of beta lactams is dependent on *f*T>MIC as opposed to peak/MIC ratios and further that continuous infusions represent an excellent option for optimizing *f*T>MIC for these agents. Similar enhancement of ceftazidime activity was noted with continuous infusions when efficacy was evaluated as reductions in bacterial densities and not mortality.[29]

More recently, studies evaluating human-simulated exposures of continuous infusions have begun to emerge. One such study evaluated the efficacy of human-simulated exposures of ceftazidime as either a 2 g every 8 hours (30-minute infusion) or a 4-g continuous infusion (steady state concentration: 30 μg/mL) for the treatment of *P aeruginosa* pneumonia in rabbits. As predicted by the simulated *f*T>MIC for the respective regimens, the continuous-infusion regimen resulted in greater efficacy, most notably in septicemia sterilization, than the intermittent infusion regimen despite a reduction in total daily dose.[31]

OPTIMIZING PHARMACODYNAMICS IN THE CLINIC

As previously discussed, there are 2 dosing strategies that will result in the most notable effects on *f*T>MIC thus optimizing beta-lactam therapy: decreasing the dosing interval and prolonging the infusion time. Although it is evident from mathematical modeling and in vivo infection models that these strategies do in fact optimize pharmacodynamic and thus efficacy, it is important to confirm that these strategies translate into clinical practice. A selection of studies examining the effects of beta-lactam dose modifications in patients follows.

Decreasing the Dosing Interval

In contemporary literature, meropenem represents the most notable example of modifying the dosing interval for pharmacodynamic optimization. Monte Carlo analysis determined that the likelihood of target attainment was similar for doses of 1 g every 8 hours (30-minute infusion) and 500 mg every 6 hours (30-minute infusion), despite the 1-g reduction in total daily dose of the 500-mg regimen.[32] Several hospitals instituted an automatic substitution of the 1 g every 8 hours regimen with 500 mg every 6 hours and published outcomes comparing preimplantation and postimplantation.[33–35] The first, conducted by the authors' group, evaluated 85 subjects receiving either the standard regimen (or renally adjusted to 1 g every 12 hours) or the optimized regimen (renally adjusted to 500 mg every 8 hours) and found no significant differences in clinical success (78% vs 82%; P = .86), microbiologic success (63% vs 79% P = .33), or infection-related length of stay (14 vs 13 days; P = .97).[34]

A similar study conducted by Patel and colleagues[35] evaluated 292 patients receiving meropenem as either standard (n = 100) or pharmacodynamically optimized regimens (n = 192) for a variety of infections. They too found no significant differences in all evaluated outcomes including: in-hospital mortality (8% vs 11.5%; P = .24), clinical success (90.9% vs 92.1%; P = .72), meropenem-related length of stay (7 vs 9 days; P = .141), and duration of meropenem therapy (5 vs 4 days; P = .055).

A final study evaluated outcomes in subjects treated for neutropenic fever refractory to cefepime with either imipenem 500 mg every 6 hours (n = 40), meropenem 1 g every 8 hours (n = 29), or meropenem 500 mg every 6 hours (n = 58).[33] The investigators noted similar findings with respect to primary outcomes of time to defervescence (2 vs 2 vs 3 days), need for additional antibiotics (20% vs 17% vs 14%; P = .71), and time to receipt of additional antibiotics (5 vs 2 vs 1 days). In addition, no significant differences were found between groups for secondary outcomes which included: treatment duration (10 vs 8 vs 8 days), in-hospital mortality (5% vs 7% vs 7%; P = .82), and 30-day mortality (13% vs 7% vs 14%; P = .64).

Prolonged Infusion

Compared with the exorbitant amount of Monte Carlo data describing the benefits of extending the infusion time for a large number of beta lactams, there are few studies evaluating the clinical outcomes associated with the use of these regimens. The first described the outcomes associated with the Monte Carlo-based adaptation of piperacillin-tazobactam dosing at Albany Medical Center Hospital as previously noted.[21,36] In this retrospective study, investigators compared clinical outcomes between subjects receiving standard 30-minute infusions of piperacillin-tazobactam to those given prolonged infusions (3.375 g every 8 hours [4-hour infusion]) for the treatment of *P aeruginosa* infections. They analyzed a total of 111 subjects, with 54 in the prolonged infusion group. As a total population, no differences were observed between the prolonged and standard infusion groups in terms of 14-day (5.6% vs 12.3%; P = .2) and 30-day mortality (7.4% vs 15.8%; P = .2) or median length of hospital stay after the start of piperacillin-tazobactam (14 vs 17 days; P = .2).[36] However, when a subset analysis was conducted on the more severely ill population (ie, Acute Physiology And Chronic Health Evaluation [APACHE] II $\geq$17), prolonged infusions resulted in a statistically lower rate of 14-day mortality (12.2% vs 31.6%; P = .04) and reduced length of hospital stay (21 vs 38 days; P = .02).[21]

As previously noted, a pharmacodynamic-based approach to empiric beta-lactam dosing in patients with VAP was instituted within the ICUs of the authors' hospital in June 2006.[20] This clinical pathway used 3-hour prolonged infusions of cefepime 2 g every 8 hours or meropenem 2 g every 8 hours to target the less susceptible population of *P aeruginosa* commonly seen in the authors' ICU patients. When comparing outcomes between 94 subjects treated for VAP after implementation of the clinical pathway and the 74 subjects treated before implementation, there was a significant reduction in infection-related mortality (8.5% vs 21.6%; $P = .29$), appropriate antibiotic therapy (71.6% vs 48.6%; $P = .007$), and infection-related length of stay (11.7 vs 26.1 days; $P<.001$). Although the clinical pathway consisted of a multifaceted approach to the treatment of VAP and included both gram-positive and gram-negative pathogens, a closer look at subjects infected with *P aeruginosa* isolates with MICs at or above the respective susceptibly breakpoints (4 and 8 µg/mL for cefepime and meropenem, respectively) revealed an important benefit of these optimized regimens. Namely, of the 9 subjects treated with these more resistant pathogens, 8 resulted in a successful outcome. Similar reports of positive outcomes in patients with cystic fibrosis being treated for lung exacerbations of *P aeruginosa* and *Burkholderia cepacia* classified as nonsusceptible (MICs 8–32 µg/mL) with high-dose prolonged infusion regimens of meropenem (2 or 3 g every 8 hours [3-hour infusion] and doripenem (2 g every 8 hours [4-hour infusion] have also been documented by the authors' group.[37,38]

Another important representation of the clinical use of prolonged infusions was during the phase III study of doripenem for the treatment of VAP. Using a noninferior study design, the investigators evaluated the efficacy of doripenem 500 mg every 8 hours (4-hour prolonged infusion) and imipenem given as either 500 mg every 6 hours (30-minute infusion) or 1 g every 8 hours (1-hour infusion). In a rather large population of subjects, prolonged-infusion doripenem resulted in clinical efficacy in 68.3% of subjects in the clinically evaluable population and was not inferior to standard infusions of imipenem (64.8%).[39]

Continuous Infusions

Relative to prolonged infusions, there are considerably more data available evaluating the use of continuous infusions in patients, many published within the last decade. Unlike most of the comparative data previously presented for prolonged infusions that used historical controls, several studies evaluating continuous infusions were randomized controlled trials. Two of these controlled studies evaluated ceftazidime for the treatment of nosocomial pneumonia. The first used a bolus of 2 g followed by a continuous infusion of 60 mg/kg;[40] whereas, the second used a 1-g bolus followed by a 3-g continuous infusion.[41] The comparator arm for each was 2 g every 8 hours (30-minute infusion) and the second study coadministered tobramycin 7 mg/kg with both treatment arms. There was no difference between groups in either study with respect to clinical outcome and several secondary endpoints, including duration of leukocytosis, duration of mechanical ventilation, and length of both hospital and ICU stay. The second study found the time it took for subjects to become afebrile in the continuous infusion arm to be statistically less than the intermittent infusion arm (3.1 vs 5.2 days; $P = .015$); whereas, the first study found no difference. It should be noted that despite similar outcomes, both of these studies administered lower total daily doses in the continuous infusion arms compared with the intermittent infusion arms. The following 3 studies evaluated equivalent total daily doses and manipulated only infusion strategies.

The first evaluated cefepime as either 2 g every 12 hours or a 4-g continuous infusion for the treatment of pneumonia or bacteremia in critically ill subjects.[42] The investigators found no significant differences between treatment arms in clinical outcome, mechanical ventilation, or bacteriologic eradication. The second study compared ceftriaxone for the treatment of sepsis given as a single 2-g bolus daily (n = 28) or a 2-g continuous infusion (n = 29); a 500-mg bolus was given on the first day of treatment in both arms. Although no significant differences were seen in any of the evaluated outcomes in the intention to treat group, in a subset of *A priori*-identified subjects receiving ceftriaxone therapy for at least 4 days, continuous infusion resulted in statistically better clinical response ($P = .04$); considerable protective effects were also noted for continuous infusion in logistic regression analysis for resolution of clinical illness and bacterial eradication.[43] The third study was the largest of the randomized studies and compared the efficacy of piperacillin-tazobactam 12/1.5 g either as a continuous infusion (n =130) or an intermittent 30-minute infusion of 3/0.375 g every 6 hours (n = 132) for the treatment of complicated intra-abdominal infections. Demographic data were similar between groups as was severity of illness. No differences were noted between the two groups in terms of clinical or microbiological success, time to defervescence, time to white blood cell normalization, or length of hospital stay.[44] It is important to note that although a majority of these analyses did not report MIC data, the pharmacodynamic advantage of optimized regimens is highly dependent on the infecting MICs (ie, lower MICs are less likely to show differences).

OTHER CONSIDERATIONS
Pathogens with Increased MICs

As previously presented, there are essentially 2 infusion-related techniques primarily used to maximize $fT>MIC$, prolonged or continuous infusion. To the authors' knowledge, there has been no clinical study comparing the efficacy of these strategies in similarly matched subjects. However, based on the current understanding of beta-lactam pharmacodynamics, there are certain theoretical scenarios when one strategy may be preferred to the other. One of the major drawbacks of both extended infusion strategies is that in prolonging administration time, peak drug concentrations are subsequently reduced. Assuming an equivalent total daily dose, the reduction in peak concentration would be more profound during continuous infusion relative to prolonged infusion. Most often, the time at peak concentrations certainly for bolus and likely with prolonged infusions are not sufficient to achieve bactericidal targets. However, in the face of salvage therapy for exceptionally pan-resistant organisms, perhaps $fT>MICs$ in the range of stasis as provided by prolonged infusions may prove useful, especially with combination therapy. On the flip side, it is theoretical that in certain patient populations, such as those with profound neutropenia, maximizing the $fT>MIC$ may be preferable to assure adequate host response.[45] Assuredly, with continuous infusion, the $fT>MIC$ will be either 100% or 0% depending on the MIC of the infecting organism coupled with the maximum total daily dose.[46] As such, although prolonged infusions may results in at or near target exposures against resistant pathogens, continuous infusions maximize pharmacodynamics, arguably beyond what is thought to be clinically relevant, against the more susceptible organisms. However, based on recognized targets and a population of clinical *P aeruginosa* isolates in the authors' hospital, they found similar optimal CFRs for 16/2 g of piperacillin-tazobactam given as either a 3-hour prolonged infusion every 6 hours or a continuous infusion, both of which were considerably higher than 30-minute infusions.[15] As a result, it is imperative that before adopting an optimized dosing strategy, the local distribution of MICs likely to be encountered in the patient population of interest is carefully considered.

Parenteral Drug Administration

Given the pharmacodynamic similarities between prolonged and continuous infusions, the decision between the two often rests on requirements of administration. Namely, for continuous infusions only a single dose of antibiotic is required per day; whereas, multiple administration times are required for prolonged infusions. The obvious tradeoff is that for continuous infusions a dedicated intravenous site is necessary for the entire hospital stay. However, patients receiving prolonged infusions will have numerous drug-free intervals to allow administration of other medications. Regardless of the chosen technique, education on the importance of adhering to administration times for the house staff is imperative. This timing is particularly important when the infusion technique allows for a reduction in the drug administered per dose (ie, a standard infusion time would result in inadequate pharmacodynamics).

Another important consideration relating to administration is the stability of the compound. This stability is particularly important for continuous infusions, but may also be of interest for prolonged infusions when consideration is given to preparation and deliver times. **Table 1** lists the reported stability at room and refrigerated temperatures of beta lactams for which alternate dosing strategies are commonly reported in the literature. Although the importance of room temperature is intuitive, the availability to chill infusion pump cassettes[47] and other refrigerated infusion devices make stability below room temperature increasingly more pertinent.

Oral Drug Administration

Although all examples of beta-lactam optimization presented thus far have centered on parenteral administration, and the likelihood of administration by other methods in critically ill patients is minimal, it should be noted that these concepts readily translate to oral therapy. When considering optimization of oral beta lactams, clearly manipulations relative to the infusion time are not possible. However, the remaining 2 methods of optimizing pharmacodynamics, namely increased doses and decreased intervals, are useful. In fact, pharmacodynamic analyses centered on oral beta-lactam optimization have been used in the development of clinical practice guidelines.[48,49] Moreover, Monte Carlo analyses similar to those produced for parenteral beta lactams have been used to compare oral agents against clinically relevant MIC distributions.[50,51]

Renal Function

Although a large proportion of the clinical data presented in the literature on beta-lactam optimization are conducted in patients with normal renal function, a significant number of patients seen within clinical practice have at least some degree of renal

Table 1
Room temperature and refrigerator stability of commonly used beta-lactam antibiotics

Antibiotic	Concentration	Room Temperature (h) (25°C)	Refrigerated (d) (4°C–5°C)
Ampicillin	<30 mg/mL	8	3
Cefepime	<280 mg/mL	24	7
Ceftazidime	20 mg/mL	24	7
Ceftriaxone	100 mg/mL	72	10
Doripenem	20 mg/mL	24	10
Imipenem	5 mg/mL	4	1
Meropenem	20 mg/mL	4	1
Nafcillin	40 mg/mL	24	4
Oxacillin	100 mg/mL	24	3
Penicillin G	500,000 units/mL	24	7
Piperacillin-tazobactam	20 mg/mL	24	7

Data from Crandon JL, Sutherland C, Nicolau DP. Stability of doripenem in polyvinyl chloride bags and elastomeric pumps. Am J Health Syst Pharm 2010;67:1539–44; and Trissel LA. Handbook of Injectable Drugs. 14th edition. Bethesda (MD): American Society of Health-System Pharmacists; 2007.

impairment. The implications of renal function are of particular importance for the beta lactams because these agents are primarily cleared through the kidneys and thus require careful consideration. With the availability of population pharmacokinetic modeling, it is possible to mathematically describe the relationship between patient renal function, most commonly reported as creatinine clearance, and antibiotic clearance. Assuming a robust pharmacokinetic data set compiled from patients with varying renal function, these data can then be applied to Monte Carlo simulation to determine dosing regimens that optimize pharmacodynamics and minimize exposure-related adverse events across a range of simulated renal functions.

An example of such an analysis is shown in **Fig. 2**. In this study, a cefepime population pharmacokinetic model was developed from subjects with VAP. The model and inherent variability surrounding each pharmacokinetic parameter was entered into a Monte Carlo simulation assuming 3 ranges in creatinine clearance (50 to 120 mL/min [see **Fig. 2A**], 30 to 49 mL/min [see **Fig. 2B**], and 10 to 29 mL/min [see **Fig. 2C**]), and the PTA for several different doses was calculated. Cefepime dosing regimens for subjects with reduced renal function were selected based on goal target attainments within each grouping of creatinine clearance.[16] In situations where pharmacokinetic targets have been shown to associate with adverse events, these analyses can also evaluate the likelihood that patients with reduced renal function would enter this toxic range. Unfortunately, no such targets have been identified for beta lactams, so the authors[52] and others[53] have compared exposure profiles in these renally impaired subsets to maximum tolerated exposures observed clinically in other patient populations (ie, normal renal function, healthy volunteers).

Pediatrics

Despite common clinical use in pediatric patients, there are little data available evaluating the clinical optimization of beta lactams in this patient population. This deficiency is important because the potential shortcomings of standard infusions are even more pronounced in pediatrics secondary to their higher rates in drug clearance relative to adults. Moreover, the resistance patterns of clinical pathogens isolated in pediatrics have also been shown to differ from adults.[54,55] However, there are a few, albeit small, pharmacokinetic analyses conducted in infected pediatric patients that have allowed the use of Monte Carlo simulation to evaluate differences in target attainments between standard and prolonged infusions of beta lactams against clinically relevant MIC distributions of *P aeruginosa*.[56,57] As might be expected, the use of optimized regimens (ie, high dose, prolonged infusions, or continuous infusions) resulted in considerable increases in PTA and CFR when compared with standard regimens. The benefits noted for optimized regimens in these studies are of utmost importance for the pediatric population given the observation that standard regimens resulted in poor PTAs against isolates well within the susceptibility range.

Economic Benefits

Throughout this article countless data are presented suggesting equivalence in the case of susceptible organisms, or enhancement in the case of resistant organisms, of the clinical and experimental efficacy for beta lactams when comparing optimized to standard regimens. Although maximizing patient outcomes is clearly the most important driver for clinical decisions, considerations of economics cannot be ignored. Assuming clinical outcomes are similar, situations where optimized regimens require less total daily doses of drug than standard regimens would result in an obvious decrease in acquisition cost, without affecting total hospital costs. In the previously described examples of administering meropenem 500 mg every 6 hours as opposed to 1 g every

8 hours at the authors' hospital and Albany Medical Center Hospital, significant reductions in costs were noted at both institutions. At Hartford Hospital, the authors saw a $406 median reduction in acquisition costs per patient ($P = .009$) and a $762 reduction in total treatment costs per patient, which included acquisition, concomitant infection-related medications, and treatment of adverse events ($P = .008$).[34] Similarly, evaluating only drug acquisition costs, investigators at Albany Medical Center Hospital saw a median $204.97 reduction in costs associated with the optimized regimen ($P<.001$).[35] Parallel examples of cost savings secondary to a reduction in total daily dose are also available for piperacillin-tazobactam as both prolonged[21] and continuous infusions,[58] as well as ceftazidime as a continuous infusion.[59]

Another not so intuitive example of economic benefits associated with beta lactam optimization is when the proposed empiric therapy results in greater drug acquisition costs than the standard regimen. There is a rather extensive compilation of data suggesting that earlier initiation of appropriate antibiotic therapy results in better patient outcomes for a variety of infections.[60–64] Given that pharmacodynamic targets are achieved against a wider range of MICs with high-dose optimized beta-lactam regimens, it seems reasonable to conclude that these empiric regimens will result in better outcomes. A pharmacoeconomic analysis was conducted based on the findings of the VAP clinical pathway instituted at Hartford Hospital as previously described.[65] Despite the empiric use of the more costly high-dose prolonged infusions of meropenem and cefepime (ie, 2 g every 8 hours [3-hour infusion]), subjects treated using the clinical pathway experienced lower hospital costs associated with the treatment of VAP ($P<.001$). Although daily hospital costs were similar for both cohorts over the first 7 days, costs declined significantly for subjects treated with the clinical pathway from that point forward ($P<.001$); this observation was likely explained by a shorter antibiotic treatment duration and shorter length of stay after the diagnosis of VAP. Importantly, median antibiotic costs were a small proportion of the total hospital costs and were similar between clinical pathway and historical control groups ($P =.45$).[65]

SUMMARY

There is an ever-growing body of literature supporting the correlation of pharmacodynamic parameters and antimicrobial efficacy. For beta lactams, there is a clear relationship between $fT>MIC$ and bacterial killing such that activity is maximized through the optimization of $fT>MIC$. With the assistance of Monte Carlo simulation, one can predict the probability that proposed dosing regimens will achieve pharmacodynamic targets against a given pathogen or a distribution of pathogens and the finding of these studies are consistent with observations in vivo. Based on mathematical, animal, and clinical data, manipulation of the infusion time offers an excellent opportunity to optimize pharmacodynamics, often in such a way that reduces cost and potential toxicities. Consideration should be given to renal function, pathogen MIC, and stability of the compound when adopting extended infusion strategies.

REFERENCES

1. America ATSatIDSo. Guidelines for the management of adults with hospital-acquired, ventilator-associated, and healthcare-associated pneumonia. Am J Respir Crit Care Med 2005;171:388–416.
2. Solomkin JS, Mazuski JE, Bradley JS, et al. Diagnosis and management of complicated intra-abdominal infection in adults and children: guidelines by the Surgical Infection Society and the Infectious Diseases Society of America. Surg Infect (Larchmt) 2010;11:79–109.

3. Stevens DL, Bisno AL, Chambers HF, et al. Practice guidelines for the diagnosis and management of skin and soft-tissue infections. Clin Infect Dis 2005;41:1373–406.
4. Eagle H, Fleischman R, Levy M. "Continuous" vs. "discontinuous" therapy with penicillin; the effect of the interval between injections on therapeutic efficacy. N Engl J Med 1953;248:481–8.
5. Eagle H, Fleischman R, Musselman AD. Effect of schedule of administration on the therapeutic efficacy of penicillin; importance of the aggregate time penicillin remains at effectively bactericidal levels. Am J Med 1950;9:280–99.
6. Craig WA. Pharmacokinetic/pharmacodynamic parameters: rationale for antibacterial dosing of mice and men. Clin Infect Dis 1998;26:1–10 [quiz: 11–2].
7. Turnidge JD. The pharmacodynamics of beta-lactams. Clin Infect Dis 1998;27: 10–22.
8. Drusano GL. Prevention of resistance: a goal for dose selection for antimicrobial agents. Clin Infect Dis 2003;36:S42–50.
9. Li C, Du X, Kuti JL, et al. Clinical pharmacodynamics of meropenem in patients with lower respiratory tract infections. Antimicrob Agents Chemother 2007;51:1725–30.
10. Crandon JL, Bulik CC, Kuti JL, et al. Clinical pharmacodynamics of cefepime in patients infected with Pseudomonas aeruginosa. Antimicrob Agents Chemother 2010;54:1111–6.
11. Craig WA, Andes D. Pharmacokinetics and pharmacodynamics of antibiotics in otitis media. Pediatr Infect Dis J 1996;15:255–9.
12. Nicolau DP, Sutherland CA, Arguedas A, et al. Pharmacokinetics of cefprozil in plasma and middle ear fluid: in children undergoing treatment for acute otitis media. Paediatr Drugs 2007;9:119–23.
13. Nicolau DP. Optimizing antimicrobial therapy and emerging pathogens. Am J Manag Care 1998;4:S525–30.
14. Lodise TP Jr, Lomaestro B, Rodvold KA, et al. Pharmacodynamic profiling of piperacillin in the presence of tazobactam in patients through the use of population pharmacokinetic models and Monte Carlo simulation. Antimicrob Agents Chemother 2004;48:4718–24.
15. Kim A, Sutherland CA, Kuti JL, et al. Optimal dosing of piperacillin-tazobactam for the treatment of Pseudomonas aeruginosa infections: prolonged or continuous infusion? Pharmacotherapy 2007;27:1490–7.
16. Nicasio AM, Ariano RE, Zelenitsky SA, et al. Population pharmacokinetics of high-dose, prolonged-infusion cefepime in adult critically ill patients with ventilator-associated pneumonia. Antimicrob Agents Chemother 2009;53:1476–81.
17. Koomanachai P, Bulik CC, Kuti JL, et al. Pharmacodynamic modeling of intravenous antibiotics against gram-negative bacteria collected in the United States. Clin Ther 2010;32:766–79.
18. Bulik CC, Fauntleroy KA, Jenkins SG, et al. Comparison of meropenem MICs and susceptibilities for carbapenemase-producing Klebsiella pneumoniae isolates by various testing methods. J Clin Microbiol 2010;48:2402–6.
19. Torres E, Villanueva R, Bou G. Comparison of different methods of determining beta-lactam susceptibility in clinical strains of Pseudomonas aeruginosa. J Med Microbiol 2009;58:625–9.
20. Nicasio AM, Eagye KJ, Nicolau DP, et al. Pharmacodynamic-based clinical pathway for empiric antibiotic choice in patients with ventilator-associated pneumonia. J Crit Care 2009;25:69–77.
21. Lodise TP Jr, Lomaestro B, Drusano GL. Piperacillin-tazobactam for Pseudomonas aeruginosa infection: clinical implications of an extended-infusion dosing strategy. Clin Infect Dis 2007;44:357–63.

22. Kim A, Banevicius MA, Nicolau DP. In vivo pharmacodynamic profiling of doripenem against Pseudomonas aeruginosa by simulating human exposures. Antimicrob Agents Chemother 2008;52:2497–502.
23. Crandon JL, Bulik CC, Nicolau DP. In vivo efficacy of 1- and 2-gram human simulated prolonged infusions of doripenem against Pseudomonas aeruginosa. Antimicrob Agents Chemother 2009;53:4352–6.
24. Bhavnani SM, Hammel JP, Cirincione BB, et al. Use of pharmacokinetic-pharmacodynamic target attainment analyses to support phase 2 and 3 dosing strategies for doripenem. Antimicrob Agents Chemother 2005;49:3944–7.
25. Van Wart SA, Andes DR, Ambrose PG, et al. Pharmacokinetic-pharmacodynamic modeling to support doripenem dose regimen optimization for critically ill patients. Diagn Microbiol Infect Dis 2009;63:409–14.
26. Roosendaal R, Bakker-Woudenberg IA, van den Berg JC, et al. Therapeutic efficacy of continuous versus intermittent administration of ceftazidime in an experimental Klebsiella pneumoniae pneumonia in rats. J Infect Dis 1985;152:373–8.
27. Roosendaal R, Bakker-Woudenberg IA, van den Berghe-van Raffe M, et al. Continuous versus intermittent administration of ceftazidime in experimental Klebsiella pneumoniae pneumonia in normal and leukopenic rats. Antimicrob Agents Chemother 1986;30:403–8.
28. Roosendaal R, Bakker-Woudenberg IA, van den Berghe-van Raffe M, et al. Impact of the dosage schedule on the efficacy of ceftazidime, gentamicin and ciprofloxacin in Klebsiella pneumoniae pneumonia and septicemia in leukopenic rats. Eur J Clin Microbiol Infect Dis 1989;8:878–87.
29. Roosendaal R, Bakker-Woudenberg IA, van den Berghe-van Raffe M, et al. Influence of dose frequency on the therapeutic efficacies of ciprofloxacin and ceftazidime in experimental Klebsiella pneumoniae pneumonia and septicemia in relation to their bactericidal activities in vitro. Pharm Weekbl Sci 1987;Suppl 9:S33–40.
30. Roosendaal R, Bakker-Woudenberg IA, van den Berghe-van Raffe M, et al. Comparative activities of ciprofloxacin and ceftazidime against Klebsiella pneumoniae in vitro and in experimental pneumonia in leukopenic rats. Antimicrob Agents Chemother 1987;31:1809–15.
31. Croisier D, Martha B, Piroth L, et al. In vivo efficacy of humanised intermittent versus continuous ceftazidime in combination with tobramycin in an experimental model of pseudomonal pneumonia. Int J Antimicrob Agents 2008;32:494–8.
32. Kuti JL, Maglio D, Nightingale CH, et al. Economic benefit of a meropenem dosage strategy based on pharmacodynamic concepts. Am J Health Syst Pharm 2003;60:565–8.
33. Arnold HM, McKinnon PS, Augustin KM, et al. Assessment of an alternative meropenem dosing strategy compared with imipenem-cilastatin or traditional meropenem dosing after cefepime failure or intolerance in adults with neutropenic fever. Pharmacotherapy 2009;29:914–23.
34. Kotapati S, Nicolau DP, Nightingale CH, et al. Clinical and economic benefits of a meropenem dosage strategy based on pharmacodynamic concepts. Am J Health Syst Pharm 2004;61:1264–70.
35. Patel GW, Duquaine SM, McKinnon PS. Clinical outcomes and cost minimization with an alternative dosing regimen for meropenem in a community hospital. Pharmacotherapy 2007;27:1637–43.
36. Lodise TP, Lomaestro BM, Drusano GL. Application of antimicrobial pharmacodynamic concepts into clinical practice: focus on beta-lactam antibiotics: insights from the Society of Infectious Diseases Pharmacists. Pharmacotherapy 2006; 26:1320–32.

37. Bulik CC, Quintiliani R Jr, Samuel Pope J, et al. Pharmacodynamics and tolerability of high-dose, prolonged infusion carbapenems in adults with cystic fibrosis – A review of 3 cases. Respir Med CME online October 14, 2009.
38. Kuti JL, Moss KM, Nicolau DP, et al. Empiric treatment of multidrug-resistant Burkholderia cepacia lung exacerbation in a patient with cystic fibrosis: application of pharmacodynamic concepts to meropenem therapy. Pharmacotherapy 2004;24: 1641–5.
39. Chastre J, Wunderink R, Prokocimer P, et al. Efficacy and safety of intravenous infusion of doripenem versus imipenem in ventilator-associated pneumonia: a multicenter, randomized study. Crit Care Med 2008;36:1089–96.
40. Hanes SD, Wood GC, Herring V, et al. Intermittent and continuous ceftazidime infusion for critically ill trauma patients. Am J Surg 2000;179:436–40.
41. Nicolau DP, McNabb J, Lacy MK, et al. Continuous versus intermittent administration of ceftazidime in intensive care unit patients with nosocomial pneumonia. Int J Antimicrob Agents 2001;17:497–504.
42. Georges B, Conil JM, Cougot P, et al. Cefepime in critically ill patients: continuous infusion vs. an intermittent dosing regimen. Int J Clin Pharmacol Ther 2005;43:360–9.
43. Roberts JA, Boots R, Rickard CM, et al. Is continuous infusion ceftriaxone better than once-a-day dosing in intensive care? A randomized controlled pilot study. J Antimicrob Chemother 2007;59:285–91.
44. Lau WK, Mercer D, Itani KM, et al. Randomized, open-label, comparative study of piperacillin-tazobactam administered by continuous infusion versus intermittent infusion for treatment of hospitalized patients with complicated intra-abdominal infection. Antimicrob Agents Chemother 2006;50:3556–61.
45. Bodey GP, Ketchel SJ, Rodriguez V. A randomized study of carbenicillin plus cefamandole or tobramycin in the treatment of febrile episodes in cancer patients. Am J Med 1979;67:608–16.
46. Moriyama B, Henning SA, Childs R, et al. High-dose continuous infusion beta-lactam antibiotics for the treatment of resistant Pseudomonas aeruginosa infections in immunocompromised patients. Ann Pharmacother 2010;44:929–35.
47. Grant EM, Zhong MK, Ambrose PG, et al. Stability of meropenem in a portable infusion device in a cold pouch. Am J Health Syst Pharm 2000;57:992–5.
48. Anon JB, Jacobs MR, Poole MD, et al. Antimicrobial treatment guidelines for acute bacterial rhinosinusitis. Otolaryngol Head Neck Surg 2004;130:1–45.
49. Dandekar PK, Nicolau DP. Pharmacodynamic considerations for the selection of oral cephalosporins in the treatment of rhinosinusitis. Otolaryngol Head Neck Surg 2002;127:S10–6.
50. Fallon RM, Kuti JL, Doern GV, et al. Pharmacodynamic target attainment of oral beta-lactams for the empiric treatment of acute otitis media in children. Paediatr Drugs 2008;10:329–35.
51. Pichichero ME, Doern GV, Kuti JL, et al. Probability of achieving requisite pharmacodynamic exposure for oral beta-lactam regimens against Haemophilus influenzae in children. Paediatr Drugs 2008;10:391–7.
52. Society of Critical Care Medicine's 39th Critical Care Congress 2010 [abstract 832]. Miami (FL), January 9–13, 2010.
53. Patel N, Scheetz MH, Drusano GL, et al. Identification of optimal renal dosage adjustments for traditional and extended-infusion piperacillin-tazobactam dosing regimens in hospitalized patients. Antimicrob Agents Chemother 2010;54:460–5.
54. Diekema DJ, Pfaller MA, Jones RN. Age-related trends in pathogen frequency and antimicrobial susceptibility of bloodstream isolates in North America: SENTRY Antimicrobial Surveillance Program, 1997–2000. Int J Antimicrob Agents 2002;20:412–8.

55. Jones RN, Biedenbach DJ, Beach ML. Influence of patient age on the susceptibility patterns of Streptococcus pneumoniae isolates in North America (2000–2001): report from the SENTRY Antimicrobial Surveillance Program. Diagn Microbiol Infect Dis 2003;46:77–80.
56. Courter JD, Kuti JL, Girotto JE, et al. Optimizing bactericidal exposure for beta-lactams using prolonged and continuous infusions in the pediatric population. Pediatr Blood Cancer 2009;53:379–85.
57. Ellis JM, Kuti JL, Nicolau DP. Use of Monte Carlo simulation to assess the pharmacodynamics of beta-lactams against Pseudomonas aeruginosa infections in children: a report from the OPTAMA program. Clin Ther 2005;27:1820–30.
58. Grant EM, Kuti JL, Nicolau DP, et al. Clinical efficacy and pharmacoeconomics of a continuous-infusion piperacillin-tazobactam program in a large community teaching hospital. Pharmacotherapy 2002;22:471–83.
59. McNabb JJ, Nightingale CH, Quintiliani R, et al. Cost-effectiveness of ceftazidime by continuous infusion versus intermittent infusion for nosocomial pneumonia. Pharmacotherapy 2001;21:549–55.
60. Ibrahim EH, Sherman G, Ward S, et al. The influence of inadequate antimicrobial treatment of bloodstream infections on patient outcomes in the ICU setting. Chest 2000;118:146–55.
61. Kollef MH, Ward S. The influence of mini-BAL cultures on patient outcomes: implications for the antibiotic management of ventilator-associated pneumonia. Chest 1998;113:412–20.
62. Luna CM, Vujacich P, Niederman MS, et al. Impact of BAL data on the therapy and outcome of ventilator-associated pneumonia. Chest 1997;111:676–85.
63. Rello J, Gallego M, Mariscal D, et al. The value of routine microbial investigation in ventilator-associated pneumonia. Am J Respir Crit Care Med 1997;156:196–200.
64. Kumar A, Zarychanski R, Light B, et al. Early combination antibiotic therapy yields improved survival compared with monotherapy in septic shock: a propensity-matched analysis. Crit Care Med 2010;38:1773–85.
65. Nicasio AM, Eagye KJ, Kuti EL, et al. Length of stay and hospital costs associated with a pharmacodynamic-based clinical pathway for empiric antibiotic choice for ventilator-associated pneumonia. Pharmacotherapy 2010;30:453–62.

Optimal Use of Fluoroquinolones in the Intensive Care Unit Setting

John C. Rotschafer, PharmD[a],*, Mary A. Ullman, PharmD[b],
Christopher J. Sullivan, MD[c]

KEYWORDS

• Fluoroquinolone antibiotics • Intensive care unit
• Pharmacodynamics

Fluoroquinolone antibiotics have been a staple in community and hospital medical practice since the mid-1980s. In many ways the fluoroquinolone antibiotics represent an ideal antibiotic. The primary agents of this class can be administered either parenterally or orally. Oral absorption essentially emulates parenteral administration in terms of the serum concentration time curve so the oral route of administration can be considered for initial therapy. If circumstances permit, parenteral to oral switch therapy even in the intensive care setting is a viable option. Dosing options and cost have made these agents easy to use and readily accessible both in the inpatient and outpatient settings. As a class, the antibacterial spectrum and level of bacterial susceptibility has held up relatively well over the years, an amazing feat considering the usage of these drugs in the community, nursing home, hospital, and animal husbandry.

Outbreaks of *Clostridium difficile* infections (CDI), increases in methicillin-/oxacillin-resistant *Staphylococcus aureus* (MRSA/ORSA), and the emergence of multidrug-resistant gram-negative infections have all been linked as collateral damage scenarios as a result of the increasing use or misuse of fluoroquinolones as well as other antibiotics.[1–3] Adverse events have, both in scope and magnitude, been heavily dependent on specific fluoroquinolones and there are clearly class-related problems that are still issues with the surviving members of the class. Although the US Food and Drug Administration (FDA) have approved a variety of fluoroquinolone antibiotics, issues primarily related to drug-induced adverse events have narrowed the class availability to primarily 3 fluoroquinolones: ciprofloxacin, levofloxacin, and moxifloxacin, and as

[a] Department of Experimental and Clinical Pharmacology, College of Pharmacy, University of Minnesota, WDH 7-189, 308 Harvard Street SE, Minneapolis, MN 55455, USA
[b] Department of Clinical Pharmacy, Regions Hospital, St Paul, MN, USA
[c] Critical Care, Fairview Hospital System, Minneapolis, MN, USA
* Corresponding author.
E-mail address: rotsc001@umn.edu

Crit Care Clin 27 (2011) 95–106
doi:10.1016/j.ccc.2010.11.005
0749-0704/11/$ – see front matter © 2011 Elsevier Inc. All rights reserved.
criticalcare.theclinics.com

a result this review discusses these 3 agents only. Ciprofloxacin is already available in generic form, levofloxacin will soon be a generic drug, and only moxifloxacin will remain a branded drug.

FLUOROQUINOLONE MECHANISM OF ACTION

Fluoroquinolones are unique antibiotics both in terms of their chemical structure and mechanism of antimicrobial action.[4-6] These agents interfere with the action of DNA gyrase. Depending on the fluoroquinolone there may be preferential activity toward DNA gyrase (gyrA and gyrB) or topoisomerase IV (parC and par E), or activity directed at both components. This interference prevents normal maintenance of the negative configuration of the supercoiled DNA helix and/or the ability of the DNA to appropriately uncoil for translation.

MICROBIOLOGY

Fluoroquinolones are active against gram-positive and gram-negative bacteria, atypical bacteria, and with select agents have anaerobic activity.[7-9] For gram-positive bacteria, action against MRSA is noticeably absent.[7-9] Of the available fluoroquinolones, levofloxacin and moxifloxacin (not ciprofloxacin) are potent antibiotics for penicillin-sensitive or -resistant *Streptococcus pneumoniae*. Usually 98% to 100% of *Streptococcus pneumoniae* using approved break points remain susceptible to moxifloxacin or levofloxacin and there is no appreciable difference in activity between the 2 fluoroquinolones **(Table 1)**.

When the fluoroquinolones were first introduced into clinical practice, these compounds offered excellent bacterial susceptibility for gram-negative pathogens. Unfortunately, over time the percent of gram-negative strains maintaining antibiotic susceptibility to fluoroquinolones has fallen off substantially. *Pseudomonas aeruginosa, Proteus mirabilis*, and *Escherichia coli* generally are less than 70% to 75% susceptible to fluoroquinolones.[3,10] Gram-negative bacteria with extended β-lactamase (ESBL) capability (despite being an unrelated mechanism of resistance)

Table 1
Select bacterial fluoroquinolone susceptibility

Pathogen	N	% of Strains Susceptible		
		Levofloxacin	Ciprofloxacin	Moxifloxacin
Serratia marcescens	287	93.7	91.3	NT
Citrobacter spp	246	94.7	92.3	NT
Enterobacter cloacae	533	91.2	89.9	NT
Klebsiella pneumoniae	1,185	91.2	90.7	NT
Proteus mirabilis	594	73.7	71.0	NT
Escherichia coli	1,306	74.3	74.3	NT
Pseudomonas aeruginosa	1,215	66.7	68.3	NT
Acinetobacter baumannii	388	49.7	48.2	NT
Streptococcus pneumoniae	2,218	99.1	NT	99.2

Abbreviation: NT, not tested.

Data from TRUST 13 study, 2009; Ortho-McNeil. Levaquin 360 information. 2010; and Ortho-McNeil-Janssen Pharmaceuticals I. Tracking resistance in the United States today (TRUST). Presented at: 100th General Meeting of the American Society of Microbiology. San Diego (CA), May 21–25. Ortho McNeil Pharmaceuticals; 2010.

are also typically fluoroquinolone resistant as a result of associated fluoroquinolone resistance mutation carriage.[11] ESBLs were primarily vectoring in *Klebsiella pneumoniae* and *Escherichia coli* but now other species of Enterobacteriaceae have demonstrated the ability to acquire and express this enzyme and the associated cross resistance pattern.[12] As ESBLs continue to spread throughout the United States the magnitude of this problem will likely get worse. Fluoroquinolones have never been proved to be a mainstay antibiotic for *Acinetobacter baumannii*, current levels of susceptibility are usually less than 50% for levofloxacin and ciprofloxacin, however antibacterial activity may depend on the specific fluoroquinolone being tested (see **Table 1**). Activity against *Stenotrophomonas maltophilia* is usually poor. Thus, for common pathogens in the intensive care unit (ICU) such as *Pseudomonas aeruginosa*, *Acinetobacter baumannii*, and *Stenotrophomonas maltophilia*, fluoroquinolones alone cannot be relied on as initial antibiotic therapy.

Ciprofloxacin is considered the most potent fluoroquinolone against gram-negative bacteria in terms of minimum inhibitory concentration (MIC) values particularly against *Pseudomonas aeruginosa*, but this advantage can be overcome with more aggressive dosing of levofloxacin, which then generates approximately the same free or unbound area under the serum concentration time curve to MIC ratio (f-AUC/MIC)[13,14] (**Tables 2** and **3**). Moxifloxacin is not considered an optimal fluoroquinolone choice for *Pseudomonas aeruginosa*. Generally the susceptibility profile of ciprofloxacin and levofloxacin against gram-negative bacteria is virtually identical including *Pseudomonas aeruginosa* (<70%–75%, see **Table 1**).

Although fluoroquinolones are not widely used for anaerobic infections, moxifloxacin does have an FDA indication for intra-abdominal infections.[8] Before the withdrawal from the market of trovafloxacin, this particular fluoroquinolone was often used for anaerobic infections. Limited data to date would suggest that to maximize the chance of clinical and microbiologic success, an f-AUC/MIC ratio of 50 or greater must be obtained when using a fluoroquinolone for anaerobic infections.[13,15,16] Suboptimal exposures can result in the rapid development of stable fluoroquinolone class resistance.[13,15,16] A possible collateral damage scenario could also result if the drug was under dosed in a previous fluoroquinolone exposure or the fluoroquinolone had modest anaerobic activity. Patients receiving fluoroquinolone therapy for a previous unrelated infection who then later required therapy for an anaerobic infection for which a fluoroquinolone with anaerobic action was going to be used could be at risk. The initial fluoroquinolone therapy could possibly convert the resident anaerobe population from fluoroquinolone sensitive to fluoroquinolone class resistant resulting in clinical failure. Presently, fluoroquinolones are not considered first-line therapy for anaerobic infections especially in the ICU and use of fluoroquinolones has been identified as a risk factor for *Clostridium difficile* colitis.

Table 2
Fluoroquinolone pharmacokinetic parameters

Fluoroquinolone	Ciprofloxacin	Levofloxacin	Moxifloxacin
Half-life (hours)[a]	4	6	12
Protein binding (%)	30	30	50
Renal elimination (%)	50	90	20
Oral bioavailability (%)	70	99	90

[a] Assumes adult patients with normal renal function.
Adapted from Wright DH, Brown GH, Peterson ML, et al. Application of fluoroquinolone pharmacodynamics. J Antimicrob Chemother 2000;46:669–83.

Table 3 f-AUC-24/MIC ratios	MIC (mg/L)				
	2.0	1.0	0.5	0.25	0.125
Ciprofloxacin 400 mg every 8 h					
Total AUC = 33	—	—	—	—	—
f-AUC = 22	11	22	44	88	177
Levofloxacin 750 mg every 24 h					
Total AUC = 72	—	—	—	—	—
f-AUC = 50	25	50	100	200	400
Moxifloxacin 400 mg every 24 h					
Total AUC = 48	—	—	—	—	—
f-AUC = 24	12	24	48	96	192

Adapted from Wright DH, Brown GH, Peterson ML, et al. Application of fluoroquinolone pharmacodynamics. J Antimicrob Chemother 2000;46:669–83.

The level of bacterial fluoroquinolone susceptibility varies depending on regional geography, the specific hospital, and hospital unit. The usefulness of fluoroquinolones against even common gram-negative bacteria but especially for *Pseudomonas aeruginosa* is usually worse in the ICU than in general patient care settings. Unfortunately, the activity of fluoroquinolones against *Escherichia coli* has also fallen to less than 70% to 75%, calling into question the ongoing usefulness of fluoroquinolones against this common gram-negative pathogen.[3] Fluoroquinolones are unlikely to play a role in the management of infections caused by gram-negative bacteria producing carbapenemases, which like the ESBLs, is a growing problem in the United States.[11,12,14]

Both levofloxacin and ciprofloxacin have an FDA indication for postexposure anthrax (*Bacillus anthracis*) and would likely be useful for exposures to *Francisella tularensis* (tularemia) and *Yersinia pestis* (plague). However, should these pathogens be engineered as bioweapons, they could be genetically altered to resist the effect of fluoroquinolone antibiotics. Many experts also consider fluoroquinolones to be very potent and invaluable second-line agents for *Mycobacterium tuberculosis* and atypical mycobacteria.[17]

MECHANISM OF BACTERIAL RESISTANCE

As with all antibiotics, widespread use of fluoroquinolones has fostered bacterial resistance.[18–21] Fluoroquinolone-resistant bacteria have mutations in gyrA, gyr B, par C, par E, and/or have 1 or more operational efflux pump. None of these mechanisms are mutually exclusive so multiple forms of resistance can be present simultaneously. Baseline resistance usually results in a 2- to 4-fold change in the bacterial MIC. As bacteria acquire additional fluoroquinolone resistance mechanisms, there is an ongoing multiplier of MIC. Generally the presence of an efflux pump and a gyr or par point mutation conveys fluoroquinolone resistance. Initially fluoroquinolone resistance was chromosomal with low mutational frequency; however, passage of fluoroquinolone resistance has now been documented via plasmid transfer.[22,23]

PHARMACODYNAMICS

Unlike pharmacokinetics, a science that studies the relationship between antibiotic concentrations and time, pharmacodynamics attempts to evaluate the antibiotic effect (bacterial killing) with time. With antibiotics, their effect on bacteria can generally be categorized as concentration dependent (time independent) or concentration independent (time dependent).[24] In the case of concentration-dependent antibiotics, the higher the free or unbound antibiotic serum concentration, the faster the rate and extent of bacterial kill.[22,23] With concentration-independent antibiotics, once an antibiotic serum concentration threshold has been exceeded, the rate and extent of bacterial kill remains essentially the same. For concentration-dependent killing antibiotics, increasing serum concentrations increases the rate and extent of kill; with a concentration-independent antibiotic the rate and extent of bacterial kill remains fixed despite increasing serum concentrations.[22,23] Maximizing dose or administering the entire daily dose as a single dose might be strategies that optimize antibiotic performance for a concentration-dependent antibiotic if performance is driven by increasing the free antibiotic peak serum concentration to MIC ratio (f-Cpmax/MIC) or the f-AUC/MIC as it is for fluoroquinolones.[22,23]

Fluoroquinolones were the first chemical class of antibiotics for which there was a real attempt to incorporate pharmacodynamics into the drug development process. Fluoroquinolones were proved to be concentration-dependent killers of gram-negative pathogens, whereas their activity against gram-positive bacteria such as *Streptococcus pneumoniae* seems to be more concentration independent.[13] Overall, f-AUC/MIC seems to be the best predictor of fluoroquinolone performance.[13,24] Although the pharmacodynamic outcome parameter may be the same for gram-positive and gram-negative pathogens, the quantitative value assigned to this outcome parameter to predict favorable outcomes differs.

An f-AUC/MIC ratio of 87.5/h or more seems to best predict clinical and microbiologic success for gram-negative infections.[24–27] Higher ratios usually ensure an acceptable clinical and microbiologic outcome with gram-negative pathogens. An f-AUC/MIC value of 33.7/h or more seems to maximize fluoroquinolone performance for gram-positive infections.[24,28] Although these data clearly can be used to predict likely clinical and microbiologic success in the patient, practically the clinician is not in a position to individualize the f-AUC/MIC value in a specific patient using commonly available hospital resources. Clinical laboratories do not routinely perform fluoroquinolone protein binding studies to estimate free drug concentrations and with limited serum sampling, most clinicians are not going to be able to accurately determine the fluoroquinolone AUC. As a result, in the antibiotic development process a pharmacodynamic tool called Monte Carlo analysis is used to simulate likely clinical experiences and then predict the probability of target attainment (reaching an adequate f-AUC/MIC ratio) for a specific antibiotic dosage regimen matched against a specific pathogen fluoroquinolone MIC value. These studies pair large data banks of patient pharmacokinetic data and large collections of bacterial susceptibility data. A computer randomly matches the individual patient f-AUC data against a randomly selected bacterial pathogen's MIC for a specific fluoroquinolone. These simulations are run 10,000 times or more. Then using the appropriate pharmacodynamic outcome parameter breakpoint value, the investigator can determine that with a particular fluoroquinolone dose and interval the probability of target attainment is say 92% in that patient population.

Efforts to increase the quantitative value for f-AUC/MIC can focus on the both the numerator and denominator of this ratio. Increasing the antibiotic dose increases the f-Cpmax and f-AUC but doubling the ratio requires a doubling of the dose. Clinically this approach has been used in the management of tuberculosis and can be monitored with fluoroquinolone serum concentrations. Higher doses especially for levofloxacin, which is almost completely eliminated by the kidneys, should be monitored using regular urinalysis specifically examining urine for evidence of crystalluria. Patients in renal failure do not clear most fluoroquinolones normally which increases f-AUC but the dose usually has to be adjusted for renal failure. Increasing the dose by 2-fold or allowing a renally compromised patient to maintain higher serum concentrations for a much longer period of time could increase the possibility of an adverse event. Thus, although dose can be manipulated to an extent, there is a limited effect on the f-AUC unless the clinician is willing to use much larger daily doses of the antibiotic.

Altering the bacterial MIC by the use of inhibitors of resistance mechanisms could dramatically alter the f-AUC/MIC ratio and likely increase the possibility of a favorable clinical and microbiologic outcome. As the MIC is found in the denominator of this ratio, reducing the MIC by 1 tube dilution increases the f-AUC/MIC ratio 2-fold. Although this maneuver would likely have the greatest effect on the fluoroquinolone f-AUC/MIC ratio, such a strategy is not practical at present. As an example of this concept, a gram-negative pathogen might normally be resistant to a particular β-lactam antibiotic but the addition of a β-lactamase inhibitor effectively reduces the core antibiotic MIC and converts the pathogen from antibiotic resistant to antibiotic susceptible. Although there have been a variety of efflux inhibitors studied that could be paired with fluoroquinolone antibiotics, none of these products have become commercially available to date.

Generally in the ICU when attempting to treat or provide empirical coverage for *Pseudomonas aeruginosa, Acinetobacter baumannii,* and so forth, fluoroquinolones should be used at their maximum dose (intravenous ciprofloxacin 400 mg every 8 hours or levofloxacin 750 mg every 24 hours) assuming no adjustments are required. Depending on circumstances, some clinicians use off-label dosing of fluoroquinolone. For example, in the management of *Mycobacterium tuberculosis*, some clinicians might use 800 mg of moxifloxacin instead of the usual 400 mg dose every 24 hours to maximize the chance of generating a f-AUC/MIC of 53 or more for this pathogen.[29] Such off-label use must be approached cautiously as the probability of adverse events may increase with dose.

ADVERSE EVENTS

Over the years a variety of adverse events have been reported with fluoroquinolones (**Box 1**). Although many of these concerns pertain to the entire fluoroquinolone class of antibiotics, some of these events were clearly associated with specific fluoroquinolones that have more or less been withdrawn from the market.

Although fluoroquinolones may be associated with a variety of drug-induced adverse events in the ICU, those of particular importance include situations with concomitant oral cation therapy or use of tube feeding that would alter oral absorption of the fluoroquinolones, the prolongation of the QTc interval, altered serum glucose blood concentration control, altered mental status, and the possibility of an associated *Clostridium difficile* infection.

Ciprofloxacin, levofloxacin, and moxifloxacin all are classified as category C agents with regard to pregnancy and caution is directed toward breastfeeding during antibiotic therapy with these agents. Initially use of fluoroquinolones in pediatric patients was cautioned but over the years, use of the agents in children has become an accepted practice. Both ciprofloxacin and levofloxacin have FDA-approved pediatric indications and dosage recommendations.

Box 1
Adverse events associated with fluoroquinolone
Central nervous system
Nausea/vomiting
Headaches
Dizziness/confusion
Insomnia
Nightmares
Paranoia
Convulsions/seizures
Peripheral neuropathy
Hypersensitivity reactions
Altered taste disturbance
Tendinitis/acute tendon rupture (FDA black-box warning)
Altered glucose homeostasis
QTc prolongation (warning if patient with uncorrected hypokalemia or receiving Class IA or III antiarrythymics)
Possible drug-drug interactions
Iron, other metal cations, some tube feeding, antacids, multiple vitamins, and sucralfate may alter fluoroquinolone absorption
Phototoxicity
Hepatotoxicity
Interstitial nephritis
Hemolytic uremic syndrome
Crystalluria
Clostridium difficile infection
Refer to product insert for appropriate dosing in renal and/or hepatic failure.

MANAGING MULTIPLE ANTIBIOTIC–RESISTANT BACTERIAL INFECTIONS

Clinical trials have demonstrated the imperative of early and effective therapy for the treatment of infectious diseases.[30–36] Inappropriate or inadequate therapy or delays in administering antibiotic therapy are associated with increased patient morbidity, mortality, length of stay, and cost of care. The difference in confronting a multiple antibiotic–resistant (MAR) infection versus an antibiotic-sensitive strain is likely vested in the limited opportunity to get it right. There are several issues that must be considered with regard to provision of effective empirical antimicrobial therapy for serious infections with fluoroquinolones. Serious infections are associated with a relatively high bacterial burden in the range of 10^7 to 10^9 colony-forming units (CFU) per milliliter or gram of infected fluid or tissue. This high organism burden likely drives the intense inflammatory responses that lead to severe sepsis and septic shock. Notably, this burden is well above the standards used to provide antibiotic susceptibility data (10^5 CFU/mL). Represented in the overall population of bacteria are subpopulations of antibiotic-susceptible and antibiotic-resistant bacteria. These bacteria may be in a stationary growth phase as opposed to an exponential growth phase, especially at the higher inoculum size. Stationary growth is more difficult to inhibit or kill as the bacteria are essentially in hibernation making antibiotics that attack active bacterial metabolic pathways pathogens ineffective. Many bacteria are capable of producing a glycocalyx or biofilm, which may present another barrier to antibiotic penetration. Glycocalyx, besides limiting antibiotic availability, may limit available nutrients, which would further contribute to the stationary growth phase and compromised antibiotic activity. The initial use of a concentration-dependent antibiotic (aminoglycoside, fluoroquinolone, or polymyxin), although effective in the short-term, may also select resistant subpopulations found in the initial bacterial inoculum especially if the dose and method of delivery is not optimized. Failure to control these resistant subsets or heteroresistant populations may provide the opportunity for these pathogens to go into exponential growth and ultimately become the problem pathogen to be confronted later in the infection.

Early therapy with effective antimicrobial therapy can have several beneficial effects. Initiation of therapy with a rapidly cidal dose of a fluoroquinolone should result in attenuation of pathogen-driven inflammatory responses with more rapid resolution of clinical manifestations including shock and organ failure. In addition, a rapid reduction of the bacterial burden has the potential to create a more favorable match between existing bacterial subpopulations and the patient's white blood cells and immune system. Lowering the bacterial burden also essentially eliminates spontaneous mutation given common bacterial mutation rates of gram-negative bacteria.

Dosing the antibiotic to optimize the value of the pharmacodynamic outcome parameter along with the method of administration (extended infusions, continuous infusions, pulse dosing, and so forth depending on the antibiotic being used) may provide the necessary incremental difference to result in clinical cure instead of failure. With concentration-dependent antibiotics including fluoroquinolones, dosing to increase f-AUC/MIC and/or the f-peak serum concentration/MIC ratios should be the goal. For MAR gram-negative infections and fluoroquinolones, this means that in adults with normal renal function, larger doses of ciprofloxacin (400 mg every 8 hours) and levofloxacin (750 mg every 24 hours) are required to maximize the probability of achieving an adequate f-AUC/MIC. Young hypermetabolic patients eliminate renally cleared antibiotics at an unusually rapid pace, which requires more frequent replacement to maintain an effective f-T>MIC.

Reduction or elimination of bacterial pathogens might also be enhanced using an appropriately chosen and administered second antibiotic. The second antibiotic should be from a different chemical class, have a different mechanism of action, and different pharmacodynamic profile than the initial antibiotic. Obviously, both drugs must have the desired spectrum of antibacterial activity. Unfortunately, in the case of fluoroquinolones the level of bacterial susceptibility especially for MAR gram-negative pathogens has fallen over the years limiting the usefulness of this class of agents.

USE OF FLUOROQUINOLONES IN THE ICU

So what happened to fluoroquinolone bacterial susceptibility? Like many new antibiotics at introduction, fluoroquinolone bacterial susceptibility initially approached 100% for many gram-negative pathogens including *Pseudomonas aeruginosa*. Overuse and misuse of the fluoroquinolones inside and outside the ICU combined with under dosing of these compounds at introduction drove bacterial resistance such that now only 50% to 60% of *Pseudomonas aeruginosa* in the ICU are still susceptible to levofloxacin and ciprofloxacin. A variety of models have been used to demonstrate that exposing bacteria to class inferior agents or under exposing bacteria to a class active agent amplifies the population of resistant strains.[15,37] With so few antibiotics in development, we must question whether we can allow potentially new and novel antibiotics of last resort to be used in environments outside the ICU for routine infectious maladies, less we forget what happened with the fluoroquinolones.

The first clinically available fluoroquinolone was norfloxacin, which was limited primarily to urinary tract infections; before levofloxacin, there was ofloxacin, a racemic mixture of enantiomers with only the l-form having biologic activity. Thus, only 50% of ofloxacin was active drug. The first offering of fluoroquinolones was limited to oral agents in a variety of underpowered dosage forms. Initial doses were not optimized from a pharmacodynamic perspective at the time of introduction. However, over time, clinical experience and the evolving science dictated that higher doses of drug were required to maximize the antibiotic effect of therapy. Even if the chosen fluoroquinolone and dose would satisfactorily concentrate at select sites such as the urinary tract, body flora elsewhere were exposed to suboptimal and potentially resistant amplifying exposures of the fluoroquinolone that over time would pose an ever-increasing clinical dilemma, the so-called collateral damage syndrome.

For community-acquired pneumonia (CAP), fluoroquinolones still cover the typical and atypical pathogens well. However, for typical gram-negative ICU pathogens, *Pseudomonas aeruginosa*, *Acinetobacter baumannii*, *Stenotrophomonas maltophilia*, and even *Escherichia coli* and *Proteus mirabilis*, the likely antibacterial coverage is not adequate.

SUMMARY

Appropriate antibiotic management of infections in the ICU requires that the clinician offer adequate antimicrobial coverage for the suspected pathogens. Antibiotic therapy should not be delayed once infection is suspected as the risk of morbidity and mortality increases with a lag in appropriate therapy. Empirical therapy with the fluoroquinolones as a primary or sole agent should be extremely limited. Once the underlying pathogen or pathogens has been identified and antibiotic susceptibility determined, antibiotic therapy can be streamlined or tailored to the specific situation. To maximize the probability of a successful clinical and microbiologic outcome, fluoroquinolones should be dosed to maximize the f-AUC/MIC ratio. A conversion from parenteral to oral therapy is almost always an option with fluoroquinolone therapy if the patient has a functioning gastrointestinal tract, the patient is not receiving concomitant agents known to interfere with oral absorption, and the patient is responding to therapy.

To provide an adequate antimicrobial spectrum or to anticipate likely patterns of antibiotic resistance, 2 or 3 antibiotics are often needed for empirical coverage, particularly in the ICU where resistant pathogens are concentrated. Over the last 20 years there has been erosion of fluoroquinolones in terms of their spectrum of coverage especially for gram-negative pathogens. Even fluoroquinolone coverage for common pathogens such as *Escherichia coli* and *Proteus mirabilis* has been reduced to the point that these agents cannot be reliably depended on by themselves to offer adequate initial empirical coverage. Typical ICU pathogens such as *Pseudomonas aeruginosa*, *Stenotrophomonas maltophilia,* and *Acinetobacter baumannii* are now often resistant not only to fluoroquinolones but often all antibiotics tested.

Although the currently available fluoroquinolones generally have an acceptable adverse event profile, ICU clinicians should always be concerned about possible changes in mental status induced by these drugs; seizures can be one manifestation of acute toxicity. Alterations in glucose metabolism (both hypoglycemia and hyperglycemia), changes in liver function, and the possibility of torsades de pointe are not common, but are possible side effects for this class of agents. Renal elimination varies among the 3 products and the dosage of levofloxacin in particular needs to be adjusted in renal failure. Oral absorption can be altered by cations and antacids. Because of the frequency with which these agents are used not only in the ICU but throughout the health care system, reports linking fluoroquinolones to increased rates of *Clostridium difficile* colitis and increases in MRSA/ORSA infections should be of concern.

Overall, fluoroquinolones have been a useful class of antibiotics in a variety of settings. However, the ongoing usefulness of these agents, particularly in the ICU, will likely continue to wane as a result of increasing bacterial resistance. It is hoped that the lesson learned with our 20 plus years of experience with fluoroquinolones is that as novel antibiotics are introduced, the optimal dose and method of presentation cannot be a work in progress if we are to stave off bacterial resistance and maximize the life cycle of new antibiotics.

REFERENCES

1. Pepin J, Saheb N, Andree-Coulombe M, et al. Emergence of fluoroquinolones as the predominant risk factor for *Clostridium difficile*-associated diarrhea: a cohort study during an epidemic in Quebec. Clin Infect Dis 2005;41(11):2365–71.
2. Graffunder EM, Venezia RA. Risk factors associated with nosocomial methicillin-resistant *Staphylococcus aureus* (MRSA) infection including previous use of antimicrobials. J Antimicrob Chemother 2002;49(6):999–1005.
3. Mihu CN, Rhomberg PR, Jones RN, et al. *Escherichia coli* resistance to quinolones at a comprehensive cancer center. Diagn Microbiol Infect Dis 2010;67:266–9.
4. Gore J, Bryant Z, Stone MD, et al. Mechanochemical analysis of DNA gyrase using rotor bead tracking. Nature 2006;439:100–4.
5. Champoux JJ. DNA topoisomerases: structure, function, and mechanism. Annu Rev Biochem 2001;70:369–413.
6. Wang JC. Cellular roles of DNA topoisomerases: a molecular perspective. Nat Rev Mol Cell Biol 2002;3(6):430–40.
7. Sicor-Pharmaceuticals. Ciprofloxacin medication Information. Irvine (CA); 2006.
8. Schering-Plough. Avelox medication information sheet. Kenilworth: Bayer Healthcare; 2008.
9. Ortho-McNeil-Janssen Pharmaceuticals I. Levaquin highlights of prescribing information. Raritan; 2009.
10. Ortho-McNeil. Levaquin 360 information. 2010.
11. Wener KM, Schechner V, Gold HS, et al. Treatment with fluoroquinolones or with β-lactam-β-lactamase inhibitor combinations is a risk factor for isolation of extended-spectrum-β-lactamase-producing *Klebsiella* species in hospitalized patients. Antimicrob Agents Chemother 2010;54(5):2010–6.
12. Potron A, Poirel L, Bernabeu S, et al. Nosocomial spread of ESBL-positive *Enterobacter cloacae* co-expressing plasmid-mediated quinolone resistance Qnr determinants in one hospital in France. J Antimicrob Chemother 2009;64(3):653–4.

13. Wright DH, Bown GH, Peterson ML, et al. Application of fluoroquinolone pharmacodynamics. J Antimicrob Chemother 2000;46:669–83.
14. Oelschlaeger P, Ai N, DaPrez KI, et al. Evolving carbapenemases: can medicinal chemists advance one step ahead of the coming storm? J Med Chem 2010;53: 3013–27.
15. Peterson ML, Houde LB, Wright DH, et al. Fluoroquinolone resistance in *Bacteroides fragilis* following sparfloxacin exposure. Antimicrob Agents Chemother 1999;43(9):2251–5.
16. Peterson ML, Houde LB, Wright DH, et al. Pharmacodynamics of trovafloxacin and levofloxacin against *B. fragilis* in an in-vitro pharmacodynamic model. Antimicrob Agents Chemother 2001;46:203–10.
17. Chan ED, Laurel V, Strand MJ, et al. Treatment and outcome analysis of 205 patients with multidrug-resistant tuberculosis. Am J Respir Crit Care Med 2004; 169:1103–9.
18. Ziha-Zarifi I, Lanes C, Kohler T, et al. In vivo emergence of multidrug-resistant mutants of *Pseudomonas aeruginosa* overexpressing the active efflux system MexA-MexB-OprM. Antimicrob Agents Chemother 1999;43(2):287–91.
19. Le Thomas I, Couetdic G, Clermont O, et al. In vivo selection of a target/efflux double mutant of *Pseudomonas aeruginosa* by ciprofloxacin therapy. J Antimicrob Chemother 2001;48(4):553–5.
20. Drlica K, Zhao X. DNA gyrase, topoisomerase IV, and the 4-quinolones. Microbiol Mol Biol Rev 1997;61(3):377–92.
21. Schmitz FJ, Hofmann B, Hansen B, et al. Relationship between ciprofloxacin, ofloxacin, levofloxacin, sparfloxacin and moxifloxacin (BAY 12-8039) MICs and mutations in grlA, grlB, gyrA and gyrB in 116 unrelated clinical isolates of *Staphylococcus aureus*. J Antimicrob Chemother 1998;41:481–4.
22. Martinez-Martinez L, Pascual A, Jacoby GA. Quinolone resistance from a transferable plasmid. Lancet 1998;351(9105):797–9.
23. Rotschafer JC, Zabinski RA, Walker KJ, et al. Pharmacotherapy and pharmacodynamics in the management of bacterial infection. J Clin Pharmacol 1992;37: 436–40.
24. Yang JC, Tsuji BT, Forrest A. Optimizing use of quinolones in the critically ill. Semin Respir Crit Care Med 2007;28:586–95.
25. Forrest A, Nix DE, Ballow CH, et al. Pharmacodynamics of intravenous ciprofloxacin in seriously ill patients. Antimicrob Agents Chemother 1993;37(5):1073–81.
26. Preston SL, Drusano GL, Berman AL, et al. Pharmacodynamics of levofloxacin: a new paradigm for early clinical trials. JAMA 1998;279(2):125–9.
27. Drusano GL, Preston S, Fowler C, et al. Relationship between fluoroquinolone area under the curve: minimum inhibitory concentration ratio and the probability of eradication of the infecting pathogen, in patients with nosocomial pneumonia. J Infect Dis 2004;189:1590–7.
28. Ambrose PG, Grasela DM, Grasela TH, et al. Pharmacodynamics of fluoroquinolones against *Streptococcus pneumoniae* in patients with community-acquired respiratory tract infections. Antimicrob Agents Chemother 2001;45(10):2793–7.
29. Gumbo T, Louie A, Deziel M, et al. Selection of a moxifloxacin dose that suppresses drug resistance in *M. tuberculosis* by use of an in-vitro pharmacodynamic model and mathematical modeling. J Infect Dis 2004;190:1642–51.
30. Alvarez-Lerma F. Modification of empiric antibiotic treatment in patients with pneumonia acquired in the intensive care unit. ICU-acquired Pneumonia Study Group. Intensive Care Med 1996;22(5):387–94.

31. Dupont H, Mentec H, Sollet JP, et al. Impact of appropriateness of initial antibiotic therapy on the outcome of ventilator-associated pneumonia. Intensive Care Med 2001;27(2):355–62.
32. Kollef M, Sherman G, Ward S, et al. Inadequate antimicrobial treatment of infections: a risk factor for hospital mortality among critically ill patients. Chest 1999; 115(2):462–74.
33. Luna C, Vujacich P, Niederman MS, et al. Impact of BAL data on the therapy and outcome of ventilator-associated pneumonia. Chest 1997;111(3):676–85.
34. Rello J, Gallego M, Mariscal D, et al. The value of routine microbial investigation in ventilator-associated pneumonia. Am J Respir Crit Care Med 1997;156(1): 196–200.
35. Ruiz M, Torres A, Ewig S, et al. Noninvasive versus invasive microbial investigation in ventilator-associated pneumonia. evaluation of outcome. Am J Respir Crit Care Med 2000;162(1):119–25.
36. Kollef M, Morrow LE, Niederman MS, et al. Clinical characteristics and treatment patterns among patients with ventilator-associated pneumonia. Chest 2006; 129(5):1210–8.
37. Madaras-Kelly KJ, Ostergaard BE, Hovde LB, et al. Twenty-four-hour area under the concentration-time curve/MIC ratio as a generic predictor of fluoroquinolone antimicrobial effect by using three strains of *Pseudomonas aeruginosa* and an in vitro pharmacodynamic model. Antimicrob Agents Chemother 1996;40(3): 627–32.

Optimizing Aminoglycoside Use

William A. Craig, MD

KEYWORDS
- Aminoglycosides • Gram-negative infections
- Combination chemotherapy
- Minimum inhibitory concentration

The aminoglycoside antibiotics have been used for treating gram-negative bacillary infections in critically ill patients for about 50 years. The main aminoglycosides still in use include gentamicin, tobramycin, amikacin, and netilmicin. However, the appearance of new third- and fourth-generation cephalosporins, carbapenems, and fluoroquinolones have decreased their usage as monotherapy for most gram-negative infections. In a large observational study of patients with gram-negative bacillary bacteremia, aminoglycosides were also shown to be less effective than β-lactams in patients with infection sites other than the urinary tract.[1] Thus, for many years, aminoglycosides were used in combination with other antibiotics to enhance bacterial killing and improve overall efficacy. However, most studies have not demonstrated improved outcomes in patients treated with antibiotic combinations when compared with those receiving monotherapy.[2,3] Only recently has early combination therapy been associated with reduced mortality in septic shock.[4] This article reviews the pharmacokinetics, pharmacodynamics, and toxicodynamics of aminoglycosides, and describes dosing strategies and other effects that could improve outcomes in critically ill patients with serious infections.

PHARMACODYNAMICS
Area Under the Curve or Peak Concentrations

As an antimicrobial class the aminoglycosides demonstrate concentration-dependent killing and produce prolonged postantibiotic effects, illustrated in **Fig. 1** (left panel) in the thighs of neutropenic mice following subcutaneous injection of increased doses of tobramycin.[5] As the dose was increased from 4 to 20 mg/kg, the rate of killing over the first few hours also increased and became steeper. When tobramycin levels fell below the minimum inhibitory concentration (MIC), regrowth was still suppressed for 3 to 7 hours. The duration of this postexposure growth suppression or postantibiotic effect also increased with higher doses. Hyperoxia also appears to prolong the tobramycin-induced postantibiotic effect with *Pseudomonas aeruginosa*, which may

Department of Medicine, University of Wisconsin School of Medicine and Public Health, 1685 Highland Avenue, Madison, WI 53705, USA
E-mail address: wac@medicine.wisc.edu

Crit Care Clin 27 (2011) 107–121
doi:10.1016/j.ccc.2010.11.006
0749-0704/11/$ – see front matter © 2011 Published by Elsevier Inc.

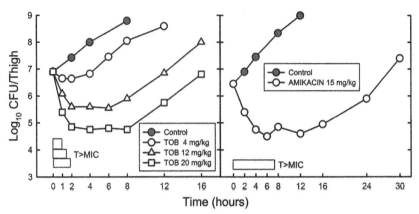

Fig. 1. The time course of killing and regrowth of *Pseudomonas aeruginosa* in thighs of neutropenic mice following 3 doses of tobramycin (TOB) in normal mice (*left panel*) and amikacin in mice with renal impairment (*right panel*). T>MIC, time above minimum inhibitory concentration.

be clinically important when patients with *P aeruginosa* infections are treated with high inspired oxygen tensions.[6] The right panel of **Fig. 1** illustrates the bactericidal activity and postantibiotic effect with a large dose of amikacin against *P aeruginosa* in the thighs of neutropenic mice that had renal impairment to delay elimination and simulate serum concentration seen in humans.[7] The duration of the postantibiotic effect was 10.2 hours for *P aeruginosa* and even longer (more than 12 hours) with a similar study using a strain of *Klebsiella pneumoniae*.

One would expect that administration of less frequent high doses would show more rapid initial killing than more frequent dosing of low doses, even when the same total amount of drug is given. Using an in vitro pharmacokinetic model, once-daily dosing of netilmicin was shown to be superior to 8-hourly dosing in initial killing of strains of Enterobacteriaceae and *Staphylococcus aureus*.[8] However, at 24 hours the bactericidal efficacy of both dosing regimens was very similar. With *P aeruginosa*, once-daily dosing also resulted in superior initial killing, but this was followed by the regrowth of resistant mutants.[9] Additional studies showed that this emergence of resistance could be prevented if the peak to MIC ratio was greater than 8.

Dose-fractionation studies reduce the independence among the various pharmacokinetic parameters and can demonstrate which pharmacokinetic parameter is most important in determining overall efficacy. In the neutropenic mouse-thigh infection the area under the curve (AUC) was the major pharmacokinetic parameter correlating with efficacy of gentamicin against *Escherichia coli* and tobramycin against *P aeruginosa* when dosing regimens varied from 1 to 6 hours.[10] At 8- to 24-hour dosing intervals, time above MIC was the major parameter correlating with efficacy. This difference in major pharmacokinetic parameters based on the frequency of drug administration is a result of the rapid elimination of aminoglycosides in small rodents. Drug half-lives in mice are only 15 to 20 minutes. Later studies with amikacin and isepamicin in mice with renal impairment that simulated human elimination of these drugs showed that AUC was also the major parameter for 6- to 24-hour dosing regimens with various strains of Enterobacteriaceae.[7,11] Drug half-lives in renal impaired mice were 90 to 120 minutes. **Fig. 2** shows one of the dose fractionation studies with amikacin against a strain of *K pneumoniae*. The 24-hour AUC/MIC ratio had the highest correlation with efficacy followed by the peak/MIC ratio. A 24-hour AUC/MIC of around 50 was associated with

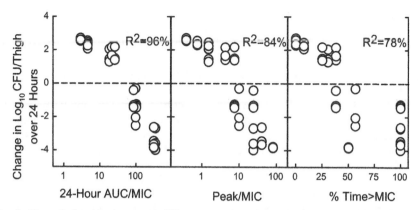

Fig. 2. The relationship between different PK?PD indices and change in the number of bacteria in the thighs of neutropenic mice. The R^2 value reflects the coefficient of determination. CFU, colony-forming units.

stasis and a value around 100 resulted in 1 to 2 logs$_{10}$ of killing. However, for *P aeruginosa* the peak/MIC ratio had the highest correlation with efficacy, resulting from "adaptive resistance" observed in strains of *P aeruginosa*, which is dependent on the Mex XY-OprM efflux pump.[11] With overexpression of this pump after initial bacterial killing, the bacteria become more resistant to killing by further doses of amikacin and other aminoglycosides. This effect has also been observed in vivo in rabbits during treatment with amikacin for *P aeruginosa* endocarditis.[12]

A combination of 4 clinical trials comparing different aminoglycosides in patients with gram-negative bacillary infections showed that the peak/MIC ratio in serum was an important determinant of clinical efficacy.[13] As shown in **Fig. 3**, an increasing response was observed between the maximal peak level/MIC and clinical response. For a peak aminoglycoside level/MIC ratio of 0 to 2, clinical efficacy was just 55%, whereas with a peak level/MIC ratio of 8 to 10, clinical efficacy rose to 90%. The AUC was not specifically measured in these studies, but it would also be expected to correlate with clinical response because all 4 aminoglycosides were administered by identical 8-hour dosing regimens. In another study in patients with severe gram-negative infections treated with tobramycin monotherapy, the 24-hour AUC/MIC value was predictive of outcome.[14] If the ratio was less than 110, the efficacy

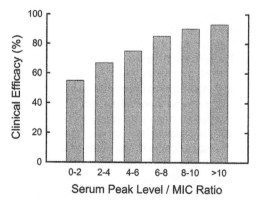

Fig. 3. The relationship between efficacy of aminoglycoside therapy in patients with gram-negative bacillary infections and the peak/MIC ratio.

was only 47%. However, when values were greater than 110 the efficacy was 80%. Two recent studies have correlated peak level/MIC and AUC/MIC to improvement in forced expiratory volume over 1 second (FEV_1) in cystic fibrosis patients with P aeruginosa infections. In one study the peak/MIC ratio produced the more significant correlation, whereas in the other the 24-hour AUC/MIC was the only index correlating with efficacy.[15,16]

Kashuba and colleagues[17] examined the role of both peak/MIC and 24-hour AUC/MIC ratios in determining rapidity of fever and leukocytosis resolution in 78 patients with pneumonia produced by various gram-negative bacilli. Both parameters were significant predictors of resolution but the peak/MIC ratio was slightly better. A peak/MIC ratio of 10 or higher was associated with a 90% resolution of fever and the leukocyte count in 7 days. The 24-hour AUC/MIC ratio to produce a 90% resolution in temperature and leukocyte count in 7 days was 150 and 175, respectively. Based on the serum levels Kashuba and colleagues obtained in these patients, these goals were reached only with organisms that had a MIC of 0.3 μg/mL or lower. However, organisms in the United States are considered susceptible up to an MIC of 4 μg/mL. With a dose of 7 mg/kg one can achieve a peak/MIC ratio of 10 or higher 90% of the time for organisms with MICs of 1 μg/mL or less. To achieve this for organisms with MICs of 2 and 4 μg/mL would require loading doses slightly more than 10 and 20 mg/kg, respectively. Synergistic activity with a β-lactam antibiotic might also allow coverage of organisms with MICs of 2 and 4 μg/mL at aminoglycoside doses of 7 mg/kg.

In summary, these studies suggest than total bacterial killing by the aminoglycosides with strains of Enterobacteriaceae correlates best with the 24-hour AUC/MIC. Peak/MIC ratios may be slightly better than the 24-hour AUC/MIC values for killing of P aeruginosa because of the phenomenon of "adaptive resistance" related to over-expression of the Mex XY-OprM efflux pump. Still the initial rate of killing, even for Enterobacteriaceae and staphylococci, is dependent on the magnitude of the dose and is enhanced when large doses are administered at widely-spaced intervals.

Dosing Regimens

Studies evaluating the efficacy of once-daily dosing of aminoglycosides in animal models have produced conflicting results. Equal efficacy of once-daily and multiple-daily dosing has been primarily observed in medium-sized, nonneutropenic animals that are usually infected with P aeruginosa.[18,19] On the other hand, studies in small neutropenic rodents infected with various strains of Enterobacteriaceae have usually shown less efficacy with once-daily dosing than with multiple-daily dosing.[20,21] This difference is due primarily to the rapid renal elimination of the aminoglycosides in small rodents compared with larger animals and humans. Furthermore, P aeruginosa is an organism that grows slower in vivo than most strains of Enterobacteriaceae, and full recovery from the postantibiotic effects takes longer with this organism. Studies of amikacin and isepamicin in neutropenic mice with normal renal function demonstrated less efficacy with once-daily dosing than with 6- and 12-hour dosing of the same total amount of drug.[7,22] However, in mice with uranyl nitrate–induced renal impairment that produced drug half-lives similar to humans, once-daily dosing was equally efficacious with 6- and 12-hour dosing of the same total amount of drug.

Aminoglycosides have also been studied in animal models in combination with various β-lactams. The combinations of tobramycin/ticarcillin and netilmicin/ceftazidime have been studied in the mouse thigh model using various dosing regimens.[23] The largest synergistic activity of the 2 combinations was observed when the aminoglycoside was administered at 12- or 24-hour dosing frequencies.

There have been at least 45 mostly prospective clinical trials comparing once-daily aminoglycoside administration with conventional 8-hourly or 12-hourly administration. These trials include more than 6500 patients receiving gentamicin, tobramycin, amikacin, and netilmicin for 7 to 14 days of therapy, and were performed primarily in nonneutropenic adults.[24–28] The studies have examined comparative efficacy and safety in a wide range of infections such as gram-negative infections, intra-abdominal infections, pneumonia, febrile neutropenia, pelvic inflammatory disease, and urinary tract infections. There are 9 formal meta-analyses of different combinations of these clinical trials.[24–32] Five of the meta-analyses have shown a small but statistically improved clinical outcome with once-daily dosing. Three meta-analyses have also shown a significantly lower incidence of nephrotoxicity with once-daily dosing. The meta-analyses have also shown equivalent ototoxicity or a trend to lower ototoxicity with once-daily dosing. Several clinical trials identified the day when toxicity developed, which demonstrated that nephrotoxicity with once-daily dosing of gentamicin develops later than with traditional 8-hourly dosing. However, with prolonged dosing out to 10 to 14 days, the incidence of nephrotoxicity was much the same with both dosing regimens.

In a model designed to correlate the serum AUC of amikacin with the probability of nephrotoxicity, Rougier and colleagues[33] showed that nephrotoxicity is delayed more by once-daily dosing than with twice-daily dosing of the same total amount of drug. The difference in nephrotoxicity between once- and twice-daily dosing of amikacin was greatest at a cumulative AUC of 2500 mg-h/L, which corresponds to 1000 mg/d for 6 days. For cumulative AUCs of amikacin above 2500 mg-h/L, the difference between the 2 regimens slowly decreases to zero. A randomized, double-blind trial of amikacin, gentamicin, and tobramycin administered once- or twice-daily also used shorter courses of therapy and demonstrated a significantly lower incidence of nephrotoxicity with once-daily dosing.[34]

Another study compared the onset of nephrotoxicity with once- and twice-daily dosing of primarily gentamicin and tobramycin. The modeling showed that nephrotoxicity started to be observed with twice-daily dosing when the daily AUC was more than 100 mg-h/L. Nephrotoxicity was not observed with once-daily dosing but it was predicted to occur if the AUC exceeded 700 mg-h/L. This study also confirmed the role of concomitant vancomycin, but not amphotericin B, in decreasing the time to onset of nephrotoxicity for both once- and twice-daily dosing regimens.

In conclusion, once-daily dosing regimens have similar efficacy or are slightly more efficacious than multiple-daily dosing regimens. Once-daily dosing can also delay the onset of nephrotoxicity compared with multiple-daily dosing if shorter courses of therapy are used. Current recommendations for once-daily dosing of all aminoglycosides are for only up to 5 to 6 days.[33,35,36] Concomitant vancomycin can also shorten the time to nephrotoxicity, but the effect is still less with once-daily administration.

A COMPARISON OF DIFFERENT AMINOGLYCOSIDES
Pharmacokinetics

The pharmacokinetics of the various aminoglycosides is very similar. Less than 1% of aminoglycosides are absorbed from the gastrointestinal (GI) tract, and they must be administered either intravascularly or intramuscularly. Serum concentrations of gentamicin, tobramycin, and netilmicin after a dose of 7 mg/kg infused over 30 minutes range from 15 to 20 µg/mL.[37,38] This corresponds to an AUC of 70 to 100 mg-h/L. A similar 30-minute infusion of amikacin at 15 mg/kg produces peak concentrations from 41 to 49 µg/mL and an AUC from 110 to 145 mg-h/L.[39,40] Binding of the aminoglycosides to serum proteins is very low and is usually less than 10%.[41] The penetration of the aminoglycosides into epithelial lining fluid ranges from 32% to 54% of serum concentrations.[42,43] The drugs distribute primarily in extracellular fluid and do not readily penetrate into cells. The volume of distribution is often higher, and therefore peak serum levels are lower, in patients with sepsis, severe burns, fever, congestive heart failure, and peritonitis.[44] The drugs are rapidly eliminated unchanged through the kidney with half-lives of 1.8 to 2.6 hours in individuals with normal renal function; elimination is very slow, with a mean half-life of 30 to 56 hours in patients with creatinine clearance less than 10 mL/min.[45]

Peak concentrations are higher and the AUCs are larger in patients with renal impairment. The suggested initial dose for the different aminoglycosides and the dosing frequency for patients with different creatinine clearances are listed in **Table 1**.[15] Dosing every 48 hours occurs when the creatinine clearance is 30 mL/min or less. About 40% to 50% of the aminoglycosides are cleared by a 6-hour hemodialysis. Many of the new techniques such as continuous venovenous hemofiltration (CVVH), continuous venovenous hemodiafiltration (CVVHDF), and continuous renal replacement therapy are extensively used in critical care units and they also remove aminoglycosides.[46] Dosing of aminoglycosides in morbidly obese patients is based on excess body weight (the difference between total body weight and ideal body weight) multiplied by 0.45 plus the ideal body weight.[47] Monitoring of aminoglycoside concentrations is very important in optimizing their use. A peak concentration obtained within the first 48 hours is important for correlating peak/MIC relationships with response. Obtaining a second value 6 to 10 hours later can be used with the peak concentration to estimate the AUC. With single-dose therapy, this can also be related to the MIC to be correlated with prior AUC/MIC related responses.

Nephrotoxicity

The aminoglycosides do accumulate in the kidney, and can account for 40% of the total drug in the body.[48] About 85% of the drug in the kidney is located in the renal cortex. The drug enters the kidney from the lumen of the renal tubules by binding to the basement membrane. The aminoglycosides actually bind to megalin, a large glycoprotein on the

Table 1
Recommended dosing schedules for adult patients with impaired renal function

Estimated Creatinine Clearance (mL/min)	Dose (mg/kg) Gentamicin, Tobramycin, Netilmicin	Amikacin	Dosing Interval (h)
100	7	20	24
90	7	20	24
80	7	20	24
70	5	15	24
60	5	15	24
50	4	12	24
40	4	12	24
30	5	15	48
20	4	12	48
10	3	10	48
<10	2.5	7.5	48

brush border of renal tubular cells, which is required for internalization of the drug by pinocytosis.[49] Animals made deficient in megalin do not accumulate aminoglycosides in the kidney cells and do not develop nephrotoxicity.[50] After pinocytosis the aminoglycoside endosomes fuse with lysosomes and continue to accumulate drug in the cell. Later permeabilization of the lysosomes occurs, and some aminoglycoside can reach the cytosol. When it reaches a critical concentration in the cytosol, the drug activates apoptosis, which causes death to the cell.[51,52] Glomerular dysfunction appears to arise subsequent to proximal tubular damage, and is caused by activation of the renin-angiotensin system and resulting vasoconstriction.[53]

There are differences among the aminoglycosides in terms of renal accumulation and activation of the apoptosis pathway. Gentamicin and netilmicin have higher renal accumulation than tobramycin and amikacin.[54] Activation of apoptosis is less with netilmicin and amikacin than with tobramycin and gentamicin[55] Still, a survey of aminoglycoside nephrotoxicity in approximately 10,000 patients described in clinical trials over a 7-year period published between 1975 and 1982 found relatively similar average frequencies: 14.0% for gentamicin, 12.9% for tobramycin, 9.4% for amikacin, and 8.7% for netilmicin.[56] Comparative nephrotoxicity appears to be relatively unimportant for choosing which aminoglycoside to use in a clinical situation.

In a large study of almost 1500 patients, risk factors for aminoglycoside nephrotoxicity included concomitant vancomycin, longer duration of therapy, pneumonia, rapidly fatal prognosis, leukemia, preexisting renal or liver disease, shock, larger volume of distribution, male sex, older age, and location in intensive care.[57] Many of these risk factors are present in patients with severe gram-negative bacillary infections, but their role in producing nephrotoxicity can be largely reduced by once-daily administration for only several days.

Ototoxicity

Gentamicin and other aminoglycosides penetrate into the endolymph and vestibular and cochlear tissue[58]; it enters the endolymph slowly and leaves the endolymph even slower. Prolonged therapy for 10 days or more, preexisting renal impairment, and prior treatment with aminoglycosides are risk factors for ototoxicity.[59] Damage is manifest as auditory (cochlear) and vestibular toxicity, but these do not always occur together. The mechanism of toxicity is damage to the sensory hair cells in the cochlea and the labyrinth.[60] The relationship between aminoglycoside pharmacokinetic parameters and auditory toxicity is unclear. Animal models suggest that ototoxicity is related to the AUC of concentrations in cochlear endolymph, which in turn are proportional to the AUC in serum.[61] This result suggests that administration of the same total daily dose will have the same incidence of ototoxicity, which accounts for the lack of significant differences in ototoxicity between once-daily and multiple-daily dosing of different aminoglycosides.[27,29–31]

One would expect an exceedingly low incidence ototoxicity with therapy restricted to 5 or 6 days. However, a rare form of auditory toxicity, often occurring after a few doses, has been described, associated with about 5 different mutations in the mitochondrial 12S ribosomal RNA gene.[62,63] A family history of this type of toxicity should be a contraindication to the use of aminoglycosides. If aminoglycosides had to be used for a longer period of time, the use of aspirin instead of placebo reduced the incidence of ototoxicity from 13% to 3% in about 100 patients in each group.[64,65]

Neuromuscular Paralysis

Neuromuscular blockade is rarely a reported adverse effect of aminoglycoside use, being more likely to occur when given intravenously in patients with renal impairment and/or administered concomitantly with neuromuscular blocking drugs or anesthetic agents.[66,67] Once-daily dosing of gentamicin at 6 mg/kg did not have any adverse effect on maximal inspiratory pressure in patients on mechanical ventilation.[67] Use of aminoglycosides was not a significant risk factor for abnormal muscle membrane excitability in patients under intensive care.[68] Amikacin is probably the safest drug, as the acute lethal dose in rats and mice is 10 times higher for amikacin than for gentamicin and tobramycin.

Antimicrobial Activity

While the aminoglycosides are active primarily against gram-negative bacilli and staphylococci, there are some important differences in potency among the agents. Tobramycin is the most active agent against *P aeruginosa* with MICs that are 2- to 4-fold more potent than for gentamicin.[69,70] This potency increases the peak/MIC and 24-hour AUC/MIC ratios and makes tobramycin the best agent for use in *Pseudomonas* infections. *Acinetobacter* species are also usually more susceptible to tobramycin than to gentamicin, but resistant strains do occur. Gentamicin is the most potent agent against most of the Enterobacteriaceae and is the preferred drug for therapy with these organisms; this is especially true for *Serratia* species.[69,70] Although MICs for amikacin against Enterobacteriaceae are 2- to 4-fold higher than for gentamicin, an important feature of amikacin is that it is active against many strains of Enterobacteriaceae (usually >80%) and also a considerable proportion of *P aeruginosa* (25%–85%), which have acquired gentamicin and tobramycin resistance.[71–73] For strains of *S aureus*, gentamicin and netilmicin have the best potency.

DIFFERENT CLINICAL INFECTIONS

As stated earlier, there are several systematic reviews that have demonstrated that monotherapy with the aminoglycosides in severe gram-negative infections is less effective than therapy with β-lactams and fluoroquinolones.[1,2] This fact is not surprising, as the peak/MIC and 24-hour AUC/MIC ratios with standard doses are effective for organisms with MICs of 0.5 μg/mL or less for gentamicin, tobramycin, and netilmicin, and MICs of 1 to 2 μg/mL and less for amikacin. However, the susceptibility breakpoints for all these drugs is about 8-fold higher. Thus, there are many organisms with higher but still susceptible MICs that are not adequately treated with these drugs. Even once-daily doses of 7 mg/kg for gentamicin, tobramycin, and netilmicin cover organisms with MICs of 1 μg/mL, whereas once-daily doses of 20 mg/kg for amikacin will treat organisms with MICs of 2 to 4 μg/mL. For these reasons, aminoglycosides should be used in combination primarily with β-lactams but also with fluoroquinolones. The recent study showing a lower incidence of early mortality with combination therapy versus monotherapy in patients with gram-negative bacillary infections with shock strongly supports their combined use in these patients.[4]

Bacteremia

There are several recent studies showing an improved outcome in patients with shock and gram-negative bacillary bacteremia treated with a combination of aminoglycoside and β-lactam.[74,75] One of the studies also shows an improved outcome in gram-negative bacillary bacteremia with combination therapy in neutropenic patients.[74] The addition of an aminoglycoside also resulted in greater initial appropriate therapy than with monotherapy.[75] This study also observed that aminoglycosides provided broader coverage of the infecting pathogen than fluoroquinolones.

Endotoxin release from large inocula of gram-negative bacteria is much lower with aminoglycosides than with β-lactam antibiotics.[76] Other studies with multiple strains of gram-negative bacilli have shown that the addition of tobramycin to cefuroxime results in a lower release of endotoxin than observed with the aminoglycoside alone.[77,78] The higher the initial tobramycin concentration, the lower the release of endotoxin with the combination. In a fibrin clot model of sepsis with *K pneumoniae*, amikacin resulted in a much smaller release of endotoxin than observed with ceftazidime and ofloxacin.[79] Reduction of endotoxin release by aminoglycosides could contribute to the decreased early mortality with combination therapy in patients with shock.

Aminoglycosides are often administered with β-lactams to treat staphylococcal bacteremia and endocarditis. A recent review was very critical of such use of aminoglycosides because of the development of nephrotoxicity without any clinical benefit.[80] Another study evaluating the use of aminoglycosides in staphylococcal endocarditis showed a significant earlier defervescence (2 days vs 4 days).[81]

Pneumonia

Hospital-acquired pneumonia is commonly caused by gram-negative bacilli such as *P aeruginosa*, *E coli*, and *Klebsiella* or *Serratia* species. Although satisfactory results have been obtained with aminoglycosides alone, combination therapy with a β-lactam gives superior results.[82] Combination therapy has not improved outcome over monotherapy with β-lactams for gram-negative bacillary pneumonia due to the Enterobacteriaceae. Nevertheless, combination therapy for a few days could be beneficial in patients with shock or hypotension. The role of combination therapy for pneumonia due to *P aeruginosa* is less clear. Some investigators have observed better results with combination therapy than with monotherapy.[83]

Aerosolized aminoglycosides have also been used in mechanically ventilated patients with pneumonia. In a retrospective case-matched study, inhaled aminoglycoside was compared mostly with combination therapy with an aminoglycoside and β-lactam antibiotic.[84] Most of the infections were caused by *P aeruginosa*. Patients treated with inhaled aminoglycosides were more likely to have complete resolution of clinical symptoms than those in the intravenous antibiotics group (81% vs 31%) and microbiologic cure group (77% vs 5%). Furthermore, none of the patients receiving inhaled aminoglycosides developed renal dysfunction, whereas the incidence in the intravenous antibiotics group was 31%. Other studies have also shown a good response in patients in intensive care with ventilator-associated pneumonia (VAP) caused by *P aeruginosa* and *Acinetobacter baumannii*.[85] Inhaled aminoglycosides seem to be a way to enhance antimicrobial activity without producing renal dysfunction. However, more controlled trials of larger numbers of patients are needed.

Intra-Abdominal Infections

There are 2 meta-analyses in patients with intra-abdominal infections that found lower clinical efficacy response for regimens with an aminoglycoside than those with a β-lactam as the anti–gram-negative bacillary drug.[86,87] Furthermore, treatment with an aminoglycoside (plus clindamycin) was associated with a higher risk of developing renal dysfunction than seen with monotherapy with β-lactams. Various clinicians have recommended that aminoglycosides not be considered as first-line therapy for intra-abdominal infection. However, in patients with sepsis and shock the addition of an aminoglycoside for a few days would still appear to be indicated.

Pyelonephritis and Complicated Urinary Tract Infections

A recent systematic review of aminoglycoside monotherapy versus other antibiotics did find aminoglycoside monotherapy to produce equal efficacy with β-lactam drugs and fluoroquinolones in urinary tract infection and pyelonephritis.[88] Nevertheless, there was a trend to more nephrotoxicity in the patients receiving the aminoglycosides. There are insufficient data to know whether 5 to 7 days of an aminoglycoside would provide equal efficacy to longer durations for pyelonephritis and complicated urinary tract infections. Aminoglycoside concentrations above the MIC of most gram-negative bacilli are still found in the urine for at least 4 days after the last dose.

SUMMARY

Despite the increasing knowledge on the pharmacodynamics of aminoglycosides and methods to use them for short periods of time, there are still publications downplaying these drugs because of their lower efficacy and nephrotoxicity.[89] The studies that have demonstrated an early survival benefit in patients with septic shock have revitalized their use.[4,75,76] Aminoglycosides should be used along with β-lactams or fluoroquinolones primarily in patients with shock or hypotension, as large single-daily doses, and very rarely for more than 5 to 6 days. The use of inhaled aminoglycosides also appears to be a rational use of these drugs in VAP patients with hard-to-treat and resistant organisms without the development of nephrotoxicity and ototoxicity. Further study will identify the overall efficacy and safety of this approach.

REFERENCES

1. Leibovici L, Paul M, Poznanski O, et al. Monotherapy versus β-lactam-aminogly-coside combination treatment for gram-negative bacteremia: a prospective, observational study. Antimicrob Agents Chemother 1997;41:1127–33.
2. Paul M, Soares-Weiser K, Leibovici L. β-lactam monotherapy versus ß-lactam-aminoglycoside combination therapy for fever with neutropenia: systematic review and meta-analysis. BMJ 2003;326:1111–20.
3. Paul M, Benuri Silbigern I, Soares-Weisern K, et al. β-lactam monotherapy versus β-lactam-aminoglycoside combination therapy for treating sepsis. BMJ 2004;328: 668–82.
4. Kumar A, Zarychanski R, Light B, et al. Early combination antibiotic therapy yields improved survival compared with monotherapy in septic shock: a propensity-matched analysis. Crit Care Med 2010;38:1773–85.
5. Craig WA, Gudmundsson S. Postantibiotic effect. In: Lorian V, editor. Antibiotics in laboratory medicine. 4th edition. Baltimore (MD): Williams and Wilkins; 1996. p. 296–329, chapter 8.
6. Park MK, Muhvich KH, Myers RAM, et al. Hyperoxia prolongs the aminoglyco-side-induced postantibiotic effect in Pseudomonas aeruginosa. Antimicrob Agents Chemother 1991;35:691–5.
7. Craig WA, Redington J, Ebert SC. Pharmacodynamics of amikacin in vitro and in mouse thigh and lung infections. J Antimicrob Chemother 1991;27(Suppl C): 29–40.
8. Blaser J, Stone BB, Zinner SH. Efficacy of intermittent versus continuous administration of netilmicin in a two-compartment in vitro model. Antimicrob Agents Chemother 1985;27:343–9.
9. Blaser J, Stone BB, Groner MC, et al. Comparative study with enoxacin and ne-tilmicin in a pharmacodynamic model to determine importance of ratio of

antibiotic peak concentration to MIC for bactericidal activity and emergence of resistance. Antimicrob Agents Chemother 1987;31:1054–60.

10. Vogelman B, Gudmundsson S, Leggett J, et al. Correlation of antimicrobial pharmacokinetic parameters with therapeutic efficacy in an animal model. J Infect Dis 1988;158:831–47.

11. Hocquet D, Vogne C, Garch El, et al. MexXY-OprM efflux pump is necessary for a adaptive resistance of *Pseudomonas aeruginosa* to aminoglycosides. Antimicrob Agents Chemother 2003;47:1371–5.

12. Xiong YQ, Caillon J, Kergueris MF, et al. Adaptive resistance of *Pseudomonas aeruginosa* induced by aminoglycosides and killing kinetics in a rabbit endocarditis model. Antimicrob Agents Chemother 1997;41:823–6.

13. Moore RD, Lietman PS, Smith CR. Clinical response to aminoglycoside therapy: importance of the ratio of peak concentration to minimal inhibitory concentration. J Infect Dis 1998;155:93–9.

14. Smith PF, Ballow CH, Booker BM, et al. Pharmacokinetics and pharmacodynamics of aztreonam and tobramycin in hospitalized patients. Clin Ther 2001;23:1231–44.

15. Mouton JW, Jacobs N, Tiddens H, et al. Pharmacodynamics of tobramycin in patients with cystic fibrosis. Diagn Microbiol Infect Dis 2005;52:123–7.

16. Burkhardt O, Lehmann C, Madabush R, et al. Once-daily tobramycin in cystic fibrosis: better for clinical outcomes than thrice-daily tobramycin but more resistance development. J Antimicrob Chemother 2006;58:822–9.

17. Kashuba AD, Nafziger AN, Drusano GL, et al. Optimizing aminoglycoside therapy for nosocomial pneumonia caused by Gram-negative bacteria. Antimicrob Agents Chemother 1999;43:623–9.

18. Powell SH, Thompson WL, Luthe MA, et al. Once-daily vs. continuous aminoglycoside dosing: efficacy and toxicity in animal and clinical studies of gentamicin, netilmicin and tobramycin. J Infect Dis 1983;147:918–32.

19. Kapusnik JE, Sande MA. Novel approaches for the use of aminoglycosides: the value of experimental models. J Antimicrob Chemother 1986;17(Suppl A):7–12.

20. Pechere M, Letarte R, Pechere JC. Efficacy of different dosing schedules of tobramycin for treating murine *Klebsiella pneumoniae* bronchopneumonia. J Antimicrob Chemother 1987;19:487–91.

21. Querioz MLS, Bathirunathan N, Mawer GE. Influence of dosage interval on the therapeutic response to gentamicin in mice infected with *Klebsiella pneumoniae*. Chemotherapy 1987;33:68–76.

22. Craig WA. Once-daily versus multiple-daily dosing of aminoglycosides. J Chemother 1995;7(Suppl 2):47–52.

23. Mouton JW, van Ogtrop ML, Andes D, et al. Use of pharmacodynamic indices to predict efficacy of combination therapy in vivo. Antimicrob Agents Chemother 1999;43:2473–8.

24. Ferriols-Lisart R, Alos-Alminana M. Effectiveness and safety of once-daily aminoglycosides: a meta-analysis. Am J Health Syst Pharm 1996;53:1141–50.

25. Freeman CD, Strayer AH. Mega-analysis of meta-analysis: and examination of meta-analysis with an emphasis on once-daily aminoglycoside comparative trials. Pharmacotherapy 1996;16:1093–102.

26. Kale-Pradhan PB, Habowski SR, Chase HC, et al. Once-daily aminoglycosides: a meta-analysis of nonneutropenic and neutropenic adults. J Pharm Technol 1998;14:22–9.

27. Galloe AM, Graudal N, Christensen HR, et al. Aminoglycosides: single or multiple daily dosing? A meta-analysis on efficacy and safety. Eur J Clin Pharmacol 1995; 48:39–43.

28. Hatala R, Dinh T, Cook DJ. Once-daily aminoglycoside dosing in immunocompetent adults: a meta-analysis. Ann Intern Med 1996;124:717–23.

29. Munckhof WJ, Grayson ML, Turnidge JD. A meta-analysis of studies on the safety and efficacy of aminoglycosides given either once daily or as divided doses. J Antimicrob Chemother 1996;37:645–63.

30. Barza M, Ioannidis JPA, Cappelleri JC, et al. Single or multiple daily doses of aminoglycosides: a meta-analysis. BMJ 1996;312:338–45.

31. Ali MZ, Goetz MB. A meta-analysis of the relative efficacy and toxicity of single daily dosing versus multiple daily dosing of aminoglycosides. Clin Infect Dis 1997;24:796–809.

32. Bailey TC, Little JR, Littenberg B, et al. A meta-analysis of extended-interval dosing versus multiple daily dosing of aminoglycosides. Clin Infect Dis 1997; 24.786–95.

33. Rougier F, Ducher M, Maurin M, et al. Aminoglycoside dosages and nephrotoxicity: quantitative relationships. Clin Pharm 2003;42:493–500.

34. Rybak MJ, Abate BJ, Kang SL, et al. Prospective evaluation of the effect of an aminoglycoside dosing regimen on rates of observed nephrotoxicity and ototoxicity. Antimicrob Agents Chemother 1999;43:1549–55.

35. Hansen M, Christrup LL, Jarlov JO, et al. Gentamicin dosing in critically ill patients. Acta Anesthesiol Scand 2001;45:734–40.

36. Drusano GL, Ambrose PG, Bhavnani SM, et al. Back to the future: using aminoglycosides again and how to dose them optimally. Clin Infect Dis 2007;45: 753–60.

37. Demczar DJ, Nafziger AN, Bertino JS Jr. Pharmacokinetics of gentamicin at traditional versus high doses: implications for once-daily aminoglycoside dosing. Antimicrob Agents Chemother 1997;41:1115–9.

38. Aroney RS, Dalley DN, Levi JA. Treatment of serious systemic infections with netilmicin in combination with other antibiotics. Med J Aust 1981;1:475–7.

39. Maller R, Ahrne H, Holmen C, et al. Once- versus twice-daily amikacin regimen: efficacy and safety in systemic Gram-negative infections. J Antimicrob Chemother 1993;31:939–48.

40. Ehrmann S, Mercier E, Vecellio L, et al. Pharmacokinetics of high-dose nebulized amikacin in mechanically ventilated healthy subjects. Intensive Care Med 2008; 34:755–62.

41. Bailey DN, Briggs JR. Gentamicin and tobramycin binding to human serum in vitro. J Anal Toxicol 2004;28:187–9.

42. Panidis D, Markantonis SL, Boutzouka E, et al. Penetration of gentamicin into the alveolar lining fluid of critically ill patients with ventilator-associated pneumonia. Chest 2005;128:545–52.

43. Carcas AJ, García-Satué JL, Zapater P, et al. Tobramycin penetration into epithelial lining fluid of patients with pneumonia. Clin Pharmacol Ther 1999;65:245–50.

44. Zaske DE, Sawchuk RJ, Gerding DN, et al. Increased dosage requirements of gentamicin in burn patients. J Trauma 1976;16:824–8.

45. Gilbert DN, Bennett WM. Use of antimicrobial agents in renal failure. Infect Dis Clin North Am 1989;3:517–31.

46. Pea F, Viale P, Pavan F, et al. Pharmacokinetic considerations for antimicrobial therapy in patients receiving renal replacement therapy. Clin Pharm 2007;46: 997–1038.

47. Traynor AM, Nafziger AN, Bertino JS. Aminoglycoside dosing weight correction factors for patients of various body sizes. Antimicrob Agents Chemother 1995; 39(2):545–8.

48. Schentag JJ, Jusko WJ. Gentamicin persistence in the body. Lancet 1977;1:486.
49. Nagai J, Tanaka H, Nakanishi N, et al. Role of megalin in renal handling of amino-glycosides. Am J Physiol Renal Physiol 2001;281:F337–44.
50. Schmitz C, Hilpert J, Jacobson C, et al. Megalin deficiency offers protection from renal aminoglycoside accumulation. J Biol Chem 2002;277:618–22.
51. El Mouedden M, Lkaurent G, Mingeot-Leclercq MP, et al. Apoptosis in renal prox-imal tubules of rats treated with low doses of aminoglycosides. Antimicrob Agents Chemother 2000;44:665–75.
52. Servais H, Jossin Y, Van Bambeke F, et al. Gentamicin causes apoptosis at low concentrations in renal LLC-PK1 cells subjected to electroporation. Antimicrob Agents Chemother 2006;50:1213–21.
53. Luft FC, Aronoff GR, Evan AP, et al. The renin-angiotensin system in aminoglyco-side-induced acute renal failure. J Pharmacol Exp Ther 1982;220:433–9.
54. Winslade NE, Adelman MH, Evans ES, et al. Single dose accumulation kinetics of tobramycin and netilmicin in normal volunteers. Antimicrob Agents Chemother 1987;31:605–9.
55. Denamur S, Van Bambeke F, Mingeot-Leclercq MP, et al. Apoptosis induced by aminoglycosides in LCC-PK1 cells: comparative study of neomycin, gentamicin, amikacin, and isepamicin using electroporation. Antimicrob Agents Chemother 2008;52:2236.
56. Kahlmeter G, Dahlager JI. Aminoglycoside toxicity—a review of clinical studies published between 1975 and 1982. J Antimicrob Chemother 1984;13(Suppl A):9–22.
57. Bertino JS Jr, Booker LA, Franck PA, et al. Incidence of and significant risk factors for aminoglycoside-associated nephrotoxicity in patients dosed by using individ-ualized pharmacokinetic monitoring. J Infect Dis 1993;167:173–9.
58. Dulon D, Aran J-M, Zajic G, et al. Comparative uptake of gentamicin, netilmicin, and amikacin in the guinea pig cochlea and vestibule. Antimicrob Agents Che-mother 1986;30:96–100.
59. Moore RD, Lerner SA, Levine DP. Nephrotoxicity and ototoxicity of aztreonam versus aminoglycoside therapy in seriously ill non-neutropenic patients. J Infect Dis 1992;165:683–8.
60. Brummett RE, Fox KE. Aminoglycoside-induced hearing loss in humans. Antimi-crob Agents Chemother 1989;33:797–800.
61. Beaubien AR, Ormsby E, Bayne A, et al. Evidence that amikacin ototoxicity is related to total perilymph area under the concentration-time curve regardless of concentration. Antimicrob Agents Chemother 1991;35:1070–4.
62. Fischel-Ghodsian N. Genetic factors in aminoglycoside toxicity. Ann N Y Acad Sci 1999;884:99–109.
63. Xing G, Chen Z, Wei Q, et al. Mitochondrial 12S rRNA A827G mutation is involved in the genetic susceptibility to aminoglycoside ototoxicity. Biochem Biophys Res Commun 2006;346:1131–5.
64. Sha S- H, Qiu JH, Schacht J. Aspirin attenuates gentamicin-induced hearing loss. N Engl J Med 2006;354:1856–7.
65. Warner WA, Sanders E. Neuromuscular blockade associated with gentamicin therapy. JAMA 1971;215:1153–4.
66. Holtzman JL. Gentamicin and neuromuscular blockade. Ann Intern Med 1976;84:55.
67. Wong J, Brown G. Does once-daily dosing of aminoglycosides affect neuromus-cular function? J Clin Pharm Ther 1996;21:401–11.
68. Weber-Carstens S, Deja M, Koch S, et al. Risk factors in critical illness myopathy during the early course of critical illness: a prospective observational study. Crit Care 2010;14:186.

69. Moellering RC Jr. In vitro antibacterial activity of the aminoglycoside antibiotics. Rev Infect Dis 1983;5(Suppl 2):212–20.
70. Guimaraes MA, Sage R, Noone P. The comparative activity of aminocyclitol antibiotics against 773 aerobic Gram-negative rods and staphylococci isolated from hospitalized patients. J Antimicrob Chemother 1985;16:555–62.
71. Price KE, Kresel PA, Farchione LA, et al. Epidemiological studies of aminoglycoside resistance in the USA. J Antimicrob Chemother 1981;8(Suppl A):89.
72. Gerding DN, Larson TA. Aminoglycoside resistance in Gram-negative bacilli during increased amikacin use. Am J Med 1985;79(1A):1–7.
73. Bengtsson S, Bernarder S, Brorson JE, et al. In vitro aminoglycoside resistance of Gram-negative bacilli and staphylococci isolated from blood in Sweden 1980-1984. Scand J Infect Dis 1986;18:257.
74. Martinez JA, Cobos-TrIqueros N, Soriano A, et al. Influence of empiric therapy with a beta-lactam alone or combined with an aminoglycoside on prognosis of bacteremia due to gram-negative microorganisms. Antimicrob Agents Chemother 2010;54:3590–6.
75. Micek ST, Welch EC, Khan J, et al. Empiric combination antibiotic therapy is associated with improved outcome against sepsis due to Gram-negative bacteria: a retrospective analysis. Antimicrob Agents Chemother 2010;54:1742–8.
76. Lepper PM, Held TK, Schneider EM, et al. Clinical implications of antibiotic-induced endotoxin release in septic shock. Intensive Care Med 2002;28:824–33.
77. Sjolin J, Goscinski G, Lundholm M, et al. Endotoxin release from Escherichia coli after exposure to tobramycin; dose-dependency and reduction in cefuroxime-induced endotoxin release. Clin Microbiol Infect 2000;6:74–81.
78. Goscinski G, Lundholm M, Odenholt I, et al. Variation in the propensity to release endotoxin after cefuroxime exposure in different gram-negative bacteria: uniform and dose-dependent reduction by the addition of tobramycin. Scand J Infect Dis 2003;35:40–6.
79. Toky V, Sharma S, Bramhne HG, et al. Antibiotic-induced release of inflammatory mediators from bacteria in experimental Klebsiella pneumoniae-induced sepsis. Folia Microbiol (Praha) 2005;50:167–71.
80. Cosgrove SE, Vigliani GA, Campion M, et al. Initial low-dose gentamicin for Staphylococcus aureus bacteremia and endocarditis is nephrotoxic. Clin Infect Dis 2009;48:713–21.
81. Hughes DW, Frei CR, Maxwell PR, et al. Continuous versus intermittent infusion of oxacillin for treatment of infectious endocarditis caused by methicillin-susceptible Staphylococcus aureus. Antimicrob Agents Chemother 2009;53:2014–9.
82. Donowitz GR, Mandell GL. Empiric therapy for pneumonia. Rev Infect Dis 1983; 5(Suppl 1):40–8.
83. Safdar N, Handelsman J, Maki DG. Does combination intravenous antibiotic therapy reduce mortality in Gram-negative bacteremia? A meta-analysis. Lancet Infect Dis 2004;4:519–27.
84. Ghannam DE, Rodrigues GH, Raad II, et al. Inhaled aminoglycosides in cancer patients with ventilator-associated Gram-negative bacterial pneumonia: safety and feasibility in the era of escalating drug resistance. Eur J Clin Microbiol Infect Dis 2009;28:253–9.
85. Czosnowski QA, Wood GC, Magnotti LJ, et al. Adjunctive aerosolized antibiotics for treatment of ventilator-associated pneumonia. Pharmacotherapy 2009;29: 1054–60.
86. Bailey JA, Virgo KS, Dipiron JT, et al. Aminoglycosides for intra-abdominal infection: equal to the challenge? Surg Infect (Larchmt) 2002;3:315–35.

87. Falagas ME, Matthaiou DK, Karveli EA, et al. Meta-analysis: randomized controlled trials of clindamicin/aminoglycoside vs. β-lactam monotherapy for the treatment of Intra-abdominal infections. Aliment Pharmacol Ther 2006;25:537–56.
88. Vidal L, Gafter-Gvili A, Borok S, et al. Efficacy and safety of aminoglycoside monotherapy: systematic review and meta-analysis of randomized controlled trials. J Antimicrob Chemother 2007;60:247–57.
89. Leibovici L, Vidal L, Paul M. Aminoglycoside drugs in clinical practice: an evidence-based approach. J Antimicrob Chemother 2009;63:246–51.

Fungal Sepsis: Optimizing Antifungal Therapy in the Critical Care Setting

Alexander Lepak, MD[a], David Andes, MD[b,c],*

KEYWORDS

- Invasive candidiasis • Pharmacokinetics-pharmacodynamics
- Therapy • Source control

Invasive fungal infections (IFI) and fungal sepsis in the intensive care unit (ICU) are increasing and are associated with considerable morbidity and mortality. In this setting, IFI are predominantly caused by *Candida* species. Currently, candidemia represents the fourth most common health care–associated blood stream infection.[1–3] With increasingly immunocompromised patient populations, other fungal species such as *Aspergillus* species, *Pneumocystis jiroveci*, *Cryptococcus*, Zygomycetes, *Fusarium* species, and *Scedosporium* species have emerged.[4–9] However, this review focuses on invasive candidiasis (IC).

Multiple retrospective studies have examined the crude mortality in patients with candidemia and identified rates ranging from 46% to 75%.[3] In many instances, this is partly caused by severe underlying comorbidities. Carefully matched, retrospective cohort studies have been undertaken to estimate mortality attributable to candidemia and report rates ranging from 10% to 49%.[10–15] Resource use associated with this infection is also significant. Estimates from numerous studies suggest the added hospital cost is as much as $40,000 per case.[10–12,16–20] Overall attributable costs are difficult to calculate with precision, but have been estimated to be close to 1 billion dollars in the United States annually.[21]

[a] University of Wisconsin, MFCB, Room 5218, 1685 Highland Avenue, Madison, WI 53705-2281, USA
[b] Department of Medicine, University of Wisconsin, MFCB, Room 5211, 1685 Highland Avenue, Madison, WI 53705-2281, USA
[c] Department of Microbiology and Immunology, University of Wisconsin, MFCB, Room 5211, 1685 Highland Avenue, Madison, WI 53705-2281, USA
* Corresponding author. Department of Microbiology and Immunology, University of Wisconsin, MFCB, Room 5211, 1685 Highland Avenue, Madison, WI 53705-2281.
E-mail address: dra@medicine.wisc.edu

Crit Care Clin 27 (2011) 123–147
doi:10.1016/j.ccc.2010.11.001
0749-0704/11/$ – see front matter. Published by Elsevier Inc.

criticalcare.theclinics.com

Understanding the management factors that affect outcome in this disease state is thus increasingly important for the critical care physician. The care strategies of demonstrated relevance include prompt suspicion of IC, rapid evaluation, diagnosis and initiation of antimicrobial therapy. In addition, the optimal agent to target these pathogens and the proper dosing regimen must be chosen, and source control should be considered. These care themes are similar to those of demonstrated importance for bacterial sepsis, yet many features are unique to IC. These issues are examined in this review.

EPIDEMIOLOGY

The incidence and epidemiology of IC in the ICU has undergone considerable change in the past 3 decades. This evolution has had a substantial effect on the therapeutic target and thus empirical treatment of IC in the ICU. The incidence of *Candida* blood stream infection (BSI) rose sharply in the 1980s with a more than 5-fold increase compared with studies a decade earlier.[22] This trend continued with a greater than 200% increase from 1979 to 2000.[23] The shift in the epidemiology of this health care–associated infection has continued in the current decade, with rates now estimated to be between 25 and 30 per 100,000 persons.[16,24] In addition to an absolute increase in disease incidence, there has also been a change in the species responsible for these infections. At least 17 *Candida* species have been reported to cause IC in humans, but 5 species (*C albicans, C glabrata, C parapsilosis, C tropicalis,* and *C krusei*) represent more than 90%. *C albicans* has historically been the predominant pathogen in IC with rates of 80% or higher in the 1980s.[3,25] Presently, *C albicans* accounts for less than 50% of all BSIs caused by the *Candida* genus.[3,26–30] The predominant non-*albicans* species in the United States is *C glabrata,* with an estimated frequency between 20% and 25%.[3] In contrast, other countries have noted dramatic increases in *C parapsilosis* and *C tropicalis.*[3,31] As *C glabrata* often exhibits reduced susceptibility to triazoles and *C parapsilosis* has reduced susceptibility to echinocandins, knowledge of the local epidemiology is imperative for selection of appropriate empirical therapy.

TIME TO THERAPY

The importance of prompt identification of IC through a combination of risk factor analysis and diagnostic assays has been demonstrated to be a key factor affecting sepsis-related mortality.[32–41] Studies on patients with IC have similarly shown excessive rates of inappropriate initial therapy and even higher mortality than infections caused by bacterial pathogens in the ICU setting.[10,14,33,34,42–47] One of the earliest studies to examine the effect of appropriate antimicrobial therapy in the ICU observed a 33% lower mortality in patients receiving adequate therapy defined by in vitro antimicrobial susceptibility testing.[33] Inappropriate treatment was most common for *Enterococcus* spp; however, inadequate coverage for IC was the second most common error and was associated with the highest mortality. Another retrospective cohort study by Kumar and colleagues[34] demonstrated that administration of adequate antimicrobial therapy within the first hour of documented hypotension was associated with a survival rate of 79.9%, and each 1-hour delay in antimicrobial therapy was linked to a 7.6% per hour decrease in survival. Subgroup analysis identified a significant relationship between hospital survival and duration of time between onset of sepsis and drug therapy for each microbial genus including *Candida* species.

Additional studies investigating the effect of time to initial appropriate therapy have specifically targeted IC. Blot and colleagues[42] reported 78% mortality in patients with IC when therapy was delayed more than 48 hours from onset of candidemia; in contrast the mortality was 44% in those who had adequate initial therapy. Another single-center retrospective cohort of 157 consecutive patients with a Candida BSI showed a trend toward improved survival when appropriate antifungal therapy was administered within 12 hours of blood culture collection (mortality 11.1% vs 33.1%; $P = .169$).[45] In multivariate analysis the odds of death was 2-fold higher if adequate therapy was delayed more than 12 hours ($P = .018$). Garey and colleagues[46] examined time to antifungal therapy in a multicenter, retrospective cohort of 230 patients with a Candida BSI who were prescribed fluconazole. Mortality was lowest (15.4%) if fluconazole therapy was started on the same day that the culture was performed and increased to 23.7% if fluconazole therapy was started on day 1, 36.4% on day 2, and 41.4% if it was started day 3 ($P = .0009$). Multivariate analysis in this study also provided a strong association between delay in therapy and mortality. In a recent publication, Patel and colleagues[48] performed a retrospective review of cases of Candida sepsis (positive blood culture within 72 hours of refractory shock) from a single center from 2003 to 2007. Using classification and regression tree analysis (CART), they found patients who received early, appropriate antifungal therapy (within 15 hours of collecting the first positive blood culture) had improved survival. Another recent publication by Taur and colleagues[49] in a cohort of patients with cancer found similar results. These data strongly support early appropriate antifungal therapy and demonstrate a need for improved disease identification.

EARLY DIAGNOSTICS

Two areas of intense investigation designed to improve early IC identification include novel laboratory assays and risk factor–based disease prediction. Unfortunately, IC lacks specific and objective clinical findings.[3,50–53] In addition, the gold standard diagnostic test for IC has been isolation of the organism in blood culture, however, blood culture for Candida is insensitive.[52–55] For example, modern blood culture systems are estimated to detect only 50% to 67% of cases of IC. Furthermore, detection of candidemia by blood culture often takes more than 24 hours. For certain species, such as C glabrata, the time to positive culture can be even longer.[56–60] In a study by Fernandez and colleagues,[56] the mean time to yeast detection in blood cultures for C albicans was 35.3 ± 18.1 hours, whereas that of C glabrata was 80.0 ± 22.4 hours. Mean time to final identification to species level for C albicans was 85.8 ± 30.9 hours compared with 154 ± 43.8 hours for C glabrata. In this study, the time to appropriate therapy for C albicans isolates was 43.3 ± 27.6 hours compared with 98.1 ± 38.3 hours for C glabrata isolates. Thus, waiting for positive blood culture results and potentially susceptibility testing leads to a significant delay in appropriate therapy and in turn higher mortality.

The relatively slow growth of these organisms in culture systems has led to the development of several non–culture-based diagnostic studies to detect fungal cell wall components, antigens, or nucleic acids secreted into the blood. Approved serologic tests in the United States or Europe include mannan antibody/antigen detection (Platelia) and β-1,3-D-glucan (Glucatell, Fungitell). In Europe, a nucleic acid identification system (SeptiFast) is approved for detection in blood of certain bacterial and fungal pathogens including the 5 most commonly encountered Candida species.

A retrospective study evaluated mannan antigen or mannan antibody detection in the sera of patients with culture proven candidemia.[61] In 36 of 43 (84%) patients with culture proven candidemia at least 1 of the 2 serologic tests was positive. The sensitivities were 40% and 98% and the specificities were 53% and 94% for mannanemia or antibody detection, respectively. These values reached 80% and 93% when the results of both tests were combined. A follow-up study of patients with candidemia revealed that 33 of 45 (73%) patients had positive serology using the Platelia assay for mannan antigen or antimannan antibodies at least 2 days before having a positive blood culture, with a mean positive serologic test 6 days before positive blood culture.[62] β-1, 3-D-Glucan detection has also been evaluated in critically ill patients, with sensitivity and specificity for diagnosis of IC estimated to be 69.9% and 87.1%, respectively.[63] Several nucleic acid detection platforms have been evaluated for detection of IC. For example, McMullan and colleagues prospectively evaluated 3 Taqman-based nested polymerase chain reaction (PCR) assays for the detection of candidemia in critical ill patients. Twenty-three of 157 patients included in the study had proven IC. The estimated clinical sensitivity, specificity, and positive and negative predictive values of the assays in this trial were 90.9%, 100%, 100%, and 99.8%, respectively.[64] Nucleic acid detection in this study identified fungal sepsis as soon as 6 hours within onset of symptoms. SeptiFast, which is able to detect DNA of 20 common bacteria and fungi, may be a helpful adjunct to blood cultures for fastidious organisms and may be advantageous in settings where patients are either already on antibiotics or have been pretreated.[65,66] An important limitation in evaluating these newer diagnostic tests is the lack a reference gold standard (blood culture) with high specificity and sensitivity. For example, in a meta-analysis of studies using PCR to diagnose IC, the sensitivity progressively decreased as the reference standard went from patients with culture proven candidemia to those with proven/probable IC, and even lower when compared with those with proven, probable, or possible IC.[67] At present, there is significant heterogeneity in assay characteristics including choice of sample, primer, nesting strategy, and nucleic acid extraction. Although promising, there is need for further prospective validation of these diagnostic tools and wider availability, as currently only a few academic centers or reference laboratories have the capability to offer these advanced diagnostic techniques. Until confirmatory results are available from ongoing studies, routine use of these new diagnostic assays will remain investigative. If the empirical trial use of the β-1, 3-D-glucan test is shown to be useful, it is reasonable to expect this assay could be adapted for use in most tertiary care centers in the near future.

EMPIRICAL AND PREEMPTIVE STRATEGIES BASED ON RISK IDENTIFICATION

The importance of prompt antifungal treatment and lack of sensitivity and timeliness of diagnostic assays has led to the development of empirical and preemptive treatment strategies. The initiation of antifungal treatment in these cases is based on a compilation of host risk factors for IC. Multiple studies have evaluated risk factors for IC.[51,68–86] Variables that have been associated with IC include high APACHE II score, exposure to broad spectrum antibiotics, cancer chemotherapy, evidence of mucosal colonization by Candida spp, pancreatitis, indwelling vascular catheters (especially central venous catheter [CVC]), administration of total parenteral nutrition, neutropenia, immune suppression therapy, prior surgery (especially gastrointestinal surgery), renal failure or hemodialysis, and prolonged ICU stay (especially in the surgical ICU). These risk factors by themselves impart limited specificity as they are present in many critically ill patients.

Attempts to enhance the predictive value of these variables have involved examining a composite of risk factors.[74,78,85,87–91] A laboratory marker used in several risk stratification schemes is culture isolation of Candida species from multiple nonblood sites. The predictive value of this laboratory marker by itself has been explored by Pittet and colleagues,[87] who examined the value of identifying Candida colonization at multiple nonblood sites, termed the Candida colonization index (CI).

This index is calculated by adding the number of nonblood sites that are culture positive for the same *Candida* species divided by the total number of sites cultured. In a single-center prospective series the group found an index greater than 0.5 to be predictive of IC in 29 patients with *Candida* colonization in either a surgical or neonatal ICU. The sensitivity and specificity of the CI was 100% and 55%, respectively, using positive blood culture as the reference. This strategy requires daily multisite *Candida* surveillance cultures, which may not be feasible or cost-effective at many centers and results would still be delayed to allow for culture growth. Additional studies have examined the usefulness of multisite colonization in the context of other risk factors. For example, Leon and colleagues[88] developed a scoring system that could be performed at the bedside termed the *Candida* score. In a large, multisite observational study they examined the incidence of IC among patients in a surgical ICU with sepsis, total parenteral nutrition (TPN) administration, multifocal *Candida* colonization. A point value was assigned to each of 4 risk factors (multifocal colonization 1 point, TPN 1 point, surgery 1 point, and sepsis 2 points). Patients with a score greater than 2.5 were nearly 8 times more likely to have proven IC (risk ratio 7.75; 95% confidence interval 4.74–12.66) than patients with a *Candida* score of 2.5 or less. The strategy was prospectively validated in a larger cohort of 1107 patients in the surgical ICU among whom 57 were diagnosed with candidemia. Patients with a *Candida* score greater than 2.5 had a 6-fold increase in relative risk for developing IC with a sensitivity of 77.6% and specificity of 66.2%.[89]

Other studies have relied solely on non–laboratory-based risk factors. Ostrosky-Zeichner and colleagues[90] performed one of the largest studies examining a clinical risk prediction rule for IC. Among 3000 patients from ICUs in the United States and Brazil, a combination of several factors was predictive of IC in patients who had been admitted to the ICU for at least 3 days. The study identified both major and minor risk factors. The 2 major risk factors included receipt of a systemic antibiotic and the presence of a CVC. Minor risk factors included TPN, dialysis, surgery in the preceding week, pancreatitis, and use of steroids or other immunosuppressive agents. Patients meeting both major risk factors and at least 2 minor risk factors constituted the high-risk group. Retrospective analysis identified a rate of invasive candidiasis among patients who fulfilled the criteria of 9.9% versus 2.3% in those who did not meet criteria. The clinical prediction rule was relatively exclusive as the total number of patients who met criteria was only 11% (n = 303) of the total population studied. The calculated sensitivity was only 34%, but specificity was 90%. A follow-up prospective validation study by the same group evaluated a modified clinical prediction rule in a medical ICU.[91] Patients meeting criteria must have been in the medical ICU for at least 3 days, have both major criteria (a CVC and antibiotic exposure), and have at least 2 minor criteria (which included mechanical ventilation in place of surgery given the study was performed in a medical ICU). Patients meeting these criteria were given fluconazole preemptively. In the year before the implementation of the rule, 9 cases of candidemia developed in the medical ICU, corresponding to a rate of 3.4 cases per 1000 CVC days. In the year of implementation, only 2 cases of candidemia were identified, a drop in the rate of *Candida* bloodstream infection to 0.8 cases per 1000 CVC days.

Further validation of risk assessment tools and assessment of the value of antifungal prophylaxis and preemptive therapy are necessary before clinical adoption of this practice. Currently, there is an ongoing multisite, randomized, double-blind, placebo-controlled trial sponsored by the Mycoses Study Group examining this risk stratification scoring system and caspofungin prophylaxis followed by preemptive therapy for IC in high-risk adults in the critical care setting.[92] The results may provide valuable insight into both risk stratification schemes and prophylaxis in the ICU.

ANTIFUNGAL DRUG CLASSES AND MECHANISM OF ACTION

Once either a definitive diagnosis occurs or risk factors trigger the initiation of therapy, the next step in management is the choice of the optimal antifungal agent and dosing regimen. Differences in the mechanism of action, spectrum of activity, pharmacokinetics, and toxicity affect this decision for a variety of clinical situations. Currently, 3 classes of antifungal drugs, a total of 8 drugs, are approved by the US Food and Drug Administration (FDA) for IC. The first class of antifungals that became available for treatment of IC is the polyene group, which includes amphotericin B deoxycholate and its 3 lipid formulations (liposomal amphotericin B, amphotericin B lipid complex, and amphotericin B cholesteryl sulfate complex). Of the 4, only amphotericin B cholesteryl sulfate does not carry an FDA indication for candidemia. The lipid formulations have been a major advance in therapeutics, providing less nephrotoxicity than that observed with conventional deoxycholate amphotericin B. All of the formulations exert their cidal effect by binding to ergosterol in the fungal cell membrane leading to depolarization, increased permeability, and ultimately cell death.[93] The second class of antifungal compounds is the triazoles; FDA-approved agents for IC include fluconazole and voriconazole. These drugs target fungal cell membrane ergosterol synthesis, the major cell membrane component, by inhibition of the fungal cytochrome P-450–dependent enzyme lanosterol 14-α-demethylase. This mechanism of action is generally considered fungistatic against Candida species.[93] The most recently developed group of antifungals is the echinocandin class, which includes caspofungin, micafungin, and anidulafungin. All 3 are FDA approved for candidemia and are cidal against Candida species.[93–95] The mechanism of action for this class is via inhibition of β-1,3-glucan synthase, an enzyme responsible for production of the major cell wall component β-1,3-D-glucan.

SPECTRUM OF ACTIVITY

Amphotericin B deoxycholate and its lipid congeners are potent against most Candida species. Among the species that are less susceptible to this drug, C glabrata and C krusei have MIC90s (minimum inhibitory concentration required to inhibit 90% of organisms) of 4 and 8 μg/mL, respectively, compared with an MIC90 of 1 μg/mL for C albicans.[3] Although the MIC for C lusitaneae is often comparable with C albicans on initial susceptibility testing, this species is notorious for development of resistance while on therapy with amphotericin B.

Fluconazole and voriconazole are also active against most Candida species including C albicans, C parapsilosis, and C tropicalis. Reduced activity is a concern for a few commonly identified species, specifically C glabrata and C krusei. C krusei is inherently resistant to fluconazole and therefore is not effective. Fluconazole resistance in C glabrata varies by geographic location with rates of 14% to 23%, with an additional 5% susceptible only to increased doses of fluconazole (susceptible dose-dependent).[3,96] Reduced C glabrata susceptibility to fluconazole is in general predictive of activity for the entire triazole class including voriconazole. However, a small subset of fluconazole resistant C glabrata isolates, approximately 17%, do remain susceptible to voriconazole.[97] A unique spectrum for voriconazole includes C krusei.

The echinocandins offer a broad spectrum that includes activity against C albicans, C glabrata, C tropicalis, and C krusei. Both C guilliermondii and C parapsilosis have reduced susceptibility to the echinocandin class. Clinical trials have not fully examined the importance of the decreased susceptibility of these 2 species, although case reports of treatment failure continue to accumulate.[98–103]

OPTIMAL DRUG CHOICE

The optimal drug choice for IC has been evaluated in numerous clinical studies and several consensus guidelines have been published.[98,104–110] Amphotericin B had long been considered the only treatment of IC before the approval of fluconazole. In 1994, Rex and colleagues[104] published the first comparative trial examining antifungal therapy (fluconazole vs amphotericin B) in non-neutropenic patients with candidemia. Similar successful clinical outcomes were noted in both groups (fluconazole 70% vs amphotericin B 79%). Significant adverse events (AE) were more common in the amphotericin B group including electrolyte imbalance and renal insufficiency. A study by Kullberg and colleagues[106] demonstrated similar successful clinical outcomes in patients with IC or candidemia treated with voriconazole compared with amphotericin B with step down to fluconazole. Significantly fewer serious AE attributable to the antifungal drug occurred in the voriconazole group versus amphotericin B. Mora-Duarte and colleagues[98] published the first comparative trial of an echinocandin and amphotericin B in 2002. This trial compared outcomes in patients with blood culture proven candidemia or IC, defined as having a positive culture from a sterile site, who received caspofungin or amphotericin B. Successful outcomes, although not significantly different, were noted in 73.4% of patients receiving caspofungin and 61.7% in those who received amphotericin B. This trial also highlighted the generally low incidence of AE and excellent tolerability for the echinocandin class. Caspofungin had significantly less clinical or laboratory AE, with only 2.6% of patients in this arm discontinuing therapy. This is in contrast to amphotericin B, which was associated with clinical AE (nausea, vomiting, chills, fever) as well as laboratory AE (electrolyte imbalances, renal insufficiency) resulting in nearly a 25% rate of drug discontinuation. In recent years, micafungin and anidulafungin have also been subjected to study in randomized controlled trials (RCTs). In a study by Kuse and colleagues,[108] micafungin was as effective and caused fewer AE than liposomal amphotericin B as first-line treatment of candidemia and invasive candidiasis. Most recently, Reboli and colleagues[107] examined anidulafungun versus fluconazole, with anidulafungin showing superiority over fluconazole. In this study, successful outcome was noted in 75.6% versus 60.2%, respectively, in patients with candidemia or IC. AEs in this trial were similar between anidulafungin and fluconazole. The sum of these studies has shown low toxicity (especially compared with amphotericin B) and equivalent or improved outcome data when echinocandins are compared with azoles or amphotericin B. Recently, a patient-level meta-analysis of RCTs for treatment of IC was performed, drawing data from 7 trials conducted from 1994 to 2007 and including more than 1800 patients.[111] The use of an echinocandin rather than another antifungal agent was associated with decreased mortality.

The Infectious Diseases Society of America (IDSA) has recently published revised recommendations for the treatment of IC.[110] In the current guidelines, first-line options include caspofungin, anidulafungin, micafungin, or fluconazole. The guideline favors an echinocandin for moderate to severe IC or any patient with previous azole exposure, with the exception of C parapsilosis for which fluconazole is suggested. Transition from an echinocandin to fluconazole is suggested when an isolate that is likely to be susceptible to fluconazole (eg, C albicans, C tropicalis, C parapsilosis) is identified and patients have clinically stabilized. Voriconazole therapy may be appropriate for C krusei and C glabrata in place of fluconazole for stable patients with laboratory-demonstrated susceptibility to this agent. Amphotericin B and its lipid formulations remain important antifungal agents for serious fungal infections including IC despite its known toxicities. With the advent of less toxic but equally effective therapy, amphotericin B is now reserved for patients who are intolerant to echinocandins, those not responding to echinocandins, or special circumstances such as meningitis with *Candida* species.

TOXICOLOGY

Although amphotericin B deoxycholate exhibits the widest spectrum of activity, administration is associated with limiting adverse effects.[95] Up to 50% of patients experience infusion-related toxicity, which includes nausea, vomiting, fever, chills, rigors, myalgias, and rarely bronchospasm and hypoxia. Electrolyte imbalance (hypokalemia, hypomagnesemia) caused by distal renal tubular toxicity and renal insufficiency secondary to vasoconstriction have been reported in up to 80% of patients. Preinfusion administration of an antipyretic and antihistamine agent may reduce infusion effects and hydration with normal saline provides some mitigation of the renal insufficiency. Some investigators have suggested that administration of deoxycholate amphotericin B by a continuous infusion may decrease nephrotoxicity, but comparative efficacy has not been studied prospectively or with a large enough sample in a retrospective manner.[112–118] Most of the data are from preemptive therapy in high-risk hematology patients with febrile neutropenia. Thus, further studies would need to examine this dosing strategy in a controlled fashion for IC before any recommendations can be made for this approach. The most affective reduction in polyene toxicity is with use of a lipid formulation, which is associated with 10- to 20-fold fewer febrile reactions and renal insufficiency.

The triazoles and echinocandins are in general well tolerated with few significant adverse effects. The most common complication of triazole use is that associated with drug interactions caused by P-450 inhibition or induction.[95] The echinocandins are associated with very few and mostly minor drug interactions.

PK CONSIDERATIONS

Consideration of infection site drug concentrations can be important when choosing the optimal antifungal. There are certain tissues for which there are pharmacokinetic differences among the antifungal agents. For most tissue sites, serum concentrations correlate closely with interstitial tissue concentrations where most fungal pathogens reside during infection. However, there are certain tissue sites for which there can be discrepancies, including the central nervous system (CNS), eye, urine, and the epithelial lining fluid of the lung.[119] The CNS, eye, and urine body sites are tissue sites of importance for a subset of patients with IC. Amphotericin B and its lipid formulations have differing tissue pharmacokinetics that are largely dependent on the carrier molecule to which they are complexed.[120–124] For example, liposomal amphotericin B is a small, unilamellar particle that exhibits high serum and CNS concentrations relative to the other amphotericin B preparations.[122] A few investigations have explored the effect/affect of these PK differences on outcomes, with a CNS candidiasis animal model in favor of the liposomal amphotericin B formulation.[121–123] This lipid formation also accumulates in the vitreal fluid, which may be attractive for endophthalmitis therapy.[95]

Fluconazole penetrates into nearly all tissue sites including CSF, vitreous fluid, and urine, and is therefore a valuable drug to treat sequestered sites of infection against susceptible *Candida* species.[95] Voriconazole also has wide tissue distribution including the CSF and vitreal fluid, but is not excreted into urine and would not be expected to be effective for *Candida* cystitis.

The echinocandins are large lipopeptide antifungal agents available only as intravenous formulations because of their chemical structure and size, which precludes adequate oral absorption. These physiochemical characteristics also affect the distribution of these compounds, which is notably low or undetectable in urine, CSF, and vitreous fluid.[95,125,126]

OPTIMAL DOSE AND REGIMEN

Treatment success following early initiation and correct drug choice will be limited if the optimal dose and dosing schedule are not considered. Numerous reports have documented the association between inadequate dosing of antifungals in patients with IC and increased length of hospital stay, health care costs, morbidity, and mortality.[10,14,20,33,42–47,127] Pharmacodynamic (PD) analyses have been crucial in developing optimal anti-infective dosing strategies. These approaches simply consider the effect of pharmacokinetics (PK) of a drug relative to the MIC of the organism on therapeutic efficacy.[128] Pharmacodynamic application has revolutionized treatment of bacterial infections in the ICU setting.[128,129] More recently, similar study results have become available for antifungal agents in this setting.[93,130]

Three PD indices have been linked to therapeutic efficacy. Each of these drug exposures indices represents a measure of drug PK relative to the MIC of the infecting organism. The indices include the peak drug concentration indexed to the MIC (C_{max}/MIC), the area under the drug concentration curve in relation to the MIC (AUC/MIC), and the time (expressed as a percentage of the dosing interval) that the drug concentrations exceed the MIC (%T>MIC). Determining which of the 3 PD indices is predictive of efficacy for an antimicrobial agent provides a framework for dosing regimen design. For example, dosing of concentration-dependent antimicrobials is optimal when large doses are administered infrequently. The concentration-dependent indices, C_{max}/MIC and AUC/MIC, are the PD indices associated with treatment efficacy for these compounds. Conversely, efficacy for antimicrobials that exhibit time-dependent activity is greatest when smaller doses are given frequently. In this scenario, maximal antimicrobial effects are observed at concentrations near the MIC. The optimal regimen design in this case would aim to keep drug concentrations higher than the organism's MIC for a longer period of time and the predictive index for these antimicrobials is the %T>MIC.

A PD study also has the ability to define the amount of antimicrobial relative to the MIC that is needed for efficacy. This drug exposure indexed to the MIC is termed the pharmacodynamic target. For example, if %T>MIC is the PD index linked to efficacy, the PD target is how much time concentrations need to exceed the MIC for optimal efficacy. These investigations have been undertaken for each of the antifungal drugs.

Amphotericin B and the Lipid Formulations

Despite the common dose-limiting toxicities, amphotericin B remains an important therapeutic option for life-threatening fungal infections, especially in resource-limited areas. In vitro and in vivo PD studies have observed increased killing of *Candida* species as the concentration of amphotericin B is escalated multiple times higher than the MIC.[120,131–133] These models have also shown that growth inhibition after amphotericin B exposure continues for long periods of time. This period of postexposure effect is called the postantifungal effect (PAFE).[131,133,134] Prolonged PAFEs should allow for wider spacing of the dosing intervals. These PD characteristics support once daily administration of maximally tolerated doses. The concentration-dependent PD index C_{max}/MIC has been most closely linked to efficacy in these infection models. The concentration relative to the MIC associated with maximal efficacy in experimental models is a C_{max}/MIC of 2 to 4.[120,131] Pharmacodynamic analyses have also been undertaken with the 3 lipid formulations of amphotericin B.[120–123] These investigations have demonstrated similar pharmacodynamic characteristics; however, for lipid preparations the C_{max}/MIC target needed for efficacy is approximately 5 times larger than for amphotericin B.[120] There is a single, small clinical PD report with liposomal amphotericin B in a pediatric population.[135] Among 39 patients, those with liposomal amphotericin B C_{max}/MIC >40 were more likely to achieve a complete or partial response. This clinical target is similar to that identified in animal model studies. No other clinical investigations with the polyenes have provided data that would allow PD analysis.

Triazoles

Extensive PD studies have been undertaken with fluconazole and voriconazole.[133,136–139] Observations from these investigations demonstrated time-dependent antifungal activity that was optimal at concentrations 1 to 2 times the MIC. In addition, in vivo studies have revealed prolonged periods of growth suppression after triazole concentrations decrease to less than the MIC (long PAFE).[139–141] These characteristics are consistent with drugs for which the AUC/MIC index is most closely linked with efficacy. In vivo animal studies against a large number of Candida strains with widely varying MICs (more than 2000-fold) show that the 24-hour AUC/MIC target associated with efficacy (50% maximal effect) for triazoles occurs at a value near 25 when free drug (non–protein bound) levels are considered.[139–141] Simplistically, this value is the average concentration at the MIC for a 24-hour dosing period (1 times the MIC times 24 hours equals a 24-hour AUC/MIC of 24).

Substantial clinical data are available for pharmacodynamic target analyses for fluconazole in the treatment of Candida infections.[142–148] The earliest and largest of these datasets included more than 1000 patients with oropharyngeal candidiasis.[146] Analysis of these trial data found that treatment efficacy was maximal with fluconazole exposures relative to the MIC of the infecting Candida species near a 24-hour AUC/MIC value of 25. When the fluconazole AUC/MIC exceeded 25, clinical success was noted in 91% to 100% of patients. However, when AUC/MIC was less than 25, clinical failure was noted in 27% to 35% of patients. A more contemporary analysis in mucosal candidiasis corroborated the earlier findings, with clinical efficacy of 92% with an AUC/MIC greater than 25 and only 9% with values less than 25.[147] Similar data are available for IC.[142,143,145,147,148] For example, Baddley and colleagues[142] examined the relationship between the fluconazole 24-hour AUC/MIC and mortality in patients with IC. Maximal survival was associated with an AUC/MIC of 25.

Calculating the AUC/MIC magnitude for fluconazole is relatively straightforward as the AUC is essentially equal to the daily dose (400 mg daily dose is approximately an AUC of 400). One can then use the PD target information to define the highest MIC for which a given dosing regimen would be expected to be adequate. For example, with a fluconazole dose of 400 mg once daily for an infection in which the MIC is 32, the AUC/MIC would be less than 25 and failure can be expected. Surveillance MIC data can then be used to estimate if a drug and dosing regimen would achieve the PD target for most organisms in the community. C albicans has the lowest wild-type MICs with 98.1% having an MIC of 0.5 µg/mL or less.[149] C parapsilosis, C tropicalis, and C lusitaneae also have low MICs of 2 µg/mL or less (93%, 98% and 96%, respectively).[149] The wild-type MICs are significantly higher for C guilliermondii (8–16 µg/mL), C glabrata (32 µg/mL), and C krusei (64–128 µg/mL).[149] Therefore, for these MIC distributions, a fluconazole regimen of 400 mg per day would be an effective empirical option for most patients infected with *C albicans*, *C parapsilosis*, and *C tropicalis*, but not *C glabrata* or *C krusei*.

Similar data are available for the triazole, voriconazole. The largest dataset includes more than 400 patients from 6 phase III clinical trials.[150] Analysis of this dataset demonstrated a strong relationship between AUC/MIC and outcome. Therapeutic success was observed in approximately 80% of patients with a 24-hour AUC/MIC greater than 25, whereas when the AUC/MIC was less than 25, clinical failure was noted in 45% of patients. Many of these studies have also highlighted the variable PK of voriconazole, and the usefulness of therapeutic drug monitoring has been suggested in the setting of invasive aspergillosis.[151–154] Treatment success in these retrospective analyses has been associated with serum trough concentrations of 1 to 2 mg/mL. If the free drug AUC associated with these trough concentrations and the MIC for voriconazole against *Aspergillus* are considered, the 24-hour AUC/MIC value would be near 25. Although not well studied in IC, the PK/PD congruency in target AUC/MIC between *Aspergillus* and *Candida* would suggest target trough concentrations should be at least 1 to 2 mg/mL for IC and concentration monitoring might be useful in the critical care setting.[155]

Echinocandins

PK/PD studies with the echinocandin class of antifungals demonstrate concentration-dependent activity with a prolonged PAFE similar to that observed with amphotericin B.[156–163] The concentration-dependent indices, C_{max}/MIC and AUC/MIC, are both closely linked to efficacy and support administration of large infrequent doses. Preclinical and clinical PK/PD investigations have sought to identify the amount of echinocandin indexed to MIC that is needed for optimal therapy. In addition to examining the effect of MIC variability, a unique feature of these studies has included examination of the potential effect of *Candida* species on the PD target.[164,165] The results of these studies demonstrated the amount of echinocandin relative to the MIC needed for efficacy was higher for *C albicans* than for *C glabrata* or *C parapsilosis*.[165] The free drug AUC/MIC target was much less for *C parapsilosis* and *C glabrata* at approximately 5 to 7, whereas for *C albicans* the target AUC/MIC was approximately 10 to 20. Identification of species variability in the PD target is not a new paradigm. For example, studies with fluoroquinolone antibacterials identified an AUC/MIC target for *Streptococcus pneumoniae* of 25, whereas for gram-negative bacteria the value was near 100.[166] Clinical trial data with all 3 echinocandins have shown that the available drugs can be used successfully to treat *C parapsilosis* infections with increased MICs.[164,167] For example, in one report 5 of 6 (83%) infections caused by *C parapsilosis* for which the MIC was 4 μg/mL were treated successfully with anidulafungin, which would support the finding that the PD target may be much lower for this species.[167] Robust PD analysis of the echinocandin class using clinical patient data is limited. One dataset has been evaluated in this manner thus far. Analysis of 2 phase III trials with micafungin for candidemia or invasive candidiasis identified similar species-specific results.[168] Results from this investigation found a free drug AUC/MIC target of greater than 7.5 was associated with favorable outcomes for all *Candida* species except *C parapsilosis,* for which a free drug AUC/MIC magnitude predictive of favorable outcome was near 1. Recognition of differences in species-specific PD targets have recently been incorporated into the Clinical Laboratory and Standards Institute antifungal susceptibility breakpoint guidelines for each of the approved echinocandins.[169] The pharmacokinetics of the present echinocandin dosing regimens would be expected to produce AUC/MIC values exceeding these pharmacodynamic target goals for most *Candida* isolates. Thus, although dose adjustments should not be needed at present, if surveillance susceptibility testing identifies the emergence of less susceptible isolates, safety studies with each of the available echinocandin compounds can be escalated without toxicity.

COMBINATION THERAPY

Combination therapy is a frequently used strategy for difficult to treat infectious diseases. However, combination antifungal therapy has not been well studied for IC. Consensus guidelines do suggest a combination of amphotericin B and flucytosine for some infection types such as *Candida* meningitis, endophthalmitis, and endocarditis.[110] A single, randomized clinical trial examined high-dose fluconazole versus standard fluconazole dosing and amphotericin B in patients with candidemia.[105] For several outcomes there was a trend in favor of the combination; however, the 2 groups had significant differences in baseline APACHE II score favoring the combination arm. Robust PK/PD analysis of combination therapy is lacking and would provide useful guidance in this area.

DURATION

There are no experimental or clinical trials designed to define the optimal duration of therapy for IC. Guidance is based on expert consensus publications. The IDSA guideline for invasive candidiasis recommends a 2-week treatment duration following clearance of *Candida* from the bloodstream and resolution of symptoms attributable to candidemia.[110] Longer durations are recommended for persistent candidemia and for metastatic infection involving other sites (ie, CNS, bone, endocarditis, joint/prosthetic joint infection).

DEESCALATION

Deescalation or step down therapy from intravenous echinocandin or polyene to oral therapy is a common strategy but has not been formally studied. In most of the randomized trials, patients treated with either an echinocandin or polyene were allowed to step down to oral therapy (fluconazole or voriconazole) after receiving at least 10 days of intravenous therapy. In 1 study, patients were allowed to step down to oral fluconazole therapy in as few as 3 to 7 days after intravenous therapy with amphotericin.[106] However, the timing of step down has not been specifically analyzed in these investigations. Treatment guidelines recommend step down to fluconazole for patients who have improved clinically after initial therapy with an echinocandin or amphotericin B and who are infected with an organism that is likely to be susceptible to fluconazole (eg, *C albicans, C parapsilosis*, and *C tropicalis*) or if there is documented susceptibility based on laboratory MIC testing.[110] It is possible that even shorter durations of parenteral therapy may be effective; however, future studies will be needed to appropriately address this important question.

SOURCE CONTROL

Source control of infectious foci is an additional measure commonly used for IC. The rationale for source control includes removal of persistent infection and decreasing the infectious burden at pharmacologically protected sites. There are 2 common IC syndromes for which a source control strategy has been useful. The first is extirpation of biofilm infections because of the high level of drug resistance associated with this form of growth.[170] This typically occurs in the setting of indwelling medical devices such as vascular and urinary catheters. Venous catheter infection and IC guidelines, including the current IDSA guidelines, recommend removal of any intravascular catheter that is positive for a fungal pathogen (ie, *Candida*) based on evidence from large retrospective and observational studies.[110,170–170] A few studies have questioned these recommendations, failing to find a significant mortality benefit with prompt removal of the line and advising that removal and placement of a new device does not come without risk and cost.[179–183] For example, a recent publication by Nucci and colleagues[183] examined the effect of early (within 24 or 48 hours) CVC removal in subgroup analysis of data pooled from 2 phase III, double-blind, multicenter RCTs of therapy for candidemia. A total of 1109 patients were included in the 2 groups. After inclusion/exclusion criteria, 842 patients were included in the analysis. The investigators found no clinical difference in microbiologic outcomes or mortality in the patient group that had the CVC removed within 48 hours versus those that had it retained for the first 48 hours. These data are in contrast to a study published in the same year using the same dataset. Horn and colleagues[178] used the same 2 phase III datasets and found that catheter retention was associated with poorer outcomes than patients who had it removed. The differences in these 2 retrospective studies using the same datasets are to the result of different methodological processes, including the definitions used, inclusion/exclusion criteria, and statistical analysis. The largest study to date examining line retention and outcome is a meta-analysis of RCTs for treatment of invasive candidiasis, drawing data from 7 trials from 1994 to 2007 and including more than 1800 patients.[111] Removal of a CVC in patients with candidemia was associated with a 13% increase in survival.

A second site for which source control can be critical is infection of the vitreous. Endophthalmitis is a not uncommon complication in patients with candidemia, with an incidence ranging from 3% to 28% in prospective studies, and carries significant morbidity.[126] The accumulation of therapeutic agents in the vitreous is limited for many compounds and there is variability among the available antifungal agents. Therefore, the current guidelines suggest ophthalmologic examination for every patient with candidemia.[110] Recommended antifungal therapies include amphotericin B, fluconazole, or voriconazole depending on the susceptibility of the isolate. Although not studied in randomized comparative trials, vitrectomy is considered an important adjunct to antifungal therapy and can be a sight-saving procedure.[184]

PROPHYLAXIS AND PREEMPTIVE THERAPY

Although it is outside the scope of this article to critically review all of the studies examining prophylaxis and preventative strategies for IC in the ICU, there are many studies and reviews on this topic.[185–191] Identification of a sufficiently high-risk group or incidence has been an issue for most studies. A few meta-analyses have suggested potential mortality benefits with fluconazole prophylaxis; however, with an incidence of 1% to 2% in most ICU populations, more than 200 patients would need to undergo prophylaxis to prevent 1 infection. Therefore, it is necessary to consider prophylaxis strategies in high-risk individuals, pointing to the need for better risk stratification schemes in the ICU. If an at-risk group with an infection rate of at least 10% could be reliably identified, the number needed to treat to prevent 1 infection would be less than 20, and certainly this can be considered a potentially useful strategy for that specific patient group. The value of preemptive therapy has been best documented in the persistently neutropenic patient, and current guidelines suggest adding a broad spectrum antifungal agent in a neutropenic patient with persistent fever for 5 days despite broad spectrum antibiotics.[192] A recent study examining non-neutropenic patients did not find a benefit for the preemptive addition of fluconazole to persistently febrile patients in the ICU.[193] Improved risk stratification schemes should allow for more directed preemptive therapy in high-risk groups. In addition, there is interest in monitoring nonculture-based diagnostic tests in critically ill patients (such as β-glucan) to identify patients on the threshold of sepsis. It is hoped that ongoing studies will help to answer these questions.

SUMMARY

Critical components in the management of antifungal sepsis that are clinician mitigated include (1) prompt antifungal therapy, (2) risk factor analysis to identify patients at higher risk than the general ICU population for IC and therefore in need of prophylactic or preemptive therapy given the current lack of prompt accurate diagnostics, (3) choice of the appropriate antifungal agent and dosing regimen, and (4) source control. Currently, until a species diagnosis or susceptibility is known, an echinocandin is recommended as first-line therapy for most patients with IC. PD studies suggest the currently recommended regimens would be useful for most infections. Once the species is identified, for C albicans, C parapsilosis, or C tropicalis and the patient is responding to initial therapy, the appropriate therapy would include step down to fluconazole. For other species, the therapy should be directed based on susceptibility data. Source control, including line removal and evaluation for endophthalmitis is recommended for all patients with IC.

REFERENCES

1. Wisplinghoff H, Bischoff T, Tallent SM, et al. Nosocomial bloodstream infections in US hospitals: analysis of 24,179 cases from a prospective nationwide surveillance study. Clin Infect Dis 2004;39(3):309–17.
2. Hidron AI, Edwards JR, Patel J, et al. NHSN annual update: antimicrobial-resistant pathogens associated with healthcare-associated infections: annual summary of data reported to the National Healthcare Safety Network at the Centers for Disease Control and Prevention, 2006–2007. Infect Control Hosp Epidemiol 2008;29(11):996–1011.
3. Pfaller MA, Diekema DJ. Epidemiology of invasive candidiasis: a persistent public health problem. Clin Microbiol Rev 2007;20(1):133–63.
4. Maschmeyer G, Haas A, Cornely OA. Invasive aspergillosis: epidemiology, diagnosis and management in immunocompromised patients. Drugs 2007; 67(11):1567–601.
5. Meersseman W, Lagrou K, Maertens J, et al. Invasive aspergillosis in the intensive care unit. Clin Infect Dis 2007;45(2):205–16.
6. Meersseman W, Vandecasteele SJ, Wilmer A, et al. Invasive aspergillosis in critically ill patients without malignancy. Am J Respir Crit Care Med 2004; 170(6):621–5.
7. Morris A, Lundgren JD, Masur H, et al. Current epidemiology of Pneumocystis pneumonia. Emerg Infect Dis 2004;10(10):1713–20.
8. Marr KA, Carter RA, Crippa F, et al. Epidemiology and outcome of mould infections in hematopoietic stem cell transplant recipients. Clin Infect Dis 2002;34(7):909–17.
9. Husain S, Alexander BD, Munoz P, et al. Opportunistic mycelial fungal infections in organ transplant recipients: emerging importance of non-Aspergillus mycelial fungi. Clin Infect Dis 2003;37(2):221–9.

10. Morgan J, Meltzer MI, Plikaytis BD, et al. Excess mortality, hospital stay, and cost due to candidemia: a case-control study using data from population-based candidemia surveillance. Infect Control Hosp Epidemiol 2005;26(6):540–7.

11. Pelz RK, Lipsett PA, Swoboda SM, et al. Candida infections: outcome and attributable ICU costs in critically ill patients. J Intensive Care Med 2000;15(5):255–61.

12. Zaoutis TE, Argon J, Chu J, et al. The epidemiology and attributable outcomes of candidemia in adults and children hospitalized in the United States: a propensity analysis. Clin Infect Dis 2005;41(9):1232–9.

13. Wey SB, Mori M, Pfaller MA, et al. Hospital-acquired candidemia. The attributable mortality and excess length of stay. Arch Intern Med 1988;148(12):2642–5.

14. Gudlaugsson O, Gillespie S, Lee K, et al. Attributable mortality of nosocomial candidemia, revisited. Clin Infect Dis 2003;37(9):1172–7.

15. Puzniak L, Teutsch S, Powderly W, et al. Has the epidemiology of nosocomial candidemia changed? Infect Control Hosp Epidemiol 2004;25(8):628–33.

16. Shorr AF, Gupta V, Sun X, et al. Burden of early-onset candidemia: analysis of culture-positive bloodstream infections from a large U.S. database. Crit Care Med 2009;37(9):2519–26 [quiz: 2535].

17. Rentz AM, Halpern MT, Bowden R. The impact of candidemia on length of hospital stay, outcome, and overall cost of illness. Clin Infect Dis 1998;27(4):781–8.

18. Arnold HM, Micek ST, Shorr AF, et al. Hospital resource utilization and costs of inappropriate treatment of candidemia. Pharmacotherapy 2010;30(4):361–8.

19. Garey KW, Turpin RS, Bearden DT, et al. Economic analysis of inadequate fluconazole therapy in non-neutropenic patients with candidaemia: a multi-institutional study. Int J Antimicrob Agents 2007;29(5):557–62.

20. Zilberberg MD, Kollef MH, Arnold H, et al. Inappropriate empiric antifungal therapy for candidemia in the ICU and hospital resource utilization: a retrospective cohort study. BMC Infect Dis 2010;10:150.

21. Miller LG, Hajjeh RA, Edwards JE Jr. Estimating the cost of nosocomial candidemia in the United States. Clin Infect Dis 2001;32(7):1110.

22. Banerjee SN, Emori TG, Culver DH, et al. Secular trends in nosocomial primary bloodstream infections in the United States, 1980–1989. National Nosocomial Infections Surveillance System. Am J Med 1991;91(3B):86S–9S.

23. Martin GS, Mannino DM, Eaton S, et al. The epidemiology of sepsis in the United States from 1979 through 2000. N Engl J Med 2003;348(16):1546–54.

24. Zilberberg MD, Shorr AF, Kollef MH. Secular trends in candidemia-related hospitalization in the United States, 2000–2005. Infect Control Hosp Epidemiol 2008;29(10):978–80.

25. Snydman DR. Shifting patterns in the epidemiology of nosocomial Candida infections. Chest 2003;123(5 Suppl):500S–3S.

26. Pfaller MA, Diekema DJ, Rinaldi MG, et al. Results from the ARTEMIS DISK Global Antifungal Surveillance Study: a 6.5-year analysis of susceptibilities of Candida and other yeast species to fluconazole and voriconazole by standardized disk diffusion testing. J Clin Microbiol 2005;43(12):5848–59.

27. Rangel-Frausto MS, Wiblin T, Blumberg HM, et al. National epidemiology of mycoses survey (NEMIS): variations in rates of bloodstream infections due to Candida species in seven surgical intensive care units and six neonatal intensive care units. Clin Infect Dis 1999;29(2):253–8.

28. Trick WE, Fridkin SK, Edwards JR, et al. Secular trend of hospital-acquired candidemia among intensive care unit patients in the United States during 1989–1999. Clin Infect Dis 2002;35(5):627–30.

29. Bouza E, Munoz P. Epidemiology of candidemia in intensive care units. Int J Antimicrob Agents 2008;32(Suppl 2):S87–91.

30. Horn DL, Neofytos D, Anaissie EJ, et al. Epidemiology and outcomes of candidemia in 2019 patients: data from the prospective antifungal therapy alliance registry. Clin Infect Dis 2009;48(12):1695–703.

31. Nucci M, Queiroz-Telles F, Tobon AM, et al. Epidemiology of opportunistic fungal infections in Latin America. Clin Infect Dis 2010;51(5):561–70.

32. Kollef MH, Sherman G, Ward S, et al. Inadequate antimicrobial treatment of infections: a risk factor for hospital mortality among critically ill patients. Chest 1999;115(2):462–74.

33. Ibrahim EH, Sherman G, Ward S, et al. The influence of inadequate antimicrobial treatment of bloodstream infections on patient outcomes in the ICU setting. Chest 2000,118(1).146–55.

34. Kumar A, Roberts D, Wood KE, et al. Duration of hypotension before initiation of effective antimicrobial therapy is the critical determinant of survival in human septic shock. Crit Care Med 2006;34(6):1589–96.

35. Kumar A, Ellis P, Arabi Y, et al. Initiation of inappropriate antimicrobial therapy results in a fivefold reduction of survival in human septic shock. Chest 2009; 136(5):1237–48.

36. Leibovici L, Shraga I, Drucker M, et al. The benefit of appropriate empirical antibiotic treatment in patients with bloodstream infection. J Intern Med 1998; 244(5):379–86.

37. MacArthur RD, Miller M, Albertson T, et al. Adequacy of early empiric antibiotic treatment and survival in severe sepsis: experience from the MONARCS trial. Clin Infect Dis 2004;38(2):284–8.

38. Garnacho-Montero J, Ortiz-Leyba C, Herrera-Melero I, et al. Mortality and morbidity attributable to inadequate empirical antimicrobial therapy in patients admitted to the ICU with sepsis: a matched cohort study. J Antimicrob Chemother 2008;61(2):436–41.

39. Garnacho-Montero J, Garcia-Garmendia JL, Barrero-Almodovar A, et al. Impact of adequate empirical antibiotic therapy on the outcome of patients admitted to the intensive care unit with sepsis. Crit Care Med 2003;31(12):2742–51.

40. Fraser A, Paul M, Almanasreh N, et al. Benefit of appropriate empirical antibiotic treatment: thirty-day mortality and duration of hospital stay. Am J Med 2006; 119(11):970–6.

41. Valles J, Rello J, Ochagavia A, et al. Community-acquired bloodstream infection in critically ill adult patients: impact of shock and inappropriate antibiotic therapy on survival. Chest 2003;123(5):1615–24.

42. Blot SI, Vandewoude KH, Hoste EA, et al. Effects of nosocomial candidemia on outcomes of critically ill patients. Am J Med 2002;113(6):480–5.

43. Harbarth S, Ferriere K, Hugonnet S, et al. Epidemiology and prognostic determinants of bloodstream infections in surgical intensive care. Arch Surg 2002; 137(12):1353–9 [discussion: 1359].

44. Almirante B, Rodriguez D, Park BJ, et al. Epidemiology and predictors of mortality in cases of Candida bloodstream infection: results from population-based surveillance, Barcelona, Spain, from 2002 to 2003. J Clin Microbiol 2005;43(4):1829–35.

45. Morrell M, Fraser VJ, Kollef MH. Delaying the empiric treatment of Candida bloodstream infection until positive blood culture results are obtained: a potential risk factor for hospital mortality. Antimicrob Agents Chemother 2005;49(9): 3640–5.

46. Garey KW, Rege M, Pai MP, et al. Time to initiation of fluconazole therapy impacts mortality in patients with candidemia: a multi-institutional study. Clin Infect Dis 2000;43(1).25–31.

47. Parkins MD, Sabuda DM, Elsayed S, et al. Adequacy of empirical antifungal therapy and effect on outcome among patients with invasive *Candida* species infections. J Antimicrob Chemother 2007;60(3):613–8.

48. Patel GP, Simon D, Scheetz M, et al. The effect of time to antifungal therapy on mortality in candidemia associated septic shock. Am J Ther 2009;16(6):508–11.

49. Taur Y, Cohen N, Dubnow S, et al. Effect of antifungal therapy timing on mortality in cancer patients with candidemia. Antimicrob Agents Chemother 2010;54(1): 184–90.

50. Alexander BD, Pfaller MA. Contemporary tools for the diagnosis and management of invasive mycoses. Clin Infect Dis 2006;43(Suppl 1):15–27.

51. Ostrosky-Zeichner L, Pappas PG. Invasive candidiasis in the intensive care unit. Crit Care Med 2006;34(3):857–63.

52. Darouiche RO. Candida in the ICU. Clin Chest Med 2009;30(2):287–93, vi–vii.

53. Zilberberg MD, Shorr AF. Fungal infections in the ICU. Infect Dis Clin North Am 2009;23(3):625–42.

54. Berenguer J, Buck M, Witebsky F, et al. Lysis-centrifugation blood cultures in the detection of tissue-proven invasive candidiasis. Disseminated versus single-organ infection. Diagn Microbiol Infect Dis 1993;17(2):103–9.

55. Pappas PG. Invasive candidiasis. Infect Dis Clin North Am 2006;20(3):485–506.

56. Fernandez J, Erstad BL, Petty W, et al. Time to positive culture and identification for *Candida* blood stream infections. Diagn Microbiol Infect Dis 2009;64(4):402–7.

57. Ben-Ami R, Weinberger M, Orni-Wasserlauff R, et al. Time to blood culture positivity as a marker for catheter-related candidemia. J Clin Microbiol 2008;46(7):2222–6.

58. George BJ, Horvath LL, Hospenthal DR. Effect of inoculum size on detection of *Candida* growth by the BACTEC 9240 automated blood culture system using aerobic and anaerobic media. J Clin Microbiol 2005;43(1):433–5.

59. Horvath LL, George BJ, Murray CK, et al. Direct comparison of the BACTEC 9240 and BacT/ALERT 3D automated blood culture systems for candida growth detection. J Clin Microbiol 2004;42(1):115–8.

60. Sogaard M, Hjort U, Hojbjerg T, et al. Detection of candidaemia in high risk patients: can yield of blood cultures be improved by blind subculture? Scand J Infect Dis 2006;38(3):187–91.

61. Sendid B, Tabouret M, Poirot JL, et al. New enzyme immunoassays for sensitive detection of circulating *Candida albicans* mannan and antimannan antibodies: useful combined test for diagnosis of systemic candidiasis. J Clin Microbiol 1999;37(5):1510–7.

62. Yera H, Sendid B, Francois N, et al. Contribution of serological tests and blood culture to the early diagnosis of systemic candidiasis. Eur J Clin Microbiol Infect Dis 2001;20(12):864–70.

63. Ostrosky-Zeichner L, Alexander BD, Kett DH, et al. Multicenter clinical evaluation of the $(1\rightarrow3)$ beta-D-glucan assay as an aid to diagnosis of fungal infections in humans. Clin Infect Dis 2005;41(5):654–9.

64. McMullan R, Metwally L, Coyle PV, et al. A prospective clinical trial of a real-time polymerase chain reaction assay for the diagnosis of candidemia in nonneutropenic, critically ill adults. Clin Infect Dis 2008;46(6):890–6.

65. Vince A, Lepej SZ, Barsic B, et al. LightCycler SeptiFast assay as a tool for the rapid diagnosis of sepsis in patients during antimicrobial therapy. J Med Microbiol 2008;57(Pt 10):1306–7.

66. Yanagihara K, Kitagawa Y, Tomonaga M, et al. Evaluation of pathogen detection from clinical samples by real-time polymerase chain reaction using a sepsis pathogen DNA detection kit. Crit Care 2010;14(4):R159.
67. Avni T, Leibovici L, Paul M. PCR diagnosis of invasive candidiasis: systematic review and meta-analysis. J Clin Microbiol 2010;48(2):489–96.
68. Wey SB, Mori M, Pfaller MA, et al. Risk factors for hospital-acquired candidemia. A matched case-control study. Arch Intern Med 1989;149(10):2349–53.
69. Blumberg HM, Jarvis WR, Soucie JM, et al. Risk factors for candidal bloodstream infections in surgical intensive care unit patients: the NEMIS prospective multicenter study. The National Epidemiology of Mycosis Survey. Clin Infect Dis 2001;33(2):177–86.
70. Diekema DJ, Pfaller MA. Nosocomial candidemia: an ounce of prevention is better than a pound of cure. Infect Control Hosp Epidemiol 2004;25(8):624–6.
71. Munoz P, Burillo A, Bouza E. Criteria used when initiating antifungal therapy against Candida spp. in the intensive care unit. Int J Antimicrob Agents 2000; 15(2):83–90.
72. Ostrosky-Zeichner L. New approaches to the risk of Candida in the intensive care unit. Curr Opin Infect Dis 2003;16(6):533–7.
73. Ostrosky-Zeichner L. Prophylaxis and treatment of invasive candidiasis in the intensive care setting. Eur J Clin Microbiol Infect Dis 2004;23(10):739–44.
74. Paphitou NI, Ostrosky-Zeichner L, Rex JH. Rules for identifying patients at increased risk for candidal infections in the surgical intensive care unit: approach to developing practical criteria for systematic use in antifungal prophylaxis trials. Med Mycol 2005;43(3):235–43.
75. Sobel JD, Rex JH. Invasive candidiasis: turning risk into a practical prevention policy? Clin Infect Dis 2001;33(2):187–90.
76. Piarroux R, Grenouillet F, Balvay P, et al. Assessment of preemptive treatment to prevent severe candidiasis in critically ill surgical patients. Crit Care Med 2004; 32(12):2443–9.
77. Wenzel RP. Nosocomial candidemia: risk factors and attributable mortality. Clin Infect Dis 1995;20(6):1531–4.
78. Wenzel RP, Gennings C. Bloodstream infections due to Candida species in the intensive care unit: identifying especially high-risk patients to determine prevention strategies. Clin Infect Dis 2005;41(Suppl 6):S389–93.
79. Guery BP, Arendrup MC, Auzinger G, et al. Management of invasive candidiasis and candidemia in adult non-neutropenic intensive care unit patients: part I. Epidemiology and diagnosis. Intensive Care Med 2009;35(1):55–62.
80. Chow JK, Golan Y, Ruthazer R, et al. Risk factors for albicans and non-albicans candidemia in the intensive care unit. Crit Care Med 2008;36(7): 1993–8.
81. Hoerauf A, Hammer S, Muller-Myhsok B, et al. Intra-abdominal Candida infection during acute necrotizing pancreatitis has a high prevalence and is associated with increased mortality. Crit Care Med 1998;26(12):2010–5.
82. Pyrgos V, Ratanavanich K, Donegan N, et al. Candida bloodstream infections in hemodialysis recipients. Med Mycol 2009;47(5):463–7.
83. Fraser VJ, Jones M, Dunkel J, et al. Candidemia in a tertiary care hospital: epidemiology, risk factors, and predictors of mortality. Clin Infect Dis 1992; 15(3):414–21.
84. Marr KA, Seidel K, White TC, et al. Candidemia in allogeneic blood and marrow transplant recipients: evolution of risk factors after the adoption of prophylactic fluconazole. J Infect Dis 2000;181(1):309–16.

85. Dupont H, Bourichon A, Paugam-Burtz C, et al. Can yeast isolation in peritoneal fluid be predicted in intensive care unit patients with peritonitis? Crit Care Med 2003;31(3):752–7.

86. Prentice HG, Kibbler CC, Prentice AG. Towards a targeted, risk-based, antifungal strategy in neutropenic patients. Br J Haematol 2000;110(2):273–84.

87. Pittet D, Monod M, Suter PM, et al. *Candida* colonization and subsequent infections in critically ill surgical patients. Ann Surg 1994;220(6):751–8.

88. Leon C, Ruiz-Santana S, Saavedra P, et al. A bedside scoring system ("Candida score") for early antifungal treatment in nonneutropenic critically ill patients with *Candida* colonization. Crit Care Med 2006;34(3):730–7.

89. Leon C, Ruiz-Santana S, Saavedra P, et al. Usefulness of the "Candida score" for discriminating between *Candida* colonization and invasive candidiasis in non-neutropenic critically ill patients: a prospective multicenter study. Crit Care Med 2009;37(5):1624–33.

90. Ostrosky-Zeichner L, Sable C, Sobel J, et al. Multicenter retrospective development and validation of a clinical prediction rule for nosocomial invasive candidiasis in the intensive care setting. Eur J Clin Microbiol Infect Dis 2007;26(4):271–6.

91. Faiz S, Neale B, Rios E, et al. Risk-based fluconazole prophylaxis of *Candida* bloodstream infection in a medical intensive care unit. Eur J Clin Microbiol Infect Dis 2009;28(6):689–92.

92. ClinicalTrials.gov. Randomized study of caspofungin prophylaxis followed by pre-emptive therapy for invasive candidiasis in the ICU (MSG-01) 2010. Available at: http://clinicaltrials.gov/ct2/show/NCT00520234. Accessed August 23, 2010.

93. Andes D. Pharmacokinetics and pharmacodynamics of antifungals. Infect Dis Clin North Am 2006;20(3):679–97.

94. Denning DW. Echinocandin antifungal drugs. Lancet 2003;362(9390):1142–51.

95. Dodds Ashley ES, Lewis R, Lewis JS, et al. Pharmacology of systemic antifungal agents. Clin Infect Dis 2006;43:S28–39.

96. Pfaller MA, Diekema DJ, Gibbs DL, et al. Geographic variation in the frequency of isolation and fluconazole and voriconazole susceptibilities of *Candida glabrata*: an assessment from the ARTEMIS DISK Global Antifungal Surveillance Program. Diagn Microbiol Infect Dis 2010;67(2):162–71.

97. Pfaller MA, Diekema DJ, Gibbs DL, et al. Results from the ARTEMIS DISK Global Antifungal Surveillance Study, 1997 to 2005: an 8.5-year analysis of susceptibilities of *Candida* species and other yeast species to fluconazole and voriconazole determined by CLSI standardized disk diffusion testing. J Clin Microbiol 2007;45(6):1735–45.

98. Mora-Duarte J, Betts R, Rotstein C, et al. Comparison of caspofungin and amphotericin B for invasive candidiasis. N Engl J Med 2002;347(25):2020–9.

99. Kabbara N, Lacroix C, Peffault de Latour R, et al. Breakthrough *C. parapsilosis* and *C. guilliermondii* blood stream infections in allogeneic hematopoietic stem cell transplant recipients receiving long-term caspofungin therapy. Haematologica 2008;93(4):639–40.

100. Brielmaier BD, Casabar E, Kurtzeborn CM, et al. Early clinical experience with anidulafungin at a large tertiary care medical center. Pharmacotherapy 2008; 28(1):64–73.

101. Forrest GN, Weekes E, Johnson JK. Increasing incidence of *Candida parapsilosis* candidemia with caspofungin usage. J Infect 2008;56(2):126–9.

102. Cheung C, Guo Y, Gialanella P, et al. Development of candidemia on caspofungin therapy: a case report. Infection 2006;34(6):345–8.

103. Pfeiffer CD, Garcia-Effron G, Zaas AK, et al. Breakthrough invasive candidiasis in patients on micafungin. J Clin Microbiol 2010;48(7):2373–80.
104. Rex JH, Bennett JE, Sugar AM, et al. A randomized trial comparing fluconazole with amphotericin B for the treatment of candidemia in patients without neutropenia. Candidemia Study Group and the National Institute. N Engl J Med 1994;331(20):1325–30.
105. Rex JH, Pappas PG, Karchmer AW, et al. A randomized and blinded multicenter trial of high-dose fluconazole plus placebo versus fluconazole plus amphotericin B as therapy for candidemia and its consequences in nonneutropenic subjects. Clin Infect Dis 2003;36(10):1221–8.
106. Kullberg BJ, Sobel JD, Ruhnke M, et al. Voriconazole versus a regimen of amphotericin B followed by fluconazole for candidaemia in non-neutropenic patients: a randomised non-inferiority trial. Lancet 2005;366(9495):1435–42.
107. Reboli AC, Rotstein C, Pappas PG, et al. Anidulafungin versus fluconazole for invasive candidiasis. N Engl J Med 2007;356(24):2472–82.
108. Kuse ER, Chetchotisakd P, da Cunha CA, et al. Micafungin versus liposomal amphotericin B for candidaemia and invasive candidosis: a phase III randomised double-blind trial. Lancet 2007;369(9572):1519–27.
109. Pappas PG, Rotstein CM, Betts RF, et al. Micafungin versus caspofungin for treatment of candidemia and other forms of invasive candidiasis. Clin Infect Dis 2007;45(7):883–93.
110. Pappas PG, Kauffman CA, Andes D, et al. Clinical practice guidelines for the management of candidiasis: 2009 update by the Infectious Diseases Society of America. Clin Infect Dis 2009;48(5):503–35.
111. Andes DR, Safdar N, Baddley J, et al. Impact of therapy on mortality across Candida spp in patients with invasive candidiasis from randomized clinical trials: a patient level analysis. Paper presented at: Interscience Conference on Antimicrobial Agents and Chemotherapy. Boston (MA), September 12–15, 2010.
112. Eriksson U, Seifert B, Schaffner A. Comparison of effects of amphotericin B deoxycholate infused over 4 or 24 hours: randomised controlled trial. BMJ 2001;322(7286):579–82.
113. Uehara RP, Sa VH, Koshimura ET, et al. Continuous infusion of amphotericin B: preliminary experience at Faculdade de Medicina da Fundacao ABC. Sao Paulo Med J 2005;123(5):219–22.
114. Speich R, Dutly A, Naef R, et al. Tolerability, safety and efficacy of conventional amphotericin B administered by 24-hour infusion to lung transplant recipients. Swiss Med Wkly 2002;132(31–32):455–8.
115. Schulenburg A, Sperr W, Rabitsch W, et al. Brief report: practicability and safety of amphotericin B deoxycholate as continuous infusion in neutropenic patients with hematological malignancies. Leuk Lymphoma 2005;46(8):1163–7.
116. Peleg AY, Woods ML. Continuous and 4 h infusion of amphotericin B: a comparative study involving high-risk haematology patients. J Antimicrob Chemother 2004;54(4):803–8.
117. Falci DR, Lunardi LW, Ramos CG, et al. Continuous infusion of amphotericin B deoxycholate in the treatment of cryptococcal meningoencephalitis: analysis of safety and fungicidal activity. Clin Infect Dis 2010;50(5):e26–9.
118. Imhof A, Walter RB, Schaffner A. Continuous infusion of escalated doses of amphotericin B deoxycholate: an open-label observational study. Clin Infect Dis 2003;36(8):943–51.
119. Kethireddy S, Andes D. CNS pharmacokinetics of antifungal agents. Expert Opin Drug Metab Toxicol 2007;3(4):573–81.

120. Andes D, Safdar N, Marchillo K, et al. Pharmacokinetic-pharmacodynamic comparison of amphotericin B (AMB) and two lipid-associated AMB preparations, liposomal AMB and AMB lipid complex, in murine candidiasis models. Antimicrob Agents Chemother 2006;50(2):674–84.

121. Groll AH, Lyman CA, Petraitis V, et al. Compartmentalized intrapulmonary pharmacokinetics of amphotericin B and its lipid formulations. Antimicrob Agents Chemother 2006;50(10):3418–23.

122. Groll AH, Giri N, Petraitis V, et al. Comparative efficacy and distribution of lipid formulations of amphotericin B in experimental *Candida albicans* infection of the central nervous system. J Infect Dis 2000;182(1):274–82.

123. Lewis RE, Liao G, Hou J, et al. Comparative analysis of amphotericin B lipid complex and liposomal amphotericin B kinetics of lung accumulation and fungal clearance in a murine model of acute invasive pulmonary aspergillosis. Antimicrob Agents Chemother 2007;51(4):1253–8.

124. Janknegt R, de Marie S, Bakker-Woudenberg IA, et al. Liposomal and lipid formulations of amphotericin B. Clinical pharmacokinetics. Clin Pharmacokinet 1992;23(4):279–91.

125. Brooks RG. Prospective study of *Candida* endophthalmitis in hospitalized patients with candidemia. Arch Intern Med 1989;149(10):2226–8.

126. Gauthier GM, Nork TM, Prince R, et al. Subtherapeutic ocular penetration of caspofungin and associated treatment failure in *Candida albicans* endophthalmitis. Clin Infect Dis 2005;41(3):e27–8.

127. Klevay MJ, Horn DL, Neofytos D, et al. Initial treatment and outcome of *Candida glabrata* versus *Candida albicans* bloodstream infection. Diagn Microbiol Infect Dis 2009;64(2):152–7.

128. Craig WA. Pharmacokinetic/pharmacodynamic parameters: rationale for antibacterial dosing of mice and men. Clin Infect Dis 1998;26(1):1–10 [quiz: 11–2].

129. Kumar A. Optimizing antimicrobial therapy in sepsis and septic shock. Crit Care Clin 2009;25(4):733–51, viii.

130. Lepak A, Andes D. Pharmacodynamics of antifungal drugs: a strategy to optimize efficacy. Curr Fungal Infect Rep 2008;2:12–9.

131. Andes D, Stamsted T, Conklin R. Pharmacodynamics of amphotericin B in a neutropenic-mouse disseminated-candidiasis model. Antimicrob Agents Chemother 2001;45(3):922–6.

132. Lewis RE, Wiederhold NP, Klepser ME. In vitro pharmacodynamics of amphotericin B, itraconazole, and voriconazole against *Aspergillus*, *Fusarium*, and *Scedosporium* spp. Antimicrob Agents Chemother 2005;49(3):945–51.

133. Ernst EJ, Klepser ME, Pfaller MA. Postantifungal effects of echinocandin, azole, and polyene antifungal agents against *Candida albicans* and *Cryptococcus neoformans*. Antimicrob Agents Chemother 2000;44(4):1108–11.

134. Turnidge JD, Gudmundsson S, Vogelman B, et al. The postantibiotic effect of antifungal agents against common pathogenic yeasts. J Antimicrob Chemother 1994;34(1):83–92.

135. Hong Y, Shaw PJ, Nath CE, et al. Population pharmacokinetics of liposomal amphotericin B in pediatric patients with malignant diseases. Antimicrob Agents Chemother 2006;50(3):935–42.

136. Andes D, van Ogtrop M. Characterization and quantitation of the pharmacodynamics of fluconazole in a neutropenic murine disseminated candidiasis infection model. Antimicrob Agents Chemother 1999;43(9):2116–20.

137. Louie A, Drusano GL, Banerjee P, et al. Pharmacodynamics of fluconazole in a murine model of systemic candidiasis. Antimicrob Agents Chemother 1998; 42(5):1105–9.

138. Klepser ME, Malone D, Lewis RE, et al. Evaluation of voriconazole pharmacodynamics using time-kill methodology. Antimicrob Agents Chemother 2000;44(7): 1917–20.
139. Andes D, Marchillo K, Stamstad T, et al. In vivo pharmacokinetics and pharmacodynamics of a new triazole, voriconazole, in a murine candidiasis model. Antimicrob Agents Chemother 2003;47(10):3165–9.
140. Andes D, Marchillo K, Stamstad T, et al. In vivo pharmacodynamics of a new triazole, ravuconazole, in a murine candidiasis model. Antimicrob Agents Chemother 2003;47(4):1193–9.
141. Andes D, Marchillo K, Conklin R, et al. Pharmacodynamics of a new triazole, posaconazole, in a murine model of disseminated candidiasis. Antimicrob Agents Chemother 2004;48(1):137–42.
142. Baddley JW, Patel M, Bhavnani SM, et al. Association of fluconazole pharmacodynamics with mortality in patients with candidemia. Antimicrob Agents Chemother 2008;52(9):3022–8.
143. Clancy CJ, Yu VL, Morris AJ, et al. Fluconazole MIC and the fluconazole dose/MIC ratio correlate with therapeutic response among patients with candidemia. Antimicrob Agents Chemother 2005;49(8):3171–7.
144. Lee SC, Fung CP, Huang JS, et al. Clinical correlates of antifungal macrodilution susceptibility test results for non-AIDS patients with severe Candida infections treated with fluconazole. Antimicrob Agents Chemother 2000;44(10):2715–8.
145. Pai MP, Turpin RS, Garey KW. Association of fluconazole area under the concentration-time curve/MIC and dose/MIC ratios with mortality in nonneutropenic patients with candidemia. Antimicrob Agents Chemother 2007;51(1):35–9.
146. Rex JH, Pfaller MA, Galgiani JN, et al. Development of interpretive breakpoints for antifungal susceptibility testing: conceptual framework and analysis of in vitro-in vivo correlation data for fluconazole, itraconazole, and candida infections. Subcommittee on Antifungal Susceptibility Testing of the National Committee for Clinical Laboratory Standards. Clin Infect Dis 1997;24(2):235–47.
147. Rodriguez-Tudela JL, Almirante B, Rodriguez-Pardo D, et al. Correlation of the MIC and dose/MIC ratio of fluconazole to the therapeutic response of patients with mucosal candidiasis and candidemia. Antimicrob Agents Chemother 2007;51(10):3599–604.
148. Takakura S, Fujihara N, Saito T, et al. Clinical factors associated with fluconazole resistance and short-term survival in patients with Candida bloodstream infection. Eur J Clin Microbiol Infect Dis 2004;23(5):380–8.
149. Pfaller MA, Andes D, Diekema DJ, et al. Wild-type MIC distributions, epidemiological cutoff values and species-specific clinical breakpoints for fluconazole and Candida: time for harmonization of CLSI and EUCAST broth microdilution methods. Paper presented at: Interscience Conference on Antimicrobial Agents and Chemotherapy. Boston (MA), September 12–15, 2010.
150. Pfaller MA, Diekema DJ, Rex JH, et al. Correlation of MIC with outcome for Candida species tested against voriconazole: analysis and proposal for interpretive breakpoints. J Clin Microbiol 2006;44(3):819–26.
151. Pascual A, Calandra T, Bolay S, et al. Voriconazole therapeutic drug monitoring in patients with invasive mycoses improves efficacy and safety outcomes. Clin Infect Dis 2008;46(2):201–11.
152. Smith J, Safdar N, Knasinski V, et al. Voriconazole therapeutic drug monitoring. Antimicrob Agents Chemother 2006;50(4):1570–2.
153. Denning DW, Ribaud P, Milpied N, et al. Efficacy and safety of voriconazole in the treatment of acute invasive aspergillosis. Clin Infect Dis 2002;34(5):563–71.

154. Trifilio S, Pennick G, Pi J, et al. Monitoring plasma voriconazole levels may be necessary to avoid subtherapeutic levels in hematopoietic stem cell transplant recipients. Cancer 2007;109(8):1532–5.

155. Andes D, Pascual A, Marchetti O. Antifungal therapeutic drug monitoring: established and emerging indications. Antimicrob Agents Chemother 2009;53(1):24–34.

156. Andes D, Marchillo K, Lowther J, et al. In vivo pharmacodynamics of HMR 3270, a glucan synthase inhibitor, in a murine candidiasis model. Antimicrob Agents Chemother 2003;47(4):1187–92.

157. Andes D, Diekema DJ, Pfaller MA, et al. In vivo pharmacodynamic characterization of anidulafungin in a neutropenic murine candidiasis model. Antimicrob Agents Chemother 2008;52(2):539–50.

158. Andes DR, Diekema DJ, Pfaller MA, et al. In vivo pharmacodynamic target investigation for micafungin against *Candida albicans* and *C. glabrata* in a neutropenic murine candidiasis model. Antimicrob Agents Chemother 2008;52(10):3497–503.

159. Ernst EJ, Roling EE, Petzold CR, et al. In vitro activity of micafungin (FK-463) against *Candida* spp.: microdilution, time-kill, and postantifungal-effect studies. Antimicrob Agents Chemother 2002;46(12):3846–53.

160. Gumbo T, Drusano GL, Liu W, et al. Anidulafungin pharmacokinetics and microbial response in neutropenic mice with disseminated candidiasis. Antimicrob Agents Chemother 2006;50(11):3695–700.

161. Gumbo T, Drusano GL, Liu W, et al. Once-weekly micafungin therapy is as effective as daily therapy for disseminated candidiasis in mice with persistent neutropenia. Antimicrob Agents Chemother 2007;51(3):968–74.

162. Louie A, Deziel M, Liu W, et al. Pharmacodynamics of caspofungin in a murine model of systemic candidiasis: importance of persistence of caspofungin in tissues to understanding drug activity. Antimicrob Agents Chemother 2005; 49(12):5058–68.

163. Walsh TJ, Lee JW, Kelly P, et al. Antifungal effects of the nonlinear pharmacokinetics of cilofungin, a 1,3-beta-glucan synthetase inhibitor, during continuous and intermittent intravenous infusions in treatment of experimental disseminated candidiasis. Antimicrob Agents Chemother 1991;35(7):1321–8.

164. Pfaller MA, Diekema DJ, Andes D, et al. Clinical breakpoints for the echinocandins and *Candida* revisited: integration of molecular, clinical, and microbiological data to arrive at species-specific interpretive criteria. Clin Microbiol Rev, in press.

165. Andes D, Diekema DJ, Pfaller MA, et al. In vivo comparison of the pharmacodynamic targets for echinocandin drugs against *Candida* species. Antimicrob Agents Chemother 2010;54(6):2497–506.

166. Ambrose PG, Bhavnani SM, Rubino CM, et al. Pharmacokinetics-pharmacodynamics of antimicrobial therapy: it's not just for mice anymore. Clin Infect Dis 2007;44(1):79–86.

167. Pfaller MA, Diekema DJ, Ostrosky-Zeichner L, et al. Correlation of MIC with outcome for *Candida* species tested against caspofungin, anidulafungin, and micafungin: analysis and proposal for interpretive MIC breakpoints. J Clin Microbiol 2008;46(8):2620–9.

168. Andes DR, Ambrose PG, Hammel JP, et al. Exposure-response (E-R) relationships for efficacy of micafungin in patients with invasive candidiasis (IC). Paper presented at: Interscience Conference on Antimicrobial Agents and Chemotherapy. San Francisco, September 12–15, 2009.

169. Clinical breakpoints for *Candida* and the echinocandins. Clinical and Laboratory Standards Institute Subcommittee on Antifungal Susceptibility Tests. Atlanta 2010.

170. Mermel LA, Allon M, Bouza E, et al. Clinical practice guidelines for the diagnosis and management of intravascular catheter-related infection: 2009 Update by the Infectious Diseases Society of America. Clin Infect Dis 2009;49(1):1–45.

171. Mermel LA, Farr BM, Sherertz RJ, et al. Guidelines for the management of intravascular catheter-related infections. Clin Infect Dis 2001;32(9):1249–72.

172. Nucci M, Colombo AL, Silveira F, et al. Risk factors for death in patients with candidemia. Infect Control Hosp Epidemiol 1998;19(11):846–50.

173. Pasqualotto AC, de Moraes AB, Zanini RR, et al. Analysis of independent risk factors for death among pediatric patients with candidemia and a central venous catheter in place. Infect Control Hosp Epidemiol 2007;28(7):799–804.

174. Labelle AJ, Micek ST, Roubinian N, et al. Treatment-related risk factors for hospital mortality in *Candida* bloodstream infections. Crit Care Med 2008; 36(11).2967–72.

175. Raad I, Hanna H, Boktour M, et al. Management of central venous catheters in patients with cancer and candidemia. Clin Infect Dis 2004;38(8):1119–27.

176. Rex JH, Bennett JE, Sugar AM, et al. Intravascular catheter exchange and duration of candidemia. NIAID Mycoses Study Group and the Candidemia Study Group. Clin Infect Dis 1995;21(4):994–6.

177. Liu CY, Huang LJ, Wang WS, et al. Candidemia in cancer patients: impact of early removal of non-tunneled central venous catheters on outcome. J Infect 2009;58(2):154–60.

178. Horn DL, Ostrosky-Zeichner L, Morris MI, et al. Factors related to survival and treatment success in invasive candidiasis or candidemia: a pooled analysis of two large, prospective, micafungin trials. Eur J Clin Microbiol Infect Dis 2010; 29(2):223–9.

179. Nucci M, Silveira MI, Spector N, et al. Risk factors for death among cancer patients with fungemia. Clin Infect Dis 1998;27(1):107–11.

180. Rodriguez D, Park BJ, Almirante B, et al. Impact of early central venous catheter removal on outcome in patients with candidaemia. Clin Microbiol Infect 2007; 13(8):788–93.

181. Velasco E, Bigni R. A prospective cohort study evaluating the prognostic impact of clinical characteristics and comorbid conditions of hospitalized adult and pediatric cancer patients with candidemia. Eur J Clin Microbiol Infect Dis 2008;27(11):1071–8.

182. Weinberger M, Leibovici L, Perez S, et al. Characteristics of candidaemia with *Candida albicans* compared with non-albicans *Candida* species and predictors of mortality. J Hosp Infect 2005;61(2):146–54.

183. Nucci M, Anaissie E, Betts RF, et al. Early removal of central venous catheter in patients with candidemia does not improve outcome: analysis of 842 patients from 2 randomized clinical trials. Clin Infect Dis 2010;51(3):295–303.

184. Essman TF, Flynn HW Jr, Smiddy WE, et al. Treatment outcomes in a 10-year study of endogenous fungal endophthalmitis. Ophthalmic Surg Lasers 1997; 28(3):185–94.

185. Rex JH, Sobel JD. Prophylactic antifungal therapy in the intensive care unit. Clin Infect Dis 2001;32(8):1191–200.

186. Viscoli C. Antifungal prophylaxis and pre-emptive therapy. Drugs 2009;69(Suppl 1): 75–8.

187. Playford EG, Lipman J, Sorrell TC. Prophylaxis, empirical and preemptive treatment of invasive candidiasis. Curr Opin Crit Care 2010;16(5):470–4.

188. Rotstein C. Invasive candidiasis in the ICU: prophylaxis versus preemptive treatment. Curr Infect Dis Rep 2008;10(6):454–8.

189. Playford EG, Webster AC, Sorrell TC, et al. Antifungal agents for preventing fungal infections in non-neutropenic critically ill and surgical patients: systematic review and meta-analysis of randomized clinical trials. J Antimicrob Chemother 2006;57(4):628–38.

190. Cruciani M, de Lalla F, Mengoli C. Prophylaxis of *Candida* infections in adult trauma and surgical intensive care patients: a systematic review and meta-analysis. Intensive Care Med 2005;31(11):1479–87.

191. Ho KM, Lipman J, Dobb GJ, et al. The use of prophylactic fluconazole in immunocompetent high-risk surgical patients: a meta-analysis. Crit Care 2005; 9(6):R710–7.

192. Hughes WT, Armstrong D, Bodey GP, et al. 2002 guidelines for the use of antimicrobial agents in neutropenic patients with cancer. Clin Infect Dis 2002; 34(6):730–51.

193. Schuster MG, Edwards JE Jr, Sobel JD, et al. Empirical fluconazole versus placebo for intensive care unit patients: a randomized trial. Ann Intern Med 2008;149(2):83–90.

Antibiotic De-Escalation

Robert G. Masterton, FRCPath, FRCP [Edin & Glas]

KEYWORDS

- De-escalation • Antimicrobial streamlining
- Antimicrobial stewardship

The present topography of clinical sepsis is a landscape populated by increasing and developing antimicrobial resistance, with a future where ever fewer new antibiotics, particularly innovative classes,[1] are becoming available to meet these challenges. This prospect has resulted in a new focus on making the best use of the antibiotics available to maximize their clinical impact and longevity. Such initiatives have become condensed into 2 main themes that are integrated, with the new treatment paradigm that deals with serious sepsis, of "hit it hard and hit early"[2] being embedded within the overall encompassing concept of antimicrobial stewardship.[3]

De-escalation forms one of the key features of the new treatment paradigm (**Box 1**). Within this paradigm de-escalation presents probably the most challenging element. Notwithstanding this, the literature shows that de-escalation has received widespread support in various review and recommendation documents[4–6] over the last decade, but in a manner that perhaps does not reflect its true standing against the difficulties attendant to its implementation. Whereas its step-down concept of changing to a more targeted antibiotic is intrinsically logical, in clinical practice it faces the natural instinct of the clinician to continue with a treatment that is proving to be effective in managing the often life-threatening infection affecting a patient. This remains true, notwithstanding the positive conclusion reached within the recently released guidelines on antimicrobial stewardship[3] stating that: "Streamlining or de-escalation of empirical antimicrobial therapy on the basis of culture results and elimination of redundant combination therapy can more effectively target the causative pathogen, resulting in decreased antimicrobial exposure and substantial cost savings."

Crucially, whereas the strength of this recommendation was assigned the top rating of an "A", it was acknowledged that the quality of the clinical evidence underpinning this was only in the middle band. This article therefore reviews the issue of de-escalation to present the current position.

Financial disclosures and/or conflicts of interest: The author has nothing to disclose against the subject matter and materials discussed in this article.
Funding support: None.
Department of Microbiology, Ayrshire & Arran NHS Board, The Ayr Hospital, Dalmellington Road, Ayr KA6 6DX, UK
E-mail address: robert.masterton@aaaht.scot.nhs.uk

Crit Care Clin 27 (2011) 149–162
doi:10.1016/j.ccc.2010.09.009
0749-0704/11/$ – see front matter

Box 1
Key principles of the new treatment paradigm

- Get effective antibiotic selection right first time
- Base antimicrobial selection, both empiric and targeted, on knowledge of local susceptibility patterns
- Use broad-spectrum antibiotics early
- Optimize the antibiotic dose and route of administration
- Administer antibiotics for the shortest possible duration

AND

- Adjust or stop antibiotic therapy as early as possible to best target the pathogen(s) and remove pressure for resistance development (ie, de-escalation)

DEFINITION OF DE-ESCALATION

The definition of antimicrobial de-escalation is that it is a mechanism whereby the provision of effective initial antibiotic treatment, particularly in cases of severe sepsis, is achieved while avoiding unnecessary antibiotic use that would promote the development of resistance. This definition therefore encompasses 2 key features. First, there is the intent to narrow the spectrum of antimicrobial coverage depending on clinical response, culture results, and susceptibilities of the pathogens identified, and second, there is the commitment to stop antimicrobial treatment if no infection is established.[7] Vidaur and colleagues[8] added to this the criterion that where possible a single rather than multiple antibiotics should be used. The problem as it relates to clinical practice is the lack of convincing trial evidence demonstrating that de-escalation does not result in a poorer clinical outcome. Solid study data establishing exactly what criteria should be used, and when, to determine changing and stopping therapy do not exist.

ANTICIPATED BENEFITS FROM DE-ESCALATION

When considering de-escalation studies, it is important to be aware of the benefits that this approach is intended to produce (**Box 2**). Perhaps, peculiarly in assessing therapeutic management lines, the key feature for the studies to date in response to the challenges described above has been to show no detriment to individual patients rather than a potential improvement in clinical outcome. The primary focus of de-escalation is actually to demonstrate longer-term benefits through a positive impact on

---

Box 2
Benefits realization in de-escalation therapy

- Treatment outcomes are unaltered from the conventional therapy approach of maintaining patients on their initially selected antimicrobials
- There is a beneficial impact observed through surveillance on the antimicrobial resistance profile for the institution at both micro and macro level
- Decrease in antibiotic related adverse events, for example, the incidence of *Clostridium difficile* infection and/or of superinfection with resistant bacteria and *Candida* organisms
- There is a reduction in overall antimicrobial costs

antibiotic resistance development, with a significant secondary goal being financial savings through improved cost effectiveness.

THE EVIDENCE FROM CLINICAL DE-ESCALATION STUDIES

The overwhelming majority of the clinical studies assessing patient outcomes performed to date have been focused on nosocomial pneumonia (NP), especially ventilator-associated pneumonia (VAP). Their findings are reviewed in **Table 1**. The table begins with the seminal short-course antibiotic treatment study of Singh and colleagues.[9] Although not normally found on a literature search for articles on de-escalation, it is among the first and strongest examples of de-escalating therapy to a stop when infection is assessed as not being present.

There are some further studies reported that are not presented in **Table 1**, which are very few and diverse. These studies demonstrate centers beginning to expand the boundaries, including the difficulties of evaluating de-escalation outside the narrow field of NP. A prospective audit among 72 hospital inpatients suffering from amoxicillin-susceptible *Escherichia coli* infection in blood and/or urine[17] found that only 19% of those who could be de-escalated to amoxicillin actually received this agent. Amongst the 54% who had their antibiotic changed 64% of these were actually moved, perversely, to an unnecessarily broad-spectrum agent, and in 10% this was actually to a drug reported to be resistant. The investigators concluded that successful implementation of de-escalation demands more than simple protocol distribution. In another recent study that explored the practical application of de-escalation,[18] data from 113 intensive care unit (ICU) meropenem prescriptions were evaluated. De-escalation was defined as the administration of an antibiotic with a narrower spectrum within 3 days of the start of meropenem. The study found a trend toward a lower mortality rate (7% vs 21%, $P = .12$) in patients who had been de-escalated. The majority of the infections were either pneumonia (46%) or intra-abdominal (31%). De-escalation was performed in 42% of patients, with the most common reasons for not doing so being the absence of conclusive microbiology or colonization with a multiresistant gram-negative bacillus. Finally, a retrospective study[19] has explored the issue of de-escalation in 102 cases of health care–associated pneumonia where high-quality samples from intubation were not available and the microbiology findings were culture negative. The Pneumonia Severity Index was used for risk adjustment. The findings were that de-escalation occurred in 75% and 77% of the culture-negative and -positive groups, respectively ($P = 1.00$). However, in culture-negative cases de-escalation took place approximately 1 day earlier (3.93 vs 5.04 days, $P = .03$) and this group also showed a shorter length of hospitalization, lower hospital costs, and lower mortality rates.

In the vast majority of the studies presented, the exact time to re-evaluation with a view to de-escalation was not set, which tended to reflect the time taken for the results to become available. In most studies, and against a continuous evaluation of the clinical response of the patient, microbiology results became available at around 48 to 72 hours, and this seems to be a pragmatic and sensible approach. However, the results[20] of a university hospital ICU are illuminating in this regard because they showed that although de-escalation was successfully implemented in 69% of patients for whom the microbiological data supported this, there was a mean interval of around 48 hours from the microbiological data being available to de-escalation action being taken.

BENEFITS REALIZATION IN DE-ESCALATION PRACTICE

Based on the clinical evidence from the now significant numbers of studies that have been performed, it is reasonable to conclude, given the consistency of these data, that

Table 1
De-escalation studies in nosocomial and ventilator-associated pneumonia

Year[Reference]	Principal Features of Study Design	Brief Methodology Overview	Principal Findings Relevant to De-Escalation
2000[9]	Randomized prospective trial involving 81 patients to minimize unnecessary antibiotic by using the clinical pulmonary infection score (CPIS) to assess ventilator-associated pneumonia (VAP) as operational tool for antibiotic therapy decision-making	Quantitative bronchoalveolar lavage (BAL) used for diagnosis. Patients with CPIS ≤6 (implying low likelihood of pneumonia) received either standard therapy (antibiotic choice and duration physician discretion) or the study group with ciprofloxacin monotherapy with reevaluation at day 3 when ciprofloxacin was discontinued if CPIS remained ≤6	Antibiotics continued beyond day 3 in 90% of those on standard approach compared with 28% in the study group ($P = .0001$). Where CPIS remained ≤6 at day 3 antibiotics were continued in 96% in standard group but 0% in the others ($P = .0001$). Mortality and length of intensive care unit (ICU) stay did not differ despite a shorter duration ($P = .0001$) and lower cost ($P = .003$) in the study arm. Antimicrobial resistance, or superinfections, or both, developed in 15% of study versus 35% of standard therapy patients ($P = .017$)
2004[10]	Prospective observational study over 43 months in a medical-surgical ICU involving 115 patients	All episodes received initial broad-spectrum coverage followed by reevaluation according to clinical response and microbiology. Quantitative cultures by bronchoscopic examination or tracheal aspirates were used to modify therapy	Change of therapy in 56.2%, including de-escalation in 31.4% (increasing to 38% if isolates were sensitive). Overall ICU mortality was 32.2%. The de-escalation mortality rate was lower than those who continued initial regimen (18% vs 43%; $P<.05$). De-escalation was lower ($P<.05$) in the presence of nonfermenting gram-negative bacillus (2.7% vs 49.3%) and in the presence of late-onset pneumonia (12.5% vs 40.7%). When the pathogen remained unknown, 50% died and de-escalation was not performed

2006[11]	An observational cohort study involving 104 patients to assess the impact of locally developed antimicrobial guidelines in the initial empiric treatment of ICU patients with severe hospital-acquired pneumonia (HAP)	Evaluation pre- and post-guideline introduction where decision to change was based on quantitative BAL. Imipenem the main guideline empiric drug	Guideline followed in 75%. Imipenem continued as directed therapy in 27 cases. De-escalation possible in 34 patients but therapy continued beyond recommendation in 16 of these. The guideline patients showed greater adequate treatment (81% vs 46%; $P<.01$) with a lower mortality rate at 14 days (8% vs 23%, respectively; $P = .03$). There was no increase in imipenem resistance related to its increased used during the study period
2006[12]	Observational prospective study conducted in 24 Spanish ICUs to assess a carbapenem-based de-escalating strategy in nosocomial pneumonia (NP) in 244 critically ill patients	NP treated empirically with imipenem ± aminoglycoside/ glycopeptide. 91% were late-onset NP where primary outcome was therapeutic success 7–9 days post therapy. Culture-positive rate 54%, based on tracheal aspirates in 82%, protected specimen brush in 33%, and BAL in 4%	Initial antibiotics inadequate for 9%. De-escalation in 23% and unchanged for 6%; 16% of patients did not receive de-escalation despite favorable microbiology. 46% therapy not altered, as no pathogen found. De-escalation implemented in only 23% with potentially multiresistant pathogens, compared with 68% in the rest ($P<.001$). Response rates were 53% and 50%, respectively in those receiving and not receiving de-escalation. No differences in superinfection rates and costs associated with de-escalation mainly dependent on the duration of hospitalization, though the duration of stay and costs in the ICU were higher for patients who were not de-escalated ($P<.001$ and $P = .001$, respectively)

(continued on next page)

Table 1
(continued)

Year[Reference] Principal Features of Study Design	Brief Methodology Overview	Principal Findings Relevant to De-Escalation
2006[13] Prospective, observational, cohort study in 20 ICUs in United States involving 398 ICU patients with suspected VAP to evaluate clinical characteristics and treatment patterns amongst VAP cases, including the implementation of and outcomes associated with de-escalation therapy	Therapy *escalation* was a switch to or addition of a drug class or classes with a broader spectrum or additional coverage. *De-escalation* was a switch to or discontinuation of a drug class resulting in a less broad spectrum of coverage. Diagnosis was by a range of methods	61.6% of patients had neither escalation nor de-escalation. Overall, escalation occurred in 15.3% and de-escalation in 22.1%. De-escalation was significantly more common where 3 or more antibiotics were prescribed. De-escalation occurred more frequently when a major pathogen was isolated (26.8% vs 6.5%). Most patients with no pathogen had no change in therapy (87.1%), compared with 57.6% when a major pathogen was isolated. In those who initially received adequate therapy de-escalation took place in 27.1%, compared with 16.6% in those whose initial therapy was not adequate ($\chi^2 = 6.15$; $P = .013$). De-escalation took place in 27.7% of BAL ($\chi^2 = 3.59$; $P = .06$); 20.5% of tracheal aspirate patients ($\chi^2 = 0.84$; $P = .36$) and 8.3% of those where neither was performed. The mortality rate was significantly reduced in de-escalated cases (17% de-escalation; 23.7% no change & 42.6% escalation [$\chi^2 = 13.25$; $P = .001$])
2007[14] Prospective observational study over 36 months to evaluate de-escalation in 115 medical-surgical ICU patients treated according to local pathway	All enrollments had positive cultures and were treated with limited-spectrum antibiotics (ie, without activity against *Pseudomonas aeruginosa*) if they had no prior hospitalization (within 21 days) or prior administration of antibiotics (within 10 days). Quantitative cultures by bronchoscopy or tracheal aspiration used to 	Limited spectrum used in 79 patients (69%). De-escalation in respectively 26% and 72% of patients with early- and late-onset ventilator-associated pneumonia; treatment escalated in 27 (23%). Overall de-escalation was feasible in 42% of patients with no differences in outcome

2007[15]	Prospective observational study involving 143 patients with VAP in a multidisciplinary ICU	Diagnosis by positive quantitative cultures of either tracheal aspirate or BAL and assessment by appropriateness of treatment for all significant isolates	Therapy de-escalated in 40.5% with decreased mortality at day 15 (5.1% vs 31.7%) and day 28 (12% vs 43.5%) and shorter intensive care unit (17.2 ± 1.2 vs 22.7 ± 6.3 days) and hospital (23.7 ± 2.8 vs 29.8 ± 11.1 days) stay ($P<.05$). In tracheal aspirate patients there was 21% de-escalation with reduced 15-day mortality (5.8% vs 34.3%), reduced 28-day mortality (11.6% vs 45.3%), and shorter intensive care unit (17.2 ± 1.6 vs 22.4 ± 6.4 days) and hospital (23.1 ± 4.4 vs 29.9 ± 11.1 days) stay ($P<.05$). In BAL patients there was 66.1% de-escalation with decreased 15-day mortality (4.8% vs 23.8%), decreased 28-day mortality (12.1% vs 38%), and shorter ICU (17.2 ± 1.1 vs 23.2 ± 6 days) and hospital (23.8 ± 2.4 vs 29.8 ± 11.4 days) stay ($P<.05$)
2009[16]	An observational study to evaluate de-escalation in 138 surgical patients, including those with septic shock	Surgical ICU patients with quantitative bronchoalveolar lavage with a positive threshold of 10,000 CFU/mL	The recurrent pneumonia rate was not significantly different at 27.3% and 35.1%, respectively in those receiving and not receiving de-escalation. Mortality did not differ (33.8% vs 42.1%, respectively). De-escalation of therapy occurred in 55% of patients with appropriate initial therapy whereas 8% required escalation

de-escalation is appropriate to implement and delivers at least the same clinical outcome as the conventional approach of maintaining the initial therapy started when this was being successful. Although the majority of these findings come from work in NP, there is now evidence for other infections including septicemia and intra-abdominal infections. With particular regard to NP, the specter of de-escalation provoking an increased incidence of relapses or recurrences has been proven not to be real. This position should now promote a scenario where further trials are used to explore how best to de-escalate rather than whether to do it.

There are several studies[10,11,13,15,19] suggesting that clinical outcome may actually be improved where de-escalation is practiced. It is difficult to hypothesize why the impact of de-escalation should be to improve clinical outcome, and therefore it remains to be determined whether this effect is genuine or merely reflects the characteristics of the patients in whom de-escalation is both feasible and chosen. Another possibility is that continued potent, broad-spectrum empiric therapy may be intrinsically detrimental in some patients. A recent meta-analysis/meta-regression demonstrated that empiric combination therapy in serious infections can be detrimental in patients at low risk of mortality even while providing significant clinical benefit in high-risk patients.[21] Patients who have already responded to potent, broad-spectrum antimicrobial therapy are similarly at a low risk of death and therefore may derive more harm than benefit from continued broad-spectrum therapy where de-escalation is not implemented, perhaps as a consequence of the modest but measurable toxicity/side effects of such regimens.

The data available on cost-effectiveness is much less in both quantity and quality. From the perspective of drug acquisition and administration, it is persuasive that de-escalation should produce savings and there is evidence to support this. As described earlier, a small number of trials that demonstrate clinical benefit appear to point to potential cost reductions through reduced complications and shorter lengths of stay, both in the ICU and in the hospital. Further determination of these aspects will clearly be linked to the future work that explores whether such clinical benefits are truly related to de-escalation as opposed to being an apparent effect.

Paradoxically, given that one of the fundamental themes underlying its promotion is the perceived potential for this intervention to positively affect antimicrobial resistance, there is a surprising lack of relevant evidence available. Indeed, this is the feature where there are the fewest data in terms of the impact of de-escalation, with very few studies exploring this aspect at all. The main question to be addressed is whether the initial use of potent broad-spectrum antibiotics in association with de-escalation will successfully protect against the development of resistance to the primary agent being used. Only one study has presented on this question[11] and, although it did demonstrate no increase in resistance to the carbapenem being used, its conclusion must be viewed with caution because of the relatively short reporting period of 6 months related to the trial. Another study[9] evaluated whether the use of de-escalation would have a positive impact on resistance development in the individual patient being treated, and concluded that it did indeed reduce the propensity to resistance development. There is clearly an overwhelming need for well-constructed de-escalation studies to identify whether short- and/or long-term benefits are truly associated with this tactic in terms of modifying the risk of resistance development.

CHALLENGES IN IMPLEMENTING DE-ESCALATION

The outcome of the adoption of de-escalation is intended to be that, based on microbiology results around the day 3 therapy point, the empiric antibiotic(s) that were started are stopped or reduced in number and/or narrowed in spectrum. Experience has shown that several factors in practice work against achieving this goal.

Adoption of De-Escalation

Rates of de-escalation range from about 10% in studies of clinical practice to about 70% in specifically designed trials; this suggests that getting clinicians to actually use de-escalation is a principal barrier. There is a natural propensity, particularly in severe sepsis when the patient who has been very seriously ill is starting to get better, to stick with a treatment regimen that is working rather than change to an alternative agent. The solution to this is to gain clinical confidence in de-escalation.

Two principal lines of attack exist to help achieve this result. First, there is the ability for the health care professional to use a robust clinical assessment so that there can be a reasonable degree of certainty about whether an infection is present. Two studies, both in respiratory tract infections,[9,19] have evaluated this type of approach, showing that it is a useful component in enabling decision-making toward de-escalation where a risk-based clinical assessment suggests that infection is very probably not present and that this is supported by negative microbiology. The potential exists to apply this type of approach in other clinical areas, for example, intra-abdominal sepsis.[22] Second, several of the trials presented in **Table 1** point to the value of diagnostic certainty where they have shown that de-escalation is most likely to take place against higher quality samples, such as bronchoalveolar lavage, when compared with less invasive tests such as tracheal aspirates. This concept was specifically explored in a study[15] where VAP was diagnosed by positive quantitative cultures of either tracheal aspirate or bronchoalveolar lavage, and where it was conclusively shown that the latter promoted the greater adherence to de-escalation.

Leaving aside the issue of what best the clinician should do in the face of uncertainty resulting from negative microbiology cultures, which is addressed later, it has also been shown that where other, more general sepsis concerns exist, physicians choose to cover these potentially pathogenic organisms rather than focus on the proven etiology. This situation is documented particularly for multiresistant gram-negative bacilli[10,12] and results in de-escalation not taking place. There are insufficient data yet available to clarify the optimum course of action in these circumstances.

It has also been shown that providing appropriate support to clinicians in the decision-making frontline can have a positive impact on action being taken when opportunities to de-escalate are present. In a before-and-after study, prescriptions of 13 selected intravenous antibiotics from surgical and medical wards were evaluated against 3 strategies over 3 consecutive 8-week periods: conventional management by the attending physician (control group); distribution of a questionnaire to the physician (questionnaire group); or distribution of the questionnaire followed by advice from an infectious disease physician (Q-IDP group).[23] The primary outcome was the percentage of modifications of antibiotic therapy at day 4, including withdrawal of therapy, de-escalation, oral switch, or reducing the planned duration of therapy. The greatest effects were seen in the Q-IDP phase where discontinuation was much more likely to happen than within the control group ($P<.001$). In addition, more prescriptions were modified in the Q-IDP group as compared with the control group ($P = .004$), and stopping therapy in the absence of apparent infection also occurred significantly more often in the Q-IDP group than in the control ($P<.0001$) or questionnaire groups ($P = .002$).

Those seeking to introduce de-escalation strategies must recognize this fundamental issue of clinician confidence, and respond positively and proactively to it in order to give implementation its greatest chance of success.

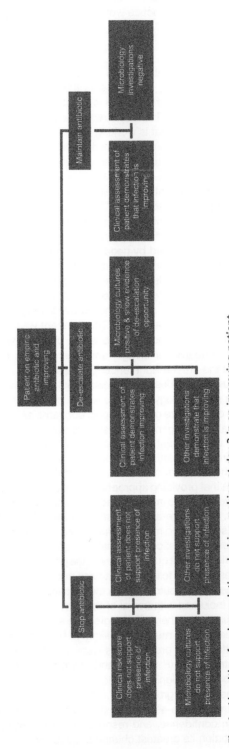

Fig. 1. Algorithm for de-escalation decision-making at day 3 in an improving patient.

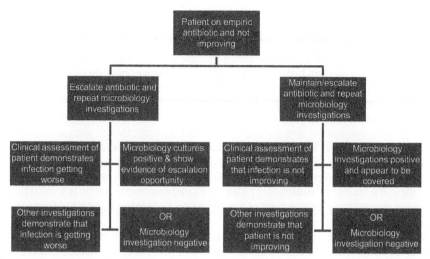

Fig. 2. Algorithm for de-escalation decision-making at day 3 in a patient not improving on the empiric antibiotic therapy.

Decision-Making in De-Escalation

One of the features that promotes clinician uncertainty is a lack of clarity about how to take decisions to de-escalate; this permeates to varying degrees each of the scenarios that the health care professional faces. However, the therapeutic approach to each setting is actually similar, though the respective contributions of the various components depend on the different clinical situations. The part that clinical risk assessments can contribute to the decision-making moment has been described in the preceding section. The other 2 features that are relevant are consideration of the clinical progress of the patient and the investigation information that is available.

Box 3

A practical clinical bedside approach to de-escalation

1. Every patient with severe sepsis on antibiotic therapy should have the need for this considered and formally documented every day

2. No later than day 3, a full assessment of investigation results and clinical progress should be performed and a positive decision should be captured to:

    Stop the treatment (eg, no infection is present)

    Narrow the spectrum of the therapy

    Reduce the number of antibiotics being used, for example, there is redundancy in the therapy or such clinical progress that multiple agents active against the same pathogen(s) are not necessary

    Not to de-escalate, for example, the specific reason for not de-escalating is documented (eg, lack of microbiology results, lack of clinical improvement)

3. Every day thereafter a positive decision to stop, change, or continue the therapy should be made against specific reasons

4. At every assessment the goal is to stop the therapy, or elements of the therapy, unless a positive and persuasive need for their continuation exists

Figs. 1 and **2** present algorithms for de-escalation decision-making at around day 3 of therapy, when the microbiology results normally first become available, in the 2 common scenarios where the patient either is improving or is not. Each of these is set against the assumptions that effective therapy with appropriate empiric antibiotic selection and dosage has been delivered and that source control for the infection has been identified and achieved. The clinical assessment of the patient incorporates not just the standard observations such as pulse, temperature, blood pressure, and oxygen saturation, but also a full physical evaluation. It is essential to consider other noninfectious causes for the patient's condition at each overall evaluation. Other investigations that can shed light on the decision-making process are evaluation of inflammatory markers such as white blood cell count, C-reactive protein, and procalcitonin as well as appropriate use of imaging modalities. Escalation of the antibiotic therapy in the face of a deteriorating patient with negative microbiology is a value judgment set against a risk assessment of the perceived gaps in the spectrum of cover and any likely potential foci of infection.

Following the initial day 3 assessment, continued consideration must be given to further opportunities for de-escalation. Key in this context is the situation where the patient is improving but microbiology cultures were negative and so the initial empiric antibiotics were continued at day 3. At a future juncture it will be necessary to decide when the treatment can be stopped at its earliest or converted to a narrower spectrum and/or oral agent. This last will be a judgment against an assessment of the clinical response, the likely source of sepsis, and also the potential pathogens to be covered. Within this envelope is the natural concern of the attending clinician to avoid making a mistake. This factor is more pressing when the patient remains seriously unwell as opposed to when the patient has improved so that organ support and mechanical ventilation are either much reduced or no longer needed. Where ongoing clinical concerns are high, it may be felt necessary to maintain the empiric antibiotic throughout the course of treatment, when it should be ensured that this is for the minimum duration possible.

Fig. 2 captures the very problematic, but by no means uncommon, midway position where the patient's condition has not improved at day 3. This scenario has never been explored in any of the clinical trials available, so it is not possible to state the best course of action. In view of this, it is probably unrealistic at present to expect de-escalation to be applied to this group of patients. Although clearly continuing clinical and investigation assessment, including microbiology tests, must be maintained, the decision whether to continue with, or escalate, the antibiotic care will be constructed on an individual patient basis depending on an overall assessment of the risks.

In summary, key elements within a successful de-escalation program at the bedside level are captured in **Box 3** as a practical aid. The formal and rigorous consideration and documentation suggested is designed to ensure that the approach is applied consistently and in a sustained way to every relevant patient every day. It is only by doing so that the benefits of such schemes can be captured.

SUMMARY

De-escalation is a critical component that lies at the center of antimicrobial stewardship programs and the "hit it hard, hit it early" serious sepsis paradigm. The data presented demonstrate that it is a clinically effective concept. However, significant and serious shortfalls in the available evidence are highlighted. These shortfalls include the need to establish the real impact of de-escalation on antimicrobial resistance development; its true cost-effectiveness profile; and, while emphasizing that it is now well demonstrated that there is no downside for patients, whether it genuinely does improve clinical outcomes. Significant work needs to be done to establish the most effective tools to implement de-escalation, particularly in terms of providing clear guidelines to clinicians to enable them to be confident in applying this maneuver. It is interesting that this concept of de-escalation is now being explored in other types of infection.[24] There is little doubt that de-escalation is now here to stay, and the issue should no longer be whether the clinician should do it but how best it can be delivered.

REFERENCES

1. Theuretzbacher U. Future antibiotics scenarios: is the tide starting to turn? Int J Antimicrob Agents 2009;34:15–20.
2. Masterton RG. The new treatment paradigm and the role of carbapenems. Int J Antimicrob Agents 2009;33:105–10.
3. Dellit TH, Owens RC, McGowan JE, et al. Infectious Diseases Society of America and the Society for Healthcare Epidemiology of America guidelines for developing an institutional program to enhance antimicrobial stewardship. Clin Infect Dis 2007;44:159–77.
4. Kollef MH. Optimizing antibiotic therapy in the intensive care unit setting. Crit Care 2001;5:189–95.
5. Lisboa T, Rello J. De-escalation in lower respiratory tract infections. Curr Opin Pulm Med 2006;12:364–8.
6. Petrosillo N, Drapeau CM, Agrafiotis M, et al. Some current issues in the pharmacokinetics/pharmacodynamics of antimicrobials in intensive care. Minerva Anestesiol 2010;76:509–24.
7. Park DR. Antimicrobial treatment of ventilator-associated pneumonia. Respir Care 2005;50:932–52.
8. Vidaur L, Sirgo G, Rodriguez AH, et al. Clinical approach to the patient with suspected ventilator-associated pneumonia. Respir Care 2005;50:965–74.
9. Singh N, Rogers P, Atwood CW, et al. Short-course empiric antibiotic therapy for patients with pulmonary infiltrates in the intensive care unit: a proposed solution for indiscriminate antibiotic prescription. Am J Respir Crit Care Med 2000;162:505–11.
10. Rello J, Vidaur L, Sandiumenge A, et al. De-escalation therapy in ventilator-associated pneumonia. Crit Care Med 2004;32:2183–90.
11. Soo Hoo GW, Wen YE, Nguyen TV, et al. Impact of clinical guidelines in the management of severe hospital acquired pneumonia. Chest 2005;128:2778–87.
12. Álvarez-Lerma F, Alvarez B, Luque P, et al. Empiric broad-spectrum antibiotic therapy of nosocomial pneumonia in the intensive care unit: a prospective observational study. Critical Care 2006;10:R78.
13. Kollef MH, Morrow LE, Niederman MS, et al. Clinical characteristics and treatment patterns among patients with ventilator-associated pneumonia. Chest 2006;129:1210–8.
14. Leone M, Garcin F, Bouvenot J, et al. Ventilator-associated pneumonia: breaking the vicious circle of antibiotic overuse. Crit Care Med 2007;35:379–85.
15. Giantsou E, Liratzopoulos N, Efraimidou E, et al. De-escalation therapy rates are significantly higher by bronchoalveolar lavage than by tracheal aspirate. Intensive Care Med 2007;33:1533–40.
16. Eachempati SR, Hydo LJ, Shou J, et al. Does de-escalation of antibiotic therapy for ventilator-associated pneumonia affect the likelihood of recurrent pneumonia or mortality in critically ill surgical patients? J Trauma 2009;66:1343–8.

17. Donaldson AD, Barkham T. De-escalation for amoxicillin-susceptible *Escherichia coli*: easier said than done. J Hosp Infect 2010;74:304–5.

18. De Waele JJ, Ravyts M, Depuydt P, et al. De-escalation after empirical meropenem treatment in the intensive care unit: fiction or reality? J Crit Care 2010. [Epub ahead of print].

19. Schlueter M, James C, Dominguez A, et al. Practice patterns for antibiotic de-escalation in culture-negative healthcare-associated pneumonia. Infection 2010;38(5):357–62.

20. Fox BC, Fish J, Zheng L, et al. Prospective study of de-escalation of antimicrobial therapy in an ICU [abstract 217]. In: Program and abstracts of the 42nd Annual Meeting of the Infectious Diseases Society of America [Boston]: Infectious Diseases Society of America, Arlington (VA), 2004: 73.

21. Kumar A, Safdar N, Kethireddy S, et al. A survival benefit of combination antibiotic therapy for serious infections associated with sepsis and septic shock is contingent only on the risk of death: a meta-analytic/meta-regression study. Crit Care Med 2010;38:1651–64.

22. Sartelli M. A focus on intra-abdominal infections. World J Emerg Surg 2010;5:9.

23. Lesprit P, Landelle C, Girou E, et al. Reassessment of intravenous antibiotic therapy using a reminder or direct counselling. J Antimicrob Chemother 2010; 65:789–95.

24. Lichtenstern C, Nguyen TH, Schemmer P, et al. Efficacy of caspofungin in invasive candidiasis and candidemia—de-escalation strategy. Mycoses 2008; 51(Suppl 1):35–46.

Antimicrobial Resistance in the Intensive Care Unit: Mechanisms, Epidemiology, and Management of Specific Resistant Pathogens

Henry S. Fraimow, MD[a],*, Constantine Tsigrelis, MD[b]

KEYWORDS

- Resistance • Mechanisms • Multidrug resistance
- Methicillin-resistant *Staphylococcus aureus*
- Vancomycin-resistant enterococci • Gram-negative bacteria

Drug-resistant and multidrug-resistant (MDR) microbial pathogens have emerged as major concerns both in and out of the hospital environment. Drug-resistant pathogens pose tremendous challenges to the health care system, including challenges related to the diagnosis, treatment, and containment of infections caused by resistant organisms.[1–3] These challenges are amplified in the intensive care unit (ICU) environment, where pressures for selection and emergence of resistance and the risks of transmission of drug-resistant pathogens are highest, and where the threat of potential drug resistance is a major driver of the selection of empiric antimicrobial regimens.[4] Critical care physicians also face the increasingly common scenario of managing infections caused by organisms, with limited or even no treatment options.[2,3] This article reviews the basic concepts of resistance to antibacterial agents including mechanisms and modes of transmission, and discusses management issues of the important drug-resistant and MDR pathogens found in the ICU.

The authors have nothing to disclose.
[a] Division of Infectious Diseases, UMDNJ-Robert Wood Johnson Medical School, Cooper University Hospital, 401 Haddon Avenue, Room 274, Camden, NJ 08103, USA
[b] Division of Infectious Diseases, UMDNJ-Robert Wood Johnson Medical School, Cooper University Hospital, 401 Haddon Avenue, Room 259, Camden, NJ 08103, USA
* Corresponding author.
E-mail address: fraimow-henry@cooperhealth.edu

Crit Care Clin 27 (2011) 163–205
doi:10.1016/j.ccc.2010.11.002
0749-0704/11/$ – see front matter © 2011 Elsevier Inc. All rights reserved.

criticalcare.theclinics.com

ANTIBACTERIAL RESISTANCE: GENERAL CONCEPTS
Definitions

Resistance is a measure of decreased ability of an antimicrobial agent to kill or inhibit the growth of a microbial organism. In practice, this is determined by testing a patient isolate against an antimicrobial in an in vitro assay system. For bacteria, the common in vitro testing systems are automated liquid media microdilution systems, disc diffusion, and the Etest. For quantitative systems like broth microdilution or Etest, the measure of drug activity is the minimum inhibitory concentration (MIC). From testing of large numbers of isolates, breakpoints that define the thresholds of susceptibility for each organism-drug combination are established by groups such as the US Clinical and Laboratory Standards Institutes (CLSI) and the European Committee on Antimicrobial Susceptibility Testing (EUCAST). Breakpoints are included in the US Food and Drug Administration (FDA)-approved product labeling for new antibacterial agents. A strain reported as *susceptible* in vitro has an MIC value at or below the defined susceptibility breakpoint, which is believed to correlate with high likelihood of therapeutic success.[5] For strains reported as *intermediate* or *indeterminate*, therapeutic effect is uncertain; for strains reported as *resistant*, use of that agent is associated with high likelihood of therapeutic failure.[5] Some resistance traits are not reliably detected by standard methods, and require additional microbiologic or molecular confirmatory testing, which may lead to delays and increased cost for correctly identifying resistant organisms.[6]

Intrinsic resistance is an inherent feature of a species resulting in the lack of activity of a drug or drug class. Intrinsic resistance may be due such factors as lack of the appropriate antimicrobial target, inability of the drug to access target, or presence of species-wide antimicrobial inactivating enzymes. An example is the intrinsic resistance of gram-negative organisms to the glycopeptides vancomycin and teicoplanin, which cannot penetrate the outer membrane to reach their target. *Circumstantial resistance* reflects the disparity between in vitro and in vivo activity. Antibiotics that are active in vitro may not be clinically effective, due to lack of drug penetration to protected sites such as the cerebrospinal fluid, or the inactivity of drug at low pH or in an anaerobic environment. The major focus of this article is *acquired resistance*: a change in phenotypic characteristics of an organism resulting in decreased effectiveness of a previously active drug. Acquired resistance is a natural consequence of genetically adaptable microorganisms responding to the selective pressure of antimicrobial agents. The phenotype of acquired resistance has a genotypic correlate, although the genetics of some resistance traits remain poorly characterized. Some important acquired resistance traits can be directly selected for in vitro and in vivo via one or several point mutations in antimicrobial target genes. Other selectable resistance traits are more complex and may involve multiple alterations in a variety of bacterial genes. There are many important resistance phenotypes, such as methicillin resistance in Staphylococci, that cannot be selected for in vitro or in vivo, and only occur through susceptible organisms acquiring exogenous genetic material.

Evolution and Spread of Antimicrobial Resistant Organisms

In a patient exposed to an antimicrobial agent, resistant organisms can emerge by selection for and expansion of subpopulations of spontaneously generated, less susceptible mutants of antimicrobial target (**Fig. 1**). The likelihood that this occurs is influenced by many factors, including the number of mutations necessary to express resistance, organism inoculum, pharmacodynamic interactions of drug and organism at the site of infection, and duration of antimicrobial exposure.[7] More commonly,

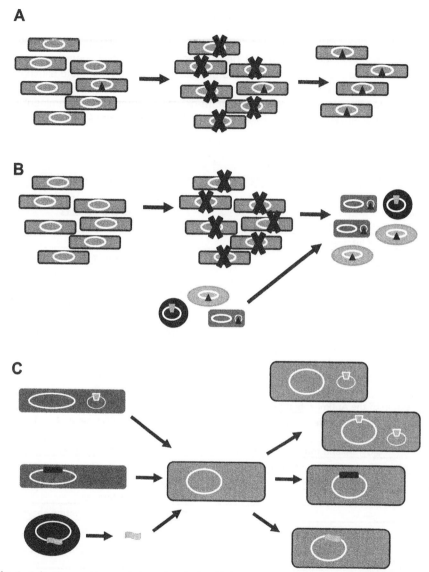

Fig. 1. Selection and transmission of antimicrobial resistance. (*A*) Selection of antibiotic resistant mutants after antibiotic exposure. (*B*) Superinfection with new antibiotic resistant bacteria after antibiotic exposure. (*C*) Horizontal transfer of resistance genes into a susceptible strain can occur through transfer of plasmids containing resistance transposons, by the direct transfer of resistance transposons from the chromosome, or by acquisition of free DNA.

colonization or infection with drug-resistant organisms results from *superinfection* rather than by evolution of resistance in the original target organism. New drug-resistant "invaders" are selected from organisms already part of the patient's endogenous flora, living on mucosal surfaces or in the gastrointestinal tract, or are newly acquired from the health care environment. Emergence of resistant organisms and superinfection are both concerns in patients failing to respond to antimicrobial therapy, but there are multiple other reasons for therapeutic failure: inadequate source control, host immune status, and pharmacologic issues of drug bioavailability and optimal dosing are only a few of these.

Bacteria employ several basic strategies for evading the effects of antibiotics,[8] including enzymatic modification and inactivation of antimicrobial agents, restriction of drug access to the cellular targets, and modification or even complete elimination of the target (**Table 1**). The most important classes of inactivating enzymes are the many β-lactamases in gram-positive and gram-negative bacteria and the aminoglycoside-modifying enzymes (AME). Restriction of drug target access can occur from

Table 1
Strategies used by bacteria to decrease the effectiveness of antimicrobial agents

General Strategy	Specific Mechanisms	Some Specific Examples, Drug Class Affected, and Genetics (if Known)
Regulation of Intracellular Drug Entry		
—	Increased efflux	Macrolide efflux pumps: *mefA, msrA*
—	—	Gram-positive fluoroquinolone/ multidrug efflux pumps: *norA, pmrA*
—	—	Gram-negative multidrug efflux pumps: *acrAB, mexAB-OprF, adeABC*
—	—	Tetracycline efflux pumps: *tetA, B, C,* and other
—	Decreased cytoplasmic transport	Aminoglycosides
—	Decreased outer membrane permeability	β-Lactams: *OmpF* and *OprD* changes via mutation or altered expression
Protection of the Antimicrobial Target		
—	Glycopeptide "trapping"	Glycopeptide resistance: VISA and heteroVISA
—	Gyrase and topoisomerase protection	Fluoroquinolones: *qnr* genes
Decreasing Concentrations of Active Drug		
—	Drug modification or destruction	Aminoglycosides: modifying enzymes
—	—	β-Lactams: β-lactamases
—	—	Chloramphenicol: inactivating enzymes
—	Decreasing drug activation	Isoniazid: *katG* mutations
—	—	Metronidazole: *rdxA* mutations
Target Modification or Bypass of Target		
—	Mutational modification	Fluoroquinolones: *gyr* and topoisomerase mutations
—	—	β-Lactams: *pbp* changes
—	—	Linezolid: 23SRNA mutations
—	—	Rifampin: *rpo* mutations
—	Acquisition of a new target	β-Lactams: *mecA*
—	Enzymatic modification of target	Ribosomal modifications
—	—	Macrolides and clindamycin: *erm* genes
—	—	Tetracyclines: *tetM, tetO*
—	—	Multiple drug classes: *cfr*
—	Novel synthetic pathways	Glycopeptides: *vanA, vanB,* and other clusters

alterations in membrane permeability to decrease drug entry, by expression of narrow- or broad-range efflux pumps to extrude antimicrobials from the cytoplasmic compartment, or by "trapping" of an antimicrobial agent before accessing the target. Target modification occurs through mutations in target genes, such as the gyrase and topoisomerase targets of fluoroquinolones, by enzymatic modification of target genes, by introduction of new, nonsusceptible targets such as the MecA protein in *Staphylococcus aureus,* or through novel synthetic pathways like the enterococcal *vanA* and *vanB* clusters that eliminate the bacteria's need for the original antimicrobial target. Levels of resistance are magnified by combining different mechanisms. For example, permeability changes and efflux pumps that decrease intracellular β-lactam concentrations enhance effectiveness of β-lactamases present in the gram-negative periplasmic space.[9]

Organisms expressing acquired resistance traits can clonally disseminate, transmitting their resistance traits to their multiple descendants. The extra "work" required for maintaining resistance traits may result in decreased fitness of the organism, thus resistance may ultimately disappear in the absence of selective pressure. However, other resistance traits are relatively stable and persist even in the absence of antibiotic exposure.[10] Resistance genes or gene clusters can also be transmitted horizontally between organisms, as well as between species.[11] Resistance genes are typically carried on transposons, which are mobile genetic elements that can move in and out of the bacterial chromosome and into plasmids, facilitating horizontal gene transfer. Unrelated resistance genes are often clustered together, enabling transfer of multiple resistances as a single package. Transfer of resistance occurs among gram-negative flora in the human gastrointestinal tract, and exchange of *vanA* resistance clusters in vivo from enterococci to *S aureus* has led to emergence of highly vancomycin-resistant *S aureus* (VRSA).[11,12]

Multidrug-Resistant Organisms

Multidrug-resistant (MDR) organisms have acquired resistance to multiple unrelated classes of antimicrobials.[1,3] Multidrug resistance can be selected by sequential exposure to different antibiotics, or by acquisition of multiple resistance traits clustered on mobile genetic elements. Some selectable resistances, such as permeability changes or upregulated broad range efflux pumps, can contribute to expression of resistance to multiple antimicrobial classes.[13] An ominous emerging threat is new gram-negative β-lactamases that cause high-level resistance to all available classes of β-lactams. Multidrug resistance is a feature of many bacterial species, but the criteria used to define an MDR organism vary.[14] MDR pathogens of greatest concern in the hospital environment include methicillin-resistant *S aureus* (MRSA), vancomycin-resistant enterococci (VRE), and drug-resistant *Streptococcus pneumoniae* (DRSP), and the MDR gram-negative organisms (MDR-GNRs) including *Pseudomonas, Acinetobacter, Klebsiella pneumoniae, Enterobacter,* and other species.[1] Criteria for defining MDR-GNRs may vary from institution to institution and are also not uniform in the published literature, although the most highly resistant strains are readily recognizable.[14]

MDR GRAM-POSITIVE ORGANISMS
Methicillin-Resistant Staphylococcus Aureus

Overview of methicillin-resistant and MDR S aureus
Since the beginning of the modern antibiotic era, *S aureus* has demonstrated the ability to progressively evolve resistance to all of the antistaphylococcal drugs introduced.[15] By the mid 1940s, the first strains of *S aureus* with plasmids encoding

for a penicillinase were identified. Within a decade, virulent penicillin-resistant *S aureus* clones had globally disseminated in and out of hospitals.[15] The challenge of penicillin-resistant staphylococci was met by the development of semisynthetic penicillins, followed quickly by the emergence of MRSA, and by the 1980s MRSA had emerged as a major nosocomial pathogen.[16] New genetic lineages of MRSA continued to circulate throughout the 1980s and 1990s, and prevalence of MRSA in hospitals and ICUs continued to increase.[17] Coincident with the relentless increase in hospital-associated MRSA (HAMRSA) infections in many, but not all countries, another trend has been the emergence of new, highly virulent MRSA clones phenotypically and genetically distinct from the predominant HAMRSA strains.[15,18] These new, community-associated MRSA (CAMRSA) have supplanted methicillin-susceptible *S aureus* (MSSA) in many regions as causes of skin and soft tissue infection (SSTI) in patients presenting to emergency rooms, and can cause serious community-onset and nosocomial infections.[18–20] The increasing incidence of MRSA resulted in major increases in glycopeptide use, but MRSA has demonstrated less susceptibility and even high-level resistance to vancomycin, as well as resistance to the newer antistaphylococcal agents linezolid and daptomycin.[21–23]

MRSA in the ICU: magnitude of the problem and consequences

MRSA infections steadily increased in United States hospitals in all regions throughout the 1990s, and peaked in the past decade. By 2003, 64.4% of ICU health care–associated *S aureus* infections in United States hospitals participating in the National Nosocomial Infections Surveillance system were caused by MRSA.[17] It is estimated that in 2005 there were 94,000 invasive MRSA infections and 19,000 hospital deaths attributable to MRSA in the United States, including 18,650 episodes of hospital-acquired MRSA bacteremia.[24] Economic costs as well as mortality rates appear to be worse for invasive MRSA than for MSSA infections.[25,26] It is unclear whether differences are attributable to less effective antimicrobials, to enhanced MRSA virulence, or to characteristics of patients who develop MRSA infections.[24] Recent surveillance data from the US Emerging Infections Program show annual decreased rates of hospital-onset and health care–associated but community-onset MRSA infections from 2005 to 2008, suggesting progress in achieving the national health care priority of preventing invasive MRSA infections.[27,28] Much of this decrease is attributable to decreased rates of central line–related MRSA bloodstream infections, but increased physician and public awareness of MRSA may have also contributed to the decline.[29,30] There are also large global differences in MRSA rates, even between countries in the same region. In Europe, MRSA rates in the United Kingdom and Greece are similar to those in the United States, whereas rates in Iceland and the Netherlands are only around 1%. Recent European surveillance data show 5-year trends similar to the United States, as many countries with traditionally high MRSA burden experience decreases in MRSA rates.[31]

Mechanisms and genetics of methicillin resistance in MRSA

Methicillin resistance in *S aureus* is almost always mediated by the *mecA* gene, which encodes a penicillin-binding protein (PBP) with decreased affinity for nearly all β-lactams.[15] The *mecA* gene is carried on large transposable chromosomal genetic elements, or SCC*mec* clusters. SCC*mec* elements include other regulatory genes and often unrelated antimicrobial resistance genes. The *mecA* gene is expressed either by all or only a small proportion of cells in a culture, depending on a variety of other regulatory genes found both inside and outside of the SCC*mec* cluster. Accurate laboratory detection of some low-level *mecA*-expressing MRSA strains can be challenging and requires use of supplemental microbiologic or genetic tests.[31] The *mecA* gene likely originated in a nonpathogenic staphylococcal species, with subsequent movement into other species including *S aureus*. Transfer of *mecA* into *S aureus* was probably an infrequent event, followed by the widespread dissemination of the most successful MRSA clones that are the progenitors of many current HAMRSA strains.[15,18] The large SCC*mec* elements of these early MRSA carried additional resistance traits such as those encoding erythromycin and clindamycin resistance, accounting for their MDR phenotype.

The worldwide appearance of CAMRSA is a more recent phenomenon. CAMRSA were first recognized in the mid 1990s when clusters of infection, including fatal infections, with non–multidrug-resistant MRSA were reported in diverse communities, including aboriginal populations in Western Australia and children and adolescents in Chicago and the rural Midwest.[32–34] CAMRSA have genetic lineages distinct from HAMRSA and carry smaller SCC*mec* elements that do not contain the other resistance genes found in older MRSA lineages.[15] Numerous CAMRSA clones emerged independently; the most successful are highly transmissible and virulent community pathogens that cause SSTIs and other infections including osteomyelitis, bacteremia, and pneumonia.[18–20,35,36] The dominant clones in the United States have been USA400 and more recently USA300, although different clones predominate in other countries.[15] CAMRSA strains express a wide array of virulence traits not found in HAMRSA that may contribute to pathogenicity.[36,37] One such trait is the Panton Valentine leukocidin (PVL). PVL is found in both CAMRSA and MSSA but is particularly prevalent among USA300, USA400, and other major CAMRSA clones.[15,36] PVL is linked to both skin infections and severe hemorrhagic necrotizing pneumonia, but its importance remains controversial.[36] Animal models support a role for PVL in severe pneumonia but not necessarily for skin infections. Other potential virulence factors, including α-hemolysin, type A phenol soluble modulins, and the arginine catabolic mobile element, may also be important in the attachment, invasiveness, and virulence of successful CAMRSA clones.[15,36,37] Clinical differentiation of HAMRSA and CAMRSA has become increasingly difficult. CAMRSA clones such as USA300 are now widely entrenched in the community in healthy individuals with no epidemiologic risks for MRSA. These individuals are hospitalized and develop nosocomial MRSA infections, and are reservoirs for cross-transmission of MRSA, contributing to the increase in USA300 as a cause of nosocomial bacteremia.[20] Many CAMRSA are no longer susceptible to fluoroquinolones and clindamycin, and display an MDR phenotype similar to HAMRSA.

Decreasing glycopeptide susceptibility in MRSA

The global dissemination of MRSA in the 1980s led to a tremendous increase in the use of glycopeptides.[38] Clinical failure of vancomycin therapy is not a recent phenomenon, but since the mid 1990s *S aureus* strains with decreased susceptibility to vancomycin have been reported with increasing frequency, including strains highly resistant to vancomycin.[12,15,39] The breakpoint for determining nonsusceptibility to vancomycin was redefined by CLSI to better reflect the clinical failure rate of vancomycin therapy for infections due to strains with higher vancomycin MICs.[40,41] There are important differences in terminology and defined susceptibility breakpoints between the United States, Europe, and Japan because of the availability of teicoplanin in some countries outside of the United States and differences in laboratory screening methods.[39] Categorization, mechanisms, prevalence, and clinical significance of strains with decreased susceptibility to vancomycin are summarized in **Table 2.**

Table 2
Categories of *S aureus* with reduced susceptibility to glycopeptides (in the United States)

Category	Vancomycin MIC (μg/ml)	Prevalence	Mechanism(s) or Genetic Association	Clinical Relevance
VRSA	≥32	Very rare ≈10 strains so far	Acquisition of enterococcal *vanA* plasmids[12]	Will fail vancomycin Rx Requires alternative Rx
VISA	4–8	Uncommon: <1%–2% in various surveys but USA data generally lower than international data	"Trapping" of vancomycin in thickened cell wall Increased cell wall precursors and turnover, increased capsule expression Altered regulation of multiple genes described	Will fail vancomycin Rx Requires alternative Rx Higher rates of daptomycin nonsusceptibility
Hetero-VISA	1–2 (subpopulations with higher MICs of 4–8)	Highly variable, depends on methodology: ranges from 0% up to 8.3% in larger studies	Same as for VISA	May fail vancomycin Rx ? Precursors of VISA
Vancomycin MIC = 2	2	Rates variable but increasing: in some recent reports up to 10% of MRSA, also can be seen in MSSA	? Same as for VISA and hetero-VISA	Higher vancomycin failure rate for bacteremia and other complicated infections

Abbreviations: Rx, treatment; VISA, vancomycin-intermediate *Staphylococcus aureus*.

VRSA strains are least frequently described, with to date only 10 isolates reported worldwide. VRSA are highly resistant to vancomycin with MICs of 32 μg/mL or more, and occur by MRSA acquiring plasmids harboring the enterococcal *vanA* gene cluster.[12] Vancomycin-intermediate *S aureus* (VISA) have MICs of 4 to 8 μg/mL and are more common than VRSA, though prevalence varies depending on methods of detection.[21,39–41] These strains evolve from *S aureus*, predominantly MRSA, by serial mutations after prolonged vancomycin exposures.[41] VISA have multiple phenotypic alterations, including a thickened cell wall and decreased peptidoglycan cross-linking, which appear to restrict access of vancomycin to its peptidoglycan target. VISA and VRSA are both associated with high likelihood of vancomycin failure.[40] Hetero-VISA (hVISA) test as vancomycin susceptible, but have small but reproducibly detectable subpopulations with MICs in a higher range similar to VISA.[39] Testing for hVISA is laborious and not available in most laboratories, and controversy persists about the prevalence as well as the therapeutic significance of this phenotype.[39,42] hVISA most likely represent either the reservoir for or an intermediate step in the evolution of VISA.[39,42] There is no specific genotypic correlate for VISA or hVISA, thus there is no molecular test for these strains. The final category includes strains with MICs of 2 μg/mL. Recent studies have described a phenomenon of "MIC creep," or increase over time in the mean vancomycin MICs of collections of clinical isolates. In some studies, mean vancomycin MICs have risen from 0.5 to 1.0 μg/mL, with increased prevalence of strains with MICs of 2 μg/mL.[42,43] MICs of 1.5 μg/mL or more are associated with slower clinical response and higher rates of failure in treating complicated bloodstream infections.[44,45] Laboratory testing for decreased glycopeptide susceptibility remains problematic.[39] The CLSI and Centers for Disease Control and Prevention (CDC) recommend use of vancomycin screening plates in addition to automated microdilution test methods.[41]

New consensus vancomycin dosing recommendations address the issue of optimal dosing for MRSA infection in the face of increasing glycopeptide resistance.[44] Vancomycin trough levels should be targeted at greater than 10 μg/mL, as exposure to lower vancomycin levels may theoretically promote emergence of VISA strains. Trough levels of 15 to 20 μg/mL are optimal for serious infections where MICs are 1 μg/mL or more. It may not be possible to achieve recommended pharmacodynamic targets when MICs are 2 μg/mL or higher using standard dosing, and alternative agents should be considered.[44] There are also reports of increased nephrotoxicity with use of aggressive vancomycin dosing regimens that target troughs of 15 to 20 μg/mL, although the exact mechanism and specific vancomycin dosing parameters that may be responsible remain poorly defined.[46] There is no evidence that targeting even higher vancomycin trough levels improves outcome, and such dosing regimens may potentially increase risks of toxicity.[44]

Newer MRSA drugs and emerging resistance: linezolid, daptomycin, tigecycline, telavancin

Resistance to the oxazalidinone antibiotic linezolid remains uncommon in *S aureus* after the first 10 years of use.[47] Resistant mutants selected in vitro and some linezolid-resistant clinical isolates contain point mutations at specific sites in the oxazalidinone ribosomal binding target in the 23S rRNA V domain. *S aureus* strains carry 5 or 6 copies of the 23S rRNA gene, and mutations in multiple gene copies are usually necessary to express resistance. More recently, transferrable linezolid resistance mediated by the ribosomal methylase *cfr* has been described in *S aureus* and coagulase-negative staphylococci.[48] The *cfr* ribosomal methylase modifies the 23S ribosome to alter binding of multiple classes of ribosomally active antibiotics. A nosocomial outbreak of linezolid-resistant MRSA caused by strains harboring *cfr* was recently reported.[22] In this ICU outbreak, several different MRSA clones as well as other staphylococci all contained the *cfr* gene, indicating horizontal transmission of this resistance trait.

Daptomycin, a lipopeptide approved in the United States in 2003 with a novel, bactericidal mechanism of activity, is increasingly used for complicated MRSA infections, especially for clinical vancomycin failure or infections due to strains with higher vancomycin MICs. MRSA with higher daptomycin MICs can be selected with very low frequency in vitro, and daptomycin resistance in large surveys of MRSA remains rare. However, resistance developed on therapy in 5.8% of patients with bacteremia and endocarditis and in 8.9% with persistent MRSA bacteremia in clinical trials.[23] Daptomycin resistance is not fully understood, but involves a variety of changes that affect cell membrane lipid composition, fluidity, and surface charge.[49] A linkage between prior glycopeptide exposure, higher glycopeptide MIC, and reduced daptomycin susceptibility has been reported, although most infections by strains with higher vancomycin MICs will respond to daptomycin therapy.[50] Isolates from patients on daptomycin should be monitored for evolution of decreased daptomycin susceptibility. Studies are ongoing to determine whether dosing daptomycin at higher than the currently FDA-approved dose of 6 mg/kg will improve outcomes and decrease emergence of resistance in serious MRSA infections. Preliminary data suggest that these higher dosing regimens of up to 10 or even 12 mg/kg are well tolerated.[51]

Many MRSA strains in the United States are susceptible to tetracyclines. Doxycycline and minocycline are often prescribed for CAMRSA SSTIs, but their role for more serious MRSA infections is uncertain. A variety of transferrable tetracycline resistance genes, including efflux pumps and ribosomal modifying enzymes, are found among gram-positive flora. Tigecycline, a glycylcycline tetracycline analogue with activity against many tetracycline-resistant *S aureus*, is FDA approved for treatment of bacterial pneumonia, SSTI, and intra-abdominal infections. In a recent United States survey, only 0.03% of more than 10,000 MRSA collected from 2004 to 2008 were nonsusceptible to tigecycline.[52] Pharmacokinetic properties of tigecycline include a large volume of distribution and low serum levels, thus there are major concerns about use of tigecycline for bacteremias, and experience with MRSA bacteremia is limited.[53]

The lipoglycopeptide telavancin, a semisynthetic vancomycin derivative with 4- to 8-fold enhanced bactericidal activity against MRSA compared with vancomycin, was recently approved in the United States for treatment of MRSA infections.[49] Telavancin is active in vitro against VISA and hVISA strains. Telavancin is currently approved only for treatment of SSTIs, and nephrotoxicity has been noted in clinical trials. There are few published reports of successful use of telavancin for MRSA bacteremia or endocarditis.[54] Quinupristin-dalfopristin is still available as a parenteral alternative for MRSA, but is not bactericidal against most strains. Another newly FDA-approved drug with activity against MRSA is the 5th generation cephalosporin ceftaroline which differs from other cephalosporins in its ability to bind to the *mecA* gene product.

Choice of agents for treatment of MRSA infections in the ICU

The availability of newer antistaphylococcal agents has improved but has also complicated the choices for treating MRSA infections in the ICU. Factors to consider include site and severity of infection, the MIC to vancomycin, and comorbidities. For bacteremia and endovascular infections including endocarditis for which bactericidal therapy is preferred, vancomycin and daptomycin are both appropriate alternatives.[55] When the vancomycin MIC is greater than 1 µg/mL, daptomycin may be preferable unless the MIC to daptomycin is also elevated.[44,45,50] The minimum daptomycin dose for MRSA at any site should be 6 mg/kg, though doses of up to 10 to 12 mg/kg are increasingly being used.[51] The bacteriostatic drug linezolid is not recommended as first-line therapy for bacteremia, but has been successfully used in salvage therapy for bacteremia and even endocarditis.[56,57]

Optimal therapy for MRSA pneumonia differs from that for bacteremia. Daptomycin is inactivated by pulmonary surfactant and was inferior to standard therapy in treatment of community acquired pneumonia.[58] Vancomycin and linezolid are both listed as options for MRSA in the American Thoracic Society-Infectious Diseases Society of America guidelines for hospital-acquired pneumonia (HAP).[59] Vancomycin has been the mainstay of therapy for nosocomial MRSA pneumonia, but linezolid was non-inferior and probably superior to vancomycin for ventilator-associated pneumonia (VAP) and HAP in recent trials.[60] Vancomycin troughs are targeted at 15 to 20 μg/mL for MRSA pneumonia, although evidence that this results in better clinical or microbiologic cure rates is lacking.[44] CAMRSA is increasingly described as a cause of primary community-acquired pneumonia (CAP) as well as secondary pneumonia in patients with influenza-like illnesses.[36,61] CAMRSA pneumonias may present as fulminate necrotizing infections complicated by empyema or abscess, and are often caused by strains containing PVL.[33,36] However, the severity of disease produced by PVL-producing MRSA strains is variable.[36] Linezolid, clindamycin, and other protein synthesis inhibitor drugs that decrease toxin production in vitro may have theoretical advantages for severe pneumonia due to PVL-producing CAMRSA.[62] These recommendations are included in the United Kingdom guidelines for management of community-onset MRSA pneumonia.[63] Tigecycline is approved for treatment of CAP and is an alternative for treatment of nonbacteremic MRSA pneumonia where broader coverage is necessary, though data is limited.

Vancomycin has traditionally been used as initial therapy for patients hospitalized with suspected or confirmed severe MRSA SSTI.[36] The newer MRSA drugs have been compared with vancomycin for complicated SSTIs in clinical trials. Linezolid, daptomycin, tigecycline, telavancin and ceftaroline are noninferior to vancomycin for complicated SSTIs, and linezolid demonstrated higher cure rates in a subgroup of patients with MRSA.[36,64–66] Linezolid may be an attractive alternative for severe soft tissue infections such as necrotizing fasciitis caused by toxin-producing strains. However, there is concern about use of this bacteriostatic agent for SSTIs complicated by secondary bacteremia. Drainage is a critical component of management of MRSA abscesses.[15,36] There are many options for less severe infections, including trimethoprim-sulfamethoxazole, doxycycline, minocycline, and clindamycin.[36] Resistance rates of CAMRSA to these agents have been low, but may be increasing.[67] Erythromycin-resistant but clindamycin-susceptible strains must be tested for inducible clindamycin resistance. CAMRSA strains may be susceptible to fluoroquinolones, but resistance develops readily on therapy. Rifampin should never be used as monotherapy for staphylococcal infections.

Combination therapy for serious MRSA infections

Combination therapy for MRSA bacteremia remains a controversial area, with only limited data to support the use of most combinations.[68] Theoretical justifications for combination therapy include more rapid clearance of bacteremia, in vitro synergy, preventing emergence of resistance, and activity in protected sites or biofilms. Recent studies found no benefit from addition of gentamicin to vancomycin for complicated MRSA bacteremia, and the combination resulted in increased nephrotoxicity.[69] Rifampin plus vancomycin is not reliably synergistic in vitro, and there is no evidence that addition of rifampin improves the outcome of bacteremia in vivo, although rifampin has a role in complicated device-associated infections.[70] Linezolid demonstrates little synergy and potential antagonism with some other agents, although there are reports on the use of linezolid plus carbapenems for refractory MRSA bacteremia.[71] Combinations of daptomycin and gentamicin or rifampin demonstrate variable effects in vitro and in animal models, and clinical data are lacking.[72] Routine use of combination therapy is not recommended for MRSA endocarditis except for prosthetic valve disease.[57]

Vancomycin-Resistant Enterococci and Multidrug-Resistant Enterococci

Epidemiology and mechanisms of resistance in VRE and MDR enterococci

Enterococci are a constituent of the normal human gastrointestinal flora and are pathogens in community-onset infections including gastrointestinal and urinary tract infections, bacteremia, and endocarditis. Enterococci are also increasingly important nosocomial pathogens, and were the third most common pathogen from nosocomial infections in United States hospitals in 2006–2007.[73] Enterococci are capable of prolonged survival on surfaces in the hospital environment. Enterococci are intrinsically resistant to many antibiotics, including cephalosporins, clindamycin, and aminoglycosides, at achievable serum levels. Intestinal concentrations of enterococci increase by several logs in patients treated with cephalosporins, which increases the risk of enterococcal superinfection and the risk of environmental contamination.[74] Enterococci are relatively tolerant to killing by penicillins and glycopeptides, although synergistic combinations of a penicillin or vancomycin with an aminoglycoside are bactericidal. Enterococcus faecalis is the most prevalent species in human infections. Enterococcus faecium is uncommon among community isolates but comprises a higher proportion of health care–associated isolates including most MDR strains.[73] The evolution of MDR enterococcus results from accumulation of genes for several different acquired resistances (**Table 3**), including penicillin resistance, glycopeptide resistance, and high-level aminoglycoside resistance (HLAR).[75] Enterococci can show all the different combinations of these 3 resistance traits.

There are 2 primary mechanisms of penicillin resistance in enterococci. Most penicillin resistance in E faecalis is mediated by a β-lactamase related to the staphylococcal β-lactamase; this remains an uncommon phenotype.[41,75,76] Most E faecium demonstrate intrinsic low-level penicillin resistance, due to presence of the PBP5 protein, with decreased affinity for penicillins.[76] Higher level resistance, with MICs of up to 256 μg/mL or more, is found among nosocomial E faecium isolates, due to either increased expression of PBP5 or additional mutations in the pbp5 gene.[77] Altered pbp5 genes are found on transferrable elements and are capable of horizontal transmission.[78] High-level ampicillin resistance is reported in other enterococcal species, although many laboratories do not reliably identify or report species other than E faecalis. Ampicillin-resistant strains are resistant to all penicillins and carbapenems.

All enterococci are intrinsically resistant to low levels of aminoglycosides because of inefficient drug entry across the bacterial cell membrane. Wild-type strains are susceptible to high levels of aminoglycosides and are identified in the laboratory by susceptibility to 500 to 1000 μg/mL of gentamicin and streptomycin. Acquired HLAR is a result of the presence of AME, most commonly AAC(6′)-APH (2″) enzymes.[75] HLAR eliminates synergistic killing of enterococci by an aminoglycoside in combination with a penicillin or vancomycin. High-level gentamicin resistance generally predicts lack of synergy with all aminoglycosides except streptomycin. Occasional isolates demonstrate high-level gentamicin but not streptomycin resistance, which is mediated by different AME.

Table 3
Important mechanisms of acquired resistance in enterococci

Drug Class	Predominant Species	Resistance Phenotype	Mechanism	Genetics and Transmission	Prevalence
Penicillins	E faecalis	Ampicillin (but difficult to detect); susceptible to ampicillin-sulbactam and imipenem	β-Lactamase	Plasmid	<1%
—	E faecium	Ampicillin MIC usually ≥64 µg/mL	Altered or new pbp5	Mutation, upregulation, or acquired on transposons	All strains have low level resistance; 90% higher level resistance in recent hospital isolates[73]
Glycopeptides	E faecalis, E faecium, Many other species	Vancomycin MIC 64–1000 µg/mL, Teicoplanin R	Target bypass with D-alanine-D-lactate intermediate	vanA cluster, Plasmids>> chromosome, Inducible	Recent US hospital isolates[73], E faecalis 6.9%, E faecium 80%
—	E faecalis, E faecium	Vancomycin MIC 4–1000 µg/mL, Teicoplanin S	Target bypass with D-alanine-D-lactate intermediate	vanB cluster, Chromosomal >>plasmid, Inducible	
—	E gallinarum, E casseliflavus	Vancomycin MIC 2–16 µg/mL	Target bypass with D-alanine-D-serine intermediate	vanC clusters, Chromosomal, Constitutive	All strains of species
Aminoglycosides (HLAR)	E faecalis, E faecium	Gentamicin MIC >1000 µg/mL	Enzymatic modification	AAC(6')-APH (2") and other enzymes, Plasmids	Only 25% in one recent survey[47] but generally 40%–60%
—	E faecium	Kanamycin, tobramycin MIC >1000 µg/mL, Gentamicin MIC 4–16 µg/mL	Enzymatic modification	AAC (6')-li, Chromosomal	All E faecium strains
Linezolid	E. faecalis, E faecium	Linezolid MIC >4 µg/mL	Ribosomal target mutation or modification	23S ribosomal mutations: G2576U, other plasmids: cfr	1.1% in recent large US surveys[47] but clusters/outbreaks
Daptomycin	E faecalis, E faecium	Daptomycin MIC >4 µg/mL	Membrane changes	?	<1% in large surveys[49], Case reports

The emergence of acquired glycopeptide resistance in enterococci after 40 years of glycopeptide use was a sentinel event in raising public awareness of the global threat of antimicrobial resistance. Vancomycin resistance was first recognized in *E faecalis* and *E faecium* in Europe and the United States in the late 1980s. Rates of VRE in United States ICUs increased from 0.3% in 1989 to more than 28% in 2003.[79] Numerous studies have assessed risk factors for VRE colonization and infection.[80,81] Acquired vancomycin resistance is predominantly found in *E faecium*, including the majority of *E faecium* from health care–associated infections, but was also found in 5% to 7% of *E faecalis* isolates from United States health care–associated infections in 2006–2007.[73] Vancomycin resistance is reported in multiple other enterococcal species, and low-level resistance is an intrinsic feature of the uncommon species *Enterococcus gallinarum* and *Enterococcus casseliflavus*. Resistance is mediated by the *van* family of structurally similar but genetically very distinct multigene clusters; the most important are the *vanA* and *vanB* clusters (see **Table 3**).[82] Glycopeptides act by avid binding of the large glycopeptide molecule to terminal D-alanine–D-alanine dipeptides in peptidoglycan precursors, blocking subsequent cell wall synthesis reactions. The *van* clusters allow enterococci to create a bypass around D-alanine–D-alanine in their peptidoglycan synthetic pathway. The *vanA* and *vanB* clusters instead use a D-alanine–D-lactate intermediate with markedly decreased affinity for glycopeptides. In some other *van* clusters, D-alanine–D-serine is the intermediate. The transferrable *vanA* and *vanB* clusters are on transposons located either on plasmids or within the chromosome. The plasmid-mediated *vanA* cluster is transferrable in vitro and in vivo into other gram-positive species, including MRSA.[12] *vanB* strains demonstrate more variable levels of resistance than *vanA* strains and are usually teicoplanin susceptible (see **Table 3**).[82] Current CLSI laboratory guidelines include use of supplemental vancomycin screening plates to improve detection of low-level expressing VRE strains.[41]

Management of infections caused by VRE and MDR enterococci

Enterococci are less virulent than *S aureus*, but are still associated with significant morbidity and mortality.[75] Differentiation of colonization from infection, especially colonization of the urinary tract, catheter tips, or chronic wounds, is essential to prevent unnecessary antibiotic usage and selection of further resistance. Some enterococcal infections resolve with measures such as removal of infected catheters without specific antibiotic therapy. When treatment is required, the site of infection and pattern of resistance are the major determinants of antibiotic selection. β-Lactamase–producing *E faecalis* can be treated with β-lactamase inhibitor drugs such as ampicillin-sulbactam, imipenem, or vancomycin. Ampicillin-resistant *E faecium* are resistant to all β-lactams including imipenem, but can be treated with vancomycin if not also vancomycin resistant. HLAR rarely impacts on management of enterococcal infections, except for endocarditis and endovascular infections, for which bactericidal therapy is recommended.[57] Vancomycin-resistant *E faecalis* are almost always susceptible to ampicillin. Treatment of ampicillin and vancomycin-resistant *E faecium* (VREF) is now less challenging with the availability of the newer agents linezolid, daptomycin, tigecycline, and telavancin. Linezolid is active against most VREF, and is used for a variety of enterococcal infections including bacteremia.[83] There are numerous reports of linezolid-resistant VREF, including outbreaks in oncology and transplant units as well as other nosocomial settings.[84] Prevalence of linezolid resistance in large surveys of enterococcal isolates remains low, but rates of nosocomial linezolid-resistant enterococci are predicted to increase with increasing levels of linezolid consumption.[47,85] Most linezolid resistance is caused by mutations in multiple copies of domain V of the 23S ribosome, most commonly at G2576U.[47,83] Tigecycline, another bacteriostatic agent, is active against most enterococci including VREF in vitro and has been used for intra-abdominal infections and SSTIs, but is not recommended for bacteremia.[83] Quinupristin-dalfopristin is a parenteral agent active against E faecium but not E faecalis and is FDA approved for VREF, but is generally bacteriostatic and is now rarely used as monotherapy for serious VREF infections.[83] Of the newer enterococcal agents, only daptomycin and telavancin demonstrate bactericidal activity against E faecalis and E faecium, including many VREF.

Acquired enterococcal resistance poses the greatest challenge in the management of enterococcal endocarditis. Addition of an aminoglycoside to ampicillin or vancomycin increases cure rates from 40% to between 70% and 80%, but this benefit is eliminated in HLAR strains.[86] Recommendations for treatment of endocarditis with ampicillin- or vancomycin-susceptible HLAR strains include prolonged duration of therapy and earlier consideration for surgery.[57] Studies have also reported the benefit of combining ampicillin with either ceftriaxone or imipenem for HLAR E faecalis endocarditis.[87] Ampicillin-resistant but vancomycin-susceptible E faecium endocarditis can be treated with vancomycin plus an aminoglycoside.[83] For endocarditis caused by VREF, cures are reported with 8 or more weeks of linezolid or quinupristin-dalfopristin treatment.[57,83] Daptomycin has also been used successfully to treat VREF endocarditis, but published experience is limited. Daptomycin MICs for enterococci are higher than for staphylococci, and doses of 10 to 12 mg/kg have been suggested for enterococcal endocarditis.[83] Resistance to daptomycin has emerged during treatment.[49] The role of combination therapy with daptomycin is uncertain, although daptomycin combined with tigecycline has been used for VREF endocarditis.[83] The new lipoglycopeptide telavancin has excellent bactericidal activity against susceptible E faecium and E faecalis, and is active against vanB VREF strains, though MICs of vanA strains are higher.[49] Clinical experience for severe enterococcal infections is limited.

Drug-Resistant Streptococcus Pneumoniae

Most pneumococcal infections are community acquired, but pneumococcal meningitis, bacteremia, and pneumonia are common causes of admission to an ICU. Data from the CDC Active Bacterial Core Surveillance Program in 2009 shows continued declines in pneumococcal susceptibility to multiple antibiotics classes, including penicillins, third-generation cephalosporins, erythromycin, and trimethoprim-sulfamethoxazole.[88] β-Lactam resistance is caused by altered PBPs with decreased affinity for penicillins and cephalosporins. PBP changes occur via point mutations and by recombination with pbp genes from other pneumococci or commensal oral streptococci.[89,90] Resistance is classified as intermediate or high level; high-level resistance cannot be overcome by increasing drug doses and leads to treatment failure, especially for meningitis. High-level penicillin resistance indicates resistance to all penicillins and to first- and second-generation cephalosporins. High-level third-generation cephalosporin resistance, found in 1.9% of United States isolates in 2009, requires additional or different PBP changes.[88–90] High-level penicillin resistance is disproportionately found in certain pneumococcal serotypes. Decline in the rate of DRSP among invasive pneumococcal isolates was observed after introduction of the 7-valent conjugate pneumococcal vaccine, although trends have reversed as new DRSP serotypes have become more prevalent.[91] Additional resistant serotypes are targeted in newer conjugate vaccines.

Penicillin-resistant pneumococci are often resistant to other drugs including macrolides, clindamycin, tetracyclines, and trimethoprim-sulfamethoxazole. Macrolide resistance caused by efflux pumps that do not confer cross-resistance to azithromycin, clindamycin, or streptogramin B (M-phenotype), to ribosomal methylases that cause cross-resistance to antibiotics that share the same target (MLSb phenotype), or to 23S ribosome mutations.[90] Fluoroquinolone resistance is caused by mutations in quinolone resistance–determining regions in gyrase and topoisomerase genes. Ciprofloxacin resistance requires a single mutation, but levofloxacin and moxifloxacin resistance requires multiple mutations and occurs less readily.[92] Risks for resistance include prior fluoroquinolone exposures and high organism load. In 2009 only 0.3% of United States isolates were levofloxacin resistant.[88] Vancomycin resistance in pneumococcus is not reported, although tolerance to vancomycin killing has been described.

ANTIMICROBIAL RESISTANCE IN GRAM-NEGATIVE BACTERIA
Introduction

Infections caused by MDR gram-negative bacteria (GNB) lead to substantial morbidity and mortality in critically ill patients; thus, it is crucial for ICU practitioners to understand key concepts related to resistant GNB. In this section, the authors review differences between structures of gram-negative and gram-positive bacterial cells, mechanisms of action and resistance of antimicrobial agents used to treat of GNB infections, and the epidemiology and management of infections caused by specific MDR GNB.

Gram-Negative Cell Structure and Antibiotic Mechanisms of Action

A major factor contributing to differences in resistance mechanisms between gram-negative and gram-positive bacteria is the difference in their cell structure. GNB possess an outer membrane (OM) not present in gram-positive bacteria (Fig. 2).[13,93–95] The OM functions as a selective barrier, and its permeability properties determine whether antimicrobials can enter into the GNB cell. In general, small hydrophilic drugs such as β-lactams, fluoroquinolones, and tetracyclines diffuse across the OM through porin proteins, whereas hydrophobic antibiotics such as aminoglycosides and polymyxins diffuse directly across the lipid membrane. Certain organisms such as *Pseudomonas aeruginosa* have a baseline low level of OM permeability because of a lack of general diffusion porins.[93] Another major structural difference between gram-negative and gram-positive bacteria is the markedly thicker peptidoglycan cell wall in gram-positive bacteria, which is 50-fold thicker than the GNB cell wall (see Fig. 2).[96] In addition, GNB have a periplasmic space in an aqueous environment that contains a large number of proteins, including β-lactamases.[94] Both gram-negative and gram-positive bacteria have efflux pumps, a cytoplasmic membrane, and similar cytoplasmic contents. The most common agents used to treat GNB infections include β-lactams, fluoroquinolones, aminoglycosides and, for some extensively drug-resistant GNB, polymyxins and tigecycline. The mechanisms of action of these antimicrobials are illustrated in Fig. 2.

Mechanisms of Antimicrobial Resistance in Gram-Negative Bacteria

β-Lactam resistance in gram-negative bacteria: an introduction to the β-lactamases
β-Lactams comprise a large group of antibiotics including the penicillins, monobactams, carbapenems, and cephalosporins. The mechanism of action of β-lactams involves inhibition of the transpeptidases (ie, PBPs) responsible for cross-linking peptidoglycan in the cell wall, ultimately resulting in destruction of the cell wall (see Fig. 2).[96] β-Lactam resistance in GNB occurs through a variety of mechanisms but most importantly by β-lactamase enzymes that hydrolyze and inactivate β-lactams

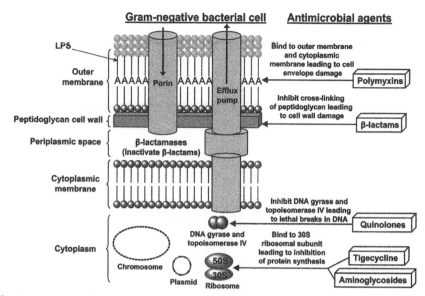

Fig. 2. A cross-sectional view of a gram-negative bacterial cell. The cell envelope is composed of: (1) the outer membrane (OM), (2) a thin cell wall composed of peptidoglycan, (3) the periplasmic space, and (4) the cytoplasmic membrane (CM). The OM functions as a barrier that allows the diffusion of nutrients and other molecules into the GNB cell. The inner portion of the OM is composed of phospholipids, while the outer portion is composed of lipopolysaccharide (LPS). The OM also contains porin proteins, which allow for diffusion of hydrophilic antibiotics across the outer membrane. Most GNB have efflux pumps that traverse both the OM and CM and remove toxic substances that accumulate in the cell, but they also function to remove antimicrobials from the cell. The periplasmic space contains a variety of proteins including β-lactamases, which hydrolyze β-lactams. The CM is composed of a phospholipid bilayer with embedded proteins, and is involved in the transport of molecules into and out of the cytoplasm, including antimicrobials. The cytoplasm contains the genome, usually consisting of a single circular chromosome, and may contain one or more plasmids, all of which may carry genes that encode antimicrobial resistance elements. Ribosomes are also located in the cytoplasm.

by disrupting the β-lactam ring.[97] In the 1960s and 1970s, resistance to early β-lactams in GNB developed through production of "broad-spectrum β-lactamases" that hydrolyzed penicillins, aminopenicillins, carboxypenicillins, ureidopenicillins, and narrow-spectrum cephalosporins.[9,98–100] These broad-spectrum β-lactamases include TEM-1, TEM-2, and SHV-1. The response to these broad-spectrum β-lactamases was development of extended-spectrum third-generation cephalosporins such as ceftriaxone, cefotaxime, and ceftazidime, monobactams like aztreonam, and carbapenems such as imipenem, which are stable in the presence of the broad-spectrum β-lactamases. By the early 1980s, GNB responded to these new antimicrobials by developing mutations in the TEM and SHV β-lactamases, resulting in the evolution of "extended-spectrum β-lactamases" (ESBLs).[101] In addition to hydrolyzing the same antimicrobials as the broad-spectrum β-lactamases, ESBLs also hydrolyze third-generation cephalosporins and aztreonam (**Table 4**). Since the 1980s, the number of ESBLs indentified has markedly increased, and new families have been described. There are now more than 300 different types of ESBL enzymes, the most common being of the TEM, SHV, CTX-M, and OXA families. Although antimicrobials such as carbapenems are available to treat ESBL-producing GNB, bacteria

Table 4
Common multidrug-resistant Enterobacteriaceae

Organism	Mechanisms of Antimicrobial Resistance[a]	Antimicrobial Treatment
ESBL-producing *Klebsiella* spp and *Escherichia coli*	Hydrolyze penicillins, aminopenicillins, carboxypenicillins, and ureidopenicillins, aztreonam, and most first-, second-, and third-generation cephalosporins. Do not hydrolyze "cephamycins" (cefoxitin and cefotetan), but may be resistant by other mechanisms ESBLs of the CTX-M and OXA families hydrolyze cefepime efficiently, whereas ESBLs of the TEM and SHV families typically have poor hydrolytic activity against cefepime Inhibited by antimicrobials containing β-lactamase inhibitors such as piperacillin-tazobactam, but resistance may develop by other mechanisms Do not hydrolyze carbapenems	*Preferred treatment:[b]* Carbapenems *Alternative treatment:[c]* For infections of low severity (such as urinary tract infection without bacteremia), consider use of: 1. Fluoroquinolones 2. Aminoglycosides 3. Trimethoprim-sulfamethoxazole Agents potentially active in vitro but of unproven efficacy: 1. Piperacillin-tazobactam 2. Cefepime (for isolates with cefepime MIC of ≤1)
AmpC producing *Enterobacter* spp, *Citrobacter freundii, Serratia marcescens, Morganella morganii*	AmpC may be "induced", or mutants hyperproducing AmpC may be "selected for," after exposure to first-, second-, and third-generation cephalosporins and other β-lactams Strains hyperproducing AmpC hydrolyze the same spectrum of β-lactams as ESBLs but also cephamycins Not inhibited by antimicrobials containing β-lactamase inhibitors Do not have significant hydrolytic activity against cefepime or carbapenems	*Preferred treatment:[b]* Carbapenems or cefepime *Alternative treatment:[c]* 1. Fluoroquinolones 2. Aminoglycosides Avoid third-generation cephalosporins even if susceptible, due to risk of clinical resistance on therapy[a]
Carbapenemase-producing *Klebsiella* and *E coli* (and other Enterobacteriaceae)	Hydrolyze the same spectrum of β-lactams as ESBLs but also hydrolyze cephamycins and carbapenems The class A KPC family of carbapenemases are only weakly inhibited by β-lactamase inhibitors and are usually resistant to β-lactamase inhibitor drugs IMP, VIM, and NDM-1 family metallo-β-lactamase do not hydrolyze aztreonam, but resistance typically develops via other mechanisms, and are not inhibited by β-lactamase inhibitors	*Preferred treatment:[b]* Aminoglycosides or polymyxins Tigecycline has been used, but consider alternative treatment for bloodstream and urinary tract infections Nebulized aminoglycosides or colistin, plus systemic therapy, for severe or highly drug-resistant pneumonia Role of combination therapy unclear *Alternative treatment:[c]* For infections of low severity, consider use of following agents: 1. Fluoroquinolones 2. Trimethoprim-sulfamethoxazole

[a] Additional changes in outer membrane permeability and overexpression of efflux pumps can enhance effectiveness of ESBL, AmpC, and carbapenemases.
[b] Choose alternative antimicrobial agent if susceptibility testing shows resistance to listed preferred agent.

responded again by the early 1990s by producing carbapenemases (see **Table 4**). These β-lactamases hydrolyze a similar spectrum of antimicrobials to ESBLs, but are also active against carbapenems.[9,98,99,102] Carbapenemase-producing organisms are frequently resistant to most other classes of antimicrobial agents, leaving limited therapeutic options.

The last major class of β-lactamases is the AmpC β-lactamase family. These β-lactamases are capable of hydrolyzing a similar spectrum of antimicrobials to ESBLs (see **Table 4**) and are present in several clinically important GNB, including *Enterobacter* spp, *Citrobacter freundii*, *Serratia marcescens*, and *Morganella morganii*, and are also found in *P aeruginosa*, *Acinetobacter* spp, and several other species.[9,98,99,103] In some of these organisms, particularly *Enterobacter* spp, mutants that hyperproduce AmpC β-lactamase may be selected for when patients are exposed to β-lactams, or "induction" of AmpC may occur after β-lactam exposure, resulting in emergence of resistance.

In addition to β-lactamases there are other mechanisms of β-lactam resistance. Altered OM permeability may contribute to β-lactam resistance, either via mutations in porins that lead to a change in shape or function of the porin, or via a loss or reduction in the number of porins.[93] For example, mutations in the OprD porin, which is important in the diffusion of carbapenems across the OM of *P aeruginosa*, is an important cause of carbapenem resistance in *P aeruginosa*. Porins such as OmpC, OmpF, and OmpK are also commonly implicated in β-lactam resistance in *K pneumoniae* and *Enterobacter* spp, as well as in *Escherichia coli*, *Proteus* spp, *S marcescens*, and *Acinetobacter baumannii*.[93,97] Efflux pumps may also contribute to resistance. In *P aeruginosa*, the MexAB-OprM and other efflux pumps may lead to resistance to multiple β-lactams, including cefepime and carbapenems.[13,95,97] In contrast to β-lactam resistance in gram-positive bacteria, β-lactam resistance in GNB is only very rarely caused by modification of penicillin-binding proteins.[97]

Fluoroquinolone resistance in gram-negative bacteria

Fluoroquinolones were introduced into clinical practice in the 1980s, and resistance was described only shortly thereafter. The mechanism of action of fluoroquinolones involves binding to DNA gyrase and topoisomerase IV, which are bacterial enzymes involved in DNA replication, transcription, and repair (see **Fig. 2**). GNB develop resistance to fluoroquinolones by developing one or more mutations in DNA gyrase or topoisomerase IV, leading to reduced fluoroquinolone binding.[104–106] GNB may also develop fluoroquinolone resistance through decreased OM permeability via mutations or decreased expression of porin proteins, and/or upregulation of efflux pumps such as the MexAB-OprM efflux pump in *P aeruginosa* or the AcrAB-TolC efflux pump in *E coli*. Enterobacteriaceae may also develop low-level fluoroquinolone resistance through 2 additional plasmid-mediated mechanisms,[104–106] namely the *qnr* genes, which encode for Qnr proteins that bind to and "protect" DNA gyrase and topoisomerase IV from inhibition by fluoroquinolones. An additional mechanism of resistance is a variant aminoglycoside acetyltransferase enzyme, AAC(6′)-Ib-cr, which binds to and diminishes the activity of ciprofloxacin and norfloxacin, but not other fluoroquinolones.

Aminoglycoside resistance in gram-negative bacteria

Aminoglycosides were introduced in the 1940s and resistance to these agents was initially described in the 1960s. The mechanism of action of aminoglycosides involves inhibition of the 30S ribosomal subunit, leading to alterations in protein synthesis (see **Fig. 2**). The most common mechanism of aminoglycoside resistance in GNB is modification of the aminoglycoside molecule via modifying enzymes, which results in poor drug binding to the 30S ribosomal subunit.[107,108] Three major families of AME have been described that result in acetylation (aminoglycoside acetyltransferases), phosphorylation (aminoglycoside phosphotransferases), or adenylation (aminoglycoside nucleotidyltransferases) of the aminoglycoside molecule. AME genes are often found on transferrable plasmids, but they are also chromosomally encoded in certain GNB species. A large number of AME are described with activity against different aminoglycosides. GNB may produce multiple AME, leading to broad aminoglycoside resistance. Aminoglycoside resistance also occurs as a result of decreased OM permeability and/or efflux pumps.[13,95,107,108] Mutations in the lipopolysaccharide (LPS) component of the OM and mutations influencing the transmembrane potential of the cytoplasmic membrane, each resulting in decreased uptake of aminoglycosides into the cell, have also been described.[107,108] Modification of the 30S ribosomal subunit antibiotic target does not play a major role in aminoglycoside resistance in GNB.

Resistance to other antimicrobials used for gram-negative bacteria: polymyxins and tigecycline

Polymyxins are cationic polypeptide antibiotics that were introduced into clinical practice in the 1950s. Colistin (polymyxin E) and polymyxin B were the 2 polymyxins available for use, but their use was abandoned in the 1970s because of toxicity.[109,110] Polymyxins were "rediscovered" in the 1990s as therapy for multidrug-resistant GNB. The mechanism of action of polymyxins involves binding to LPS in the OM and binding to the cytoplasmic membrane, leading to cell envelope damage, altered membrane permeability, and cell death (see **Fig. 2**). Resistance to polymyxins is uncommon, but may occur by modification of the lipid A component of the LPS polymyxin-binding target.[110]

Tigecycline is a glycylcycline tetracycline analogue introduced for clinical use in 2005. Tigecycline binds to the 30S bacterial ribosomal subunit, leading to inhibition of protein synthesis (see **Fig. 2**). It is active against most Enterobacteriaceae and *Acinetobacter* spp. Tigecycline has poor activity against *P aeruginosa*, *Proteus* spp, *Morganella* spp, and *Providencia* spp, due to expression of efflux pumps.[111,112] Acquired tigecycline resistance has now been reported in multiple other GNB via expression of efflux pumps, including the AcrAB efflux pump in *E coli*, *K pneumoniae*, and *Enterobacter cloacae*, and the AdeABC multidrug-efflux pump in *Acinetobacter* spp.[112]

Extended-Spectrum β-Lactamase–Producing Enterobacteriaceae

Introduction to ESBL-producing enterobacteriaceae

ESBLs are most commonly found in clinical *K pneumoniae* and *E coli* isolates, but are also described in many other Enterobacteriaceae and even in nonfermenting GNB such as *P aeruginosa*.[9,97,99] There are several ESBL families, the most common being the TEM and SHV families found in both *Klebsiella* and *E coli* and the CTX-M family, predominantly in *E coli*. There are many members of each family, with more than 300 different ESBLs described to date.[99,101] A variety of other less common ESBL families such as OXA-type ESBLs have also been described.[9,97] Most ESBLs hydrolyze a similar spectrum of β-lactams (see **Table 4**), but there are some differences among the various ESBLs.[9,101] For example, ESBLs may have variable activity against cefepime. ESBLs are inhibited by β-lactamase inhibitors such as tazobactam and clavulanic acid, but resistance may develop to these agents via other mechanisms. Resistance to non–β-lactam antimicrobials such as aminoglycosides and fluoroquinolones is common in ESBL-producing strains. Carbapenems retain good activity against ESBL-producing Enterobacteriaceae, as do tigecycline and the polymyxins.

Detection of ESBL-producing enterobacteriaceae
The CLSI and other groups that establish standards for susceptibility testing have for the past decade recommended screening for ESBL-producing Enterobacteriaceae. An ESBL screen is positive when MIC values to any third-generation cephalosporin or aztreonam are greater than 1 µg/mL, even if still within the susceptible range of 8 µg/mL or less.[101,113] In these settings, a confirmatory "phenotypic" ESBL test is performed. This procedure most commonly has included testing for susceptibility to third-generation cephalosporins with and without the β-lactamase inhibitor clavulanate. Presence of an ESBL is detected by increased susceptibility to the third-generation cephalosporin combined with clavulanate. According to previous CLSI guidelines, if an ESBL confirmatory test is positive, all penicillins, aztreonam, and all cephalosporins including cefepime are automatically reported as resistant, even if their MIC values are in the susceptible range. Interpretations for β-lactam-β-lactamase inhibitors such as piperacillin-tazobactam are not changed. A "genotypic" test using the polymerase chain reaction (PCR) for ESBL genes is not routinely performed in clinical laboratories.

As of 2010, CLSI no longer recommends ESBL screening and confirmatory testing of Enterobacteriaceae, which has significant clinical implications for treating these pathogens.[41] Instead, CLSI has lowered the cephalosporin MIC breakpoints for Enterobacteriaceae, which obviates the need for ESBL testing. The "susceptible" MIC breakpoints for cefotaxime and ceftriaxone were decreased from 8 µg/mL or less to 1 µg/mL or less; thus, organisms that were previously considered susceptible to cefotaxime or ceftriaxone with an MIC between 2 and 8 µg/mL will now be reported as either intermediate or resistant, with no further screening for or reporting of an ESBL result. If the MIC for any single third- or fourth-generation cephalosporin is within the susceptible range, it will no longer automatically be reported as resistant even if another drug is reported as resistant. Clinicians will then have the option to treat the patient with one of these alternative cephalosporins. Adopting this method should have a profound impact on selection of antibiotics for these pathogens. This dramatic change will likely take several years to fully implement in clinical laboratories that follow CLSI guidelines, especially those with automated susceptibility testing systems.

Epidemiology of ESBL-producing enterobacteriaceae
Rates of infections caused by ESBL-producing Enterobacteriaceae in ICUs vary widely depending on location. In a study from 42 ICUs in the United States from 2000 to 2002, 13.7% of K pneumoniae and 3.6% of E coli were ESBL producers. The most common ESBLs were SHV enzymes, but TEM and CTX-M were also found.[114] The CDC collected data on predominantly ICU-related United States health care–associated infections in 2006–2007. ESBL confirmatory testing was not performed, but the proportion of K pneumoniae and E coli that were ceftriaxone or ceftazidime resistant and likely ESBL producers was between 21% to 27% and 6% to 11%, respectively.[73] Similar data were collected on ICU health care–associated infections from 2003 to 2008 in Latin America, Asia, Africa, and Europe. Here, between 70% to 76% of K pneumoniae and 42% to 68% of E coli were probable ESBL producers, much higher than found in the United States.[115] In another study from ICUs in Canada in from 2005 and 2006, only 3.7% of E coli isolates and 1.8% of K pneumoniae were ESBL producers, significantly lower than the other recent studies.[116,117] This Canadian study was one of the few to report a higher proportion of ESBL E coli than

K pneumoniae. All ESBL *E coli* isolates were of the CTX-M type and 72% were CTX-M-15, the most widely distributed CTX-M enzyme worldwide.[118] These ESBL *E coli* isolates were frequently resistant to other antimicrobials, including ciprofloxacin (78%), cefepime (88% with MIC >1 µg/mL), and gentamicin (28%). No ESBL *E coli* isolates were carbapenem or tigecycline resistant and only 11% were resistant to piperacillin-tazobactam.

Management of infections caused by ESBL-producing enterobacteriaceae

There are no data from randomized controlled clinical trials comparing antibiotic treatments for ESBL-producing Enterobacteriaceae. Carbapenems have been considered the treatment of choice, because they are not hydrolyzed by ESBLs, are highly active in vitro, and high rates of successful outcome have been reported in the literature (see **Table 4**).[101,118,122] Although recommended by some investigators, there are only limited published data to support use of piperacillin-tazobactam for infections caused by susceptible ESBL-producing strains.[119,123–126] In one series of infections caused by piperacillin-tazobactam susceptible ESBL-producing *E coli* and *Klebsiella* spp, successful outcomes were reported in 10 of 11 patients treated for non-urinary tract infections and in 6 of 6 treated for urinary tract infections.[124] Further data are needed before recommending the use of piperacillin-tazobactam as a treatment of choice for ESBL-producing Enterobacteriaceae.[101,118]

The use of any third- and fourth-generation cephalosporin for the treatment of serious infections due to ESBL-producing Enterobacteriaceae had not been recommended because of high failure rates for infections caused by strains with MIC values of 2 to 8 µg/mL, which were elevated but still within the previous susceptible range.[119,121,122,127–129] For ESBL-producing Enterobacteriaceae treated with third- and fourth-generation cephalosporins where MICs are 1 or less, failure rates are much lower.[121,127,130] For laboratories that are implementing the new 2010 CLSI guidelines, the question will arise as to whether cefepime or other agents can now be used for an ESBL-producing organism if it is susceptible with an MIC of less than 1 µg/mL.[41] Certain ESBLs hydrolyze cefepime poorly, and MIC values to cefepime for these strains may test within the susceptible range. In a recent study, 11 of 12 patients with ESBL-producing *K pneumoniae* and *E coli* infections with cefepime MIC values of 2 µg/mL or less treated with cefepime had clinical cure or improvement.[131] In another recent study of 22 patients with bacteremia due to ESBL-producing CTX-M type *E coli* resistant to cefotaxime but susceptible to ceftazidime, clinical success rates were similar for ceftazidime (86%) and imipenem (88%).[132] Thus, cefepime and ceftazidine may be potential therapeutic options for some infections, although further data are needed. When the cefepime MIC is between 2 and 8 µg/mL, higher cefepime dosages of up to 2 g every 8 hours would likely be needed to achieve adequate serum antibiotic levels.[41,101,133–135] Another theoretical concern for use of cefepime for the treatment of ESBL-producing organisms is the "inoculum effect".[136] In vitro, concentrations of ESBL-producing bacteria higher than those used in routine susceptibility testing produce more β-lactamase and hydrolyze cefepime more effectively, and MIC values are higher with these higher organism concentrations. Whether this has importance clinically for treating "high inoculum" infections is uncertain.[137] The inoculum effect is less important with piperacillin-tazobactam or carbapenems.

There is limited information on use of fluoroquinolones or aminoglycosides for serious infections caused by ESBL-producing Enterobacteriaceae. Rates of fluoroquinolone resistance in ESBL-producing organisms are high, and aminoglycoside resistance is common.[118] Even for susceptible organisms, several studies have shown that outcome of infections treated with fluoroquinolones is worse than outcome with carbapenems.[119,120] Some studies have also reported poor efficacy of aminoglycosides for serious infections such as bacteremia.[138] For infections that are of low severity and of "low inoculum", fluoroquinolones and aminoglycosides can be considered (see **Table 4**). Trimethoprim-sulfamethoxazole resistance rates are also high, but this agent can be considered for infections of low severity such as uncomplicated urinary tract infections due to susceptible isolates (see **Table 4**).[118] Although cephamycins such as cefoxitin are not inactivated by ESBLs, they are not recommended as treatment options because of development of resistance by loss of porin proteins.[101,118]

AmpC β-Lactamase-Producing Enterobacteriaceae

Mechanism of antimicrobial resistance and epidemiology of AmpC β-lactamases

AmpC β-lactamases are present in numerous bacterial species and are most commonly described in *Enterobacter* spp, *C freundii*, *S marcescens*, and *M morganii*, but are also found in strains of *P aeruginosa*, *Acinetobacter* spp, and several other Enterobacteriaceae.[103] Plasmid-mediated AmpC β-lactamases have also been reported infrequently in *Klebsiella* and *E coli*. AmpC β-lactamases hydrolyze the same spectrum of antimicrobials as ESBLs but also hydrolyze cephamycins and are not inhibited by β-lactamase inhibitors (see **Table 4**). AmpC β-lactamases have poor hydrolytic activity against carbapenems and cefepime. A unique characteristic of many AmpC β-lactamases is that baseline expression may be low, but increases after exposure to β-lactams.[103] One explanation for this is "induction" of AmpC. Induction occurs following a β-lactam exposure, which stimulates transcription of the *ampC* gene and production of AmpC. Although some β-lactams such as penicillins, aminopenicillins, and early-generation cephalosporins may be stronger inducers, most β-lactams can induce AmpC hyperproduction.[103] An additional explanation for AmpC hyperproduction after β-lactam exposure is selection of spontaneous mutants that hyperproduce AmpC.[139] Thus, an isolate initially susceptible to a β-lactam may develop resistance during or after exposure.

Development of resistance on therapy is most commonly reported with *Enterobacter* spp infections treated with third-generation cephalosporins. Third-generation cephalosporin resistance developed in 19% of 129 patients with *Enterobacter* spp bacteremia.[140] In another cohort of 477 patients with *Enterobacter* infections, resistance developed in 19% of patients, with highest risk (29%) in those with bloodstream infections.[139] Risk of developing resistance appears higher for *Enterobacter* spp than for other AmpC-containing species. In one large study, resistance occurred in 8.3% of patients with *Enterobacter* spp infection, but in only 2.6% with *C. freundii* and in 0% of those with *S marcescens* or *M morganii*, with highest rates in those with *Enterobacter* bacteremia.[141] In this study, no patients who received cefepime, carbapenems, or fluoroquinolones developed resistance during therapy.

Management of infections caused by AmpC β-lactamase–producing enterobacteriaceae

Use of third-generation cephalosporins should be avoided for GNB that produce AmpC, especially *Enterobacter* spp, even if they test as susceptible in vitro, due to risk for emergence of resistance (see **Table 4**).[103,139–141] Carbapenems and cefepime are not readily hydrolyzed by AmpC, and these are the treatments of choice for susceptible strains. Fluoroquinolones are acceptable options for susceptible strains, and aminoglycosides can also be considered.

Carbapenemase-Producing Enterobacteriaceae

Nomenclature and epidemiology of carbapenemase-producing enterobacteriaceae

Carbapenemase-producing GNB are a major emerging problem. They are often also resistant to most available antimicrobial agents, leaving limited therapeutic options. Carbapenemases hydrolyze the same spectrum of antimicrobials as do ESBLs but also hydrolyze cephamycins and carbapenems. Most are also generally poorly inhibited by β-lactamase inhibitors. There are also some differences between different carbapenemase families in their ability to hydrolyze various β-lactams (see **Table 4**).[9,102]

The class A carbapenemases encompass several families, the most prevalent being the KPC family.[102] The KPC carbapenemases (KPCs) are plasmid-mediated and hydrolyze all currently available β-lactams (see **Table 4**). KPCs are only weakly inhibited by β-lactamase inhibitors such as tazobactam, and KPC strains often carry additional mechanisms for resistance to β-lactamase inhibitors. KPC-producing GNB also frequently harbor other resistance traits including aminoglycoside and fluoroquinolone resistance.[142,143] Since their first appearance in the United States in 1996, at least 7 slightly different KPCs have been described, though the majority of United States clinical isolates contain KPC-2 or KPC-3. KPCs are found mainly in *K pneumoniae*, but are also described in other Enterobacteriaceae including *E coli* and *Klebsiella oxytoca*, and in *P aeruginosa*.[102,142] KPC-producing GNB are now found throughout the United States, Europe, China, and South America, with major epidemic/endemic areas in the United States east coast, Greece, Israel, and the Zhejiang province of China.[102,142]

The metallo-β-lactamases include several families of carbapenemases, the most common being the plasmid-mediated IMP and VIM families, which have now been detected worldwide.[102] These metallo-β-lactamases hydrolyze all β-lactams with the exception of aztreonam, but most are also resistant to aztreonam via other resistance determinants; they are also not inhibited by β-lactamase inhibitors. The metallo-β-lactamases have been described in a variety of GNB, including *P aeruginosa*, *A baumannii*, *K pneumoniae*, *E coli*, and several other species. One novel metallo-β-lactamase, NDM-1, was initially described in a *K pneumoniae* isolate in a patient in India in 2008.[144] Reports of NDM-1-producing Enterobacteriaceae have increased markedly since 2008 throughout India, Pakistan, and the United Kingdom in both hospital- and community-acquired infections, predominantly in *K pneumoniae* and *E coli* but also in other Enterobacteriaceae.[145] NDM-1-producing Enterobacteriaceae are now reported in patients worldwide, including many European countries, the United States, Canada,, Australia, Japan, Oman, and Kenya.[146,147] There is significant concern that NDM-1–producing Enterobacteriaceae will continue to spread and become endemic globally. The NDM-1 gene is carried on plasmids, facilitating horizontal transfer. NDM-1-producing isolates are generally resistant to all β-lactams including aztreonam, as well as aminoglycosides and fluoroquinolones.

The OXA-type carbapenemases have mostly been described in *A baumannii*, and are rare in other organisms.[102] This family of carbapenemases has been found in *Acinetobacter* throughout the world, including in Europe, South America, Korea, the United States, and in military and civilian personnel in Iraq and Afghanistan. OXA-type carbapenemases hydrolyze penicillins, most cephalosporins (except some extended-spectrum cephalosporins), and carbapenems, but not aztreonam.

Management of infections caused by carbapenemase-producing enterobacteriaceae

Treatment options for carbapenemase-producing Enterobacteriaceae are limited because of the presence of multiple other resistance traits including resistance to fluoroquinolones, aminoglycosides, and trimethoprim-sulfamethoxazole (see **Table 4**).[142] Colistin (ie, polymyxin E) and polymyxin B are increasingly used for KPC-producing Enterobacterlaceae.[142,140] Ninety percent to 100% of KPC-producing *K pneumoniae* remain susceptible to polymyxins, but there are increasing reports of resistance.[142,143,149–152] Understanding of pharmacokinetics and dosing of polymyxins is incomplete. A loading dose has been recommended to more rapidly achieve drug levels above the MIC, although data are limited.[110] Aminoglycosides are potential treatment options, but rates of resistance to all aminoglycosides of from 45% to as high as 90% are reported.[143,150] Fluoroquinolone resistance is reported in approximately 90% to 100% of isolates.[143,150] Tigecycline has good in vitro susceptibility against most isolates, but tigecycline serum and urine levels are low, and there are reports of bacteremia developing during therapy.[142,148,153–156] Inhaled nebulized antibiotics such as tobramycin or colistin have been used as adjunctive treatment for pneumonia in combination with systemic antimicrobials.[148]

Combination therapy, including combinations comprising drugs that may be inactive in vitro, are increasingly employed for these infections, but there are few clinical data and no comparative trials for any regimens, and routine use is not currently recommended.[142,148] Rifampin is often used in combination with other agents. Rifampin is inactive against most GNB due to its inability to penetrate the OM, but may be able to reach its cytoplasmic target when combined with cell wall active drugs. In one in vitro study, polymyxin B plus rifampin was synergistic for 15 of 16 KPC-producing *K pneumoniae*, including 2 polymyxin-resistant isolates.[143] In this study, polymyxin B was bactericidal whereas tigecycline was bacteriostatic. Treatment options for metallo-β-lactamase–producing GNB are similar to those for KPC-producing strains. Ninety percent to 100% of NDM-1–producing Enterobacteriaceae isolates have been susceptible to colistin and 55% to 65% to tigecycline.[145] NDM-1 organisms have high rates of resistance to most other antimicrobials, including aztreonam, aminoglycosides, and fluoroquinolones.[145]

Multidrug-Resistant Nonfermenting Gram-Negative Bacteria: Pseudomonas aeruginosa, Acinetobacter spp, and Stenotrophomonas maltophilia

"Nonfermenting" gram-negative bacteria are found in soil and water and are also widely found in the health care environment, including on respiratory therapy/ventilator equipment, environmental surfaces, and as colonizers of patients and health care workers.[157–160] The most important nonfermenting GNB in clinical practice include *P aeruginosa*, *Acinetobacter* spp, and *Stenotrophomonas maltophilia*. *P aeruginosa* is by far the most common of these pathogens, while *Acinetobacter* spp is less common but is often reported from ICU outbreaks. *S maltophilia* is also less common, but arises in the setting of broad-spectrum antimicrobial exposure, usually in the respiratory tract.[160,161]

Mechanisms of antimicrobial resistance in P aeruginosa, Acinetobacter spp, and S maltophilia

P aeruginosa and *Acinetobacter* spp are intrinsically resistant to many antimicrobials but also have an impressive arsenal of mechanisms facilitating further emergence of acquired resistance to essentially all antimicrobials (**Table 5**).[158,159,162,163] *S maltophilia* are intrinsically resistant to most agents, including carbapenems and other β-lactams, but are usually susceptible to trimethoprim-sulfamethoxazole and ticarcillin-clavulanate (see **Table 5**). Resistance to trimethoprim-sulfamethoxazole in *S maltophilia* is rare, but may occur via *sul* genes or other poorly characterized mechanisms.[164]

Table 5
Common multidrug-resistant nonfermenting gram-negative bacteria

Organism	Mechanisms of Antimicrobial Resistance	Antimicrobial Treatment[a,b]
MDR *Pseudomonas aeruginosa*	*Decrease in intracellular drug entry:* • Alteration in outer membrane porin proteins: β-lactams, fluoroquinolones, aminoglycosides • Efflux pumps: β-lactams, fluoroquinolones, aminoglycosides *Drug destruction or modification:* • Early broad-spectrum β-lactamases, extended-spectrum β-lactamases, AmpC β-lactamases, carbapenemases (KPC family, metallo-β-lactamases) • Aminoglycoside-modifying enzymes *Modification of the antibiotic target:* • DNA gyrase and topoisomerase mutations: fluoroquinolones • Modification of lipopolysaccharide: polymyxins	*Preferred treatment:* Limited options for isolates resistant to all β-lactams and fluoroquinolones Aminoglycosides or polymyxins Nebulized aminoglycosides or colistin plus systemic therapy for severe or highly drug-resistant pneumonia Role of combination therapy unclear
MDR *Acinetobacter*	*Decrease in intracellular drug entry:* • Alteration in outer membrane porin proteins: β-lactams, fluoroquinolones, aminoglycosides • Efflux pumps: β-lactams, fluoroquinolones, aminoglycosides, tigecycline *Drug destruction or modification:* • Early broad-spectrum β-lactamases, extended-spectrum β-lactamases, AmpC β-lactamases, carbapenemases (OXA family, metallo-β-lactamases) • Aminoglycoside-modifying enzymes *Modification of the antibiotic target:* • DNA gyrase and topoisomerase mutations: fluoroquinolones • Presumed modification of lipopolysaccharide: polymyxins	*Preferred treatment:* Limited options for isolates resistant to all β-lactams and fluoroquinolones Ampicillin-sulbactam, carbapenems, aminoglycosides, polymyxins Tigecycline has been used, but consider alternative treatment for bloodstream and urinary tract infections Nebulized aminoglycosides or colistin plus systemic therapy for severe or highly drug-resistant pneumonia Role of combination therapy unclear
Stenotrophomonas maltophilia	*Decrease in intracellular drug entry:* • Alteration in outer membrane porin proteins: β-lactams, fluoroquinolones, aminoglycosides • Efflux pumps: fluoroquinolones, tetracycline *Drug destruction or modification:* • Carbapenemases (metallo-β-lactamases) and other β-lactamases • Aminoglycoside-modifying enzymes	*Preferred treatment:* 1. Trimethoprim-sulfamethoxazole 2. Ticarcillin-clavulanate (if cannot tolerate trimethoprim-sulfamethoxazole) *Alternative treatment:* Fluoroquinolones

[a] If susceptible.
[b] Choose alternative antimicrobial agent if susceptibility testing shows resistance to listed preferred and/or alternative antibiotic treatments.

Epidemiology of infections caused by MDR P aeruginosa, Acinetobacter spp, and S maltophilia

Antimicrobial resistance is very common in nonfermenting GNB, especially in ICUs, but rates vary depending on location. Resistance rates in the United States for isolates from ICU and other health care–associated infections were recently reported.[73] Thirty-one percent of *P aeruginosa* isolates were resistant to fluoroquinolones, 25% to carbapenems, 18% to piperacillin or piperacillin-tazobactam, 13% to 19% to ceftazidime, 11% to cefepime, and 6% to amikacin. Among *A baumannii* isolates, resistance to carbapenems ranged from 26% to 37%. Rates of multidrug resistance among United States health care and ICU associated infections are also high.[165] Ten percent of *P aeruginosa* were resistant to 3 classes of antimicrobials and 2% to 4 classes; 60% of *A baumannii* were resistant to 3 classes and 34% to 4 classes. Resistance among *P aeruginosa* in a Canadian ICU survey were similar but slightly lower than those in the United States, including moderate levels of resistance to levofloxacin, meropenem, piperacillin-tazobactam, cefepime, and gentamicin.[117] Thirteen percent of *P aeruginosa* were resistant to 3 or more antimicrobial classes. In an international study from ICUs in Latin America, Asia, Africa, and Europe from 2003 to 2008, resistance rates were even higher than in North America.[115] Fifty percent of *P aeruginosa* were resistant to fluoroquinolones, 44% to carbapenems, 78% to piperacillin or piperacillin-tazobactam, 73% to cefepime, and 13% to amikacin. Forty-six percent of *A baumannii* isolates were carbapenem resistant.

Management of infections caused by MDR P aeruginosa, Acinetobacter spp, and S maltophilia

Treatment options are often very limited for infections caused by nonfermenting GNB, especially for MDR *P aeruginosa* and *Acinetobacter* spp (see **Table 5**).[148] Most isolates of MDR *P aeruginosa* and *Acinetobacter* spp are susceptible to polymyxins, and colistin and polymyxin B are frequently used for these infections.[109,110,152] Aminoglycosides have also been used for *P aeruginosa* and *Acinetobacter* spp, when they are susceptible. Inhaled nebulized antibiotics, usually tobramycin or colistin, can be considered as an adjunctive treatment for severe drug-resistant *P aeruginosa* and *Acinetobacter* spp pneumonia, in combination with systemic antimicrobials.[148] *P aeruginosa* isolates with low-level resistance to imipenem or meropenem should be tested for susceptibility to doripenem, which may be more active against some carbapenem resistant *P aeruginosa*.[112,166] *P aeruginosa* is intrinsically resistant to tigecycline. Tigecycline is an option for *Acinetobacter* spp infections but is not recommended for bloodstream and urinary tract infections.[148,154,167] Ampicillin-sulbactam is a preferred option for susceptible MDR *Acinetobacter* spp infections.[148,168] Sulbactam alone has high intrinsic activity against *Acinetobacter* spp.[159]

The role of combination therapy for infections caused by MDR and extensively drug-resistant *P aeruginosa* and *Acinetobacter* spp is unclear. As with infections caused by MDR carbapenemase-producing organisms, rifampin has been used in combination with cell wall active agents. The combination of rifampin plus a polymyxin has consistently shown in vitro synergism, although clinical studies of benefit are lacking.[110,169] Combinations of carbapenems and polymyxins have shown both synergism and antagonism in vitro.[110,169] Use of combination therapy is not routinely recommended, but may be considered in individual cases of serious extensively drug-resistant infections.

Most *S maltophilia* isolates are susceptible to trimethoprim-sulfamethoxazole, which is the treatment of choice.[160,170] Ticarcillin-clavulanate is an alternative when trimethoprim-sulfamethoxazole cannot be used. Fluoroquinolones are also an alternative for susceptible isolates.[170,171] Tigecycline has excellent in vitro activity against *S. maltophilia* but clinical data supporting its use are lacking.[172]

RESISTANCE TO ANAEROBIC AGENTS IN THE ICU

Bacteroides spp are among the most common anaerobes in the lower gastrointestinal tract, and are an important component of intra-abdominal infections.[173] Nearly all *Bacteroides* spp produce a chromosomally encoded β-lactamase (ie, a class 2e cephalosporinase) that hydrolyzes penicillins and cephalosporins.[98,173,174] Class 2e cephalosporinases are not able to hydrolyze the cephamycins cefoxitin and cefotetan or carbapenems, and are inhibited by β-lactamase inhibitors. Resistance to cephamycins occurs due to other β-lactamases such as *cfxA*. The β-lactam–β-lactamase inhibitors such as ampicillin-sulbactam and piperacillin-tazobactam and the carbapenems remain active against most *Bacteroides* spp but resistance has been reported, due to the production of metallo-β-lactamases.[173] Resistance to clindamycin occurs via modification (ie, methylation) of the 50S ribosomal subunit target.[173] Metronidazole is a prodrug that is converted to its active form by anaerobic bacteria. Resistance to metronidazole is rare, but may occur through genes or mutations that prevent the conversion of prodrug to its active form.[173,174] Fluoroquinolone resistance may occur through mutations in DNA gyrase and topoisomerase IV, and also through efflux pumps.

Resistance to clindamycin increased from 5% to 6% in 1981–1989 and 23% in 1990–1999 to more than 30% in 2000–2007 in one United States study.[175] Rates of resistance to moxifloxacin ranged from 32% to 56%. These data support recent recommendations that clindamycin and moxifloxacin are not reliable empiric options for intra-abdominal and other infections for which *Bacteroides* spp is a consideration. Resistance rates to cefoxitin were 9% in 2000–2007, although rates of resistance to imipenem, piperacillin-tazobactam, and ampicillin-sulbactam all remained at less than 1% to 4% for most species. Rates of resistance to tigecycline ranged from 0% to 7%, but less than 0.1% were resistant to metronidazole. Recent European susceptibility data for the *Bacteroides fragilis* group also showed increasing resistance to clindamycin, cefoxitin, and moxifloxacin.[176]

MANAGEMENT OF ANTIMICROBIAL RESISTANCE IN THE ICU

The ICU remains at the epicenter of the crisis of antimicrobial resistance in hospitalized patients.[1,3,73] Although rates of hospital MRSA infections may be declining, rates of MDR gram-negative rods, including pan-resistant *Klebsiella*, *Pseudomonas*, and *Acinetobacter*, continue to increase.[1,27,73,148] Several new drugs for gram-positive infections have been approved within the past decade, but the pipeline of novel drugs to meet the challenge of MDR gram-negative pathogens remains limited.[1,3] There is no single solution to containing the spread of antimicrobial resistant pathogens, but multiple interventions have demonstrated potential benefit and many others are being evaluated. An essential component of all strategies to prevent spread of antimicrobial resistance is physician and societal recognition of the magnitude of the problem, and commitment to take aggressive steps to intervene. There are many guidelines from national and international agencies that address resistant organisms, but guidelines alone are not adequate to change behaviors.[80,81] The heightened societal concern about resistance has led to enactment of legislation for controlling antibiotic-resistant bacteria, including hospital-based screening of specific pathogens and reporting of hand washing and infection rates.[177] In the United States, hospital reimbursement by Medicare and other payers may be withheld for specific potentially preventable events, including hospital-acquired infections caused by resistant pathogens.

Strategies for preventing antimicrobial resistance are outlined in the CDC Campaign to Prevent Antimicrobial Resistance in Healthcare Settings.[178] These approaches include preventing health care–associated infections, optimizing the specific diagnosis and treatment of infections, optimizing use of antimicrobial agents including improving the choice, dose, and duration of therapy, and preventing cross-transmission of resistant pathogens.[178] The strategies are based on premises that emergence of resistance is directly linked to antimicrobial use, and that nosocomial infections and transmission of resistant pathogens are preventable events.[179,180] Control of resistance requires the support of clinical microbiology, an active infection prevention program, and effective processes for information exchange between microbiologists, infection prevention practitioners, and clinicians.

REGULATION OF ANTIMICROBIAL USAGE IN THE ICU

The primary challenge to regulating antibiotics in the ICU is balancing the compelling data that timely administration of appropriate antibiotics decreases mortality from severe infections along with the evidence that indiscriminant and unnecessary antibiotic use leads to increased resistance.[180–182] This challenge is more complex when an institution's antibiotic resistance profile worsens, necessitating use of broader initial empiric treatment regimens. There are multiple components to a comprehensive program for antimicrobial usage in the ICU, which are often integrated in an Antimicrobial Stewardship Program, supervised by Infectious Disease practitioners and clinical pharmacists.[183] Selection of initial empiric antimicrobial regimens relies on accurate information on local antibiotic resistance patterns, contained in the hospital antibiogram. A whole hospital antibiogram may not adequately reflect the resistance profiles of ICU pathogens, and more useful information is provided by an ICU-specific antibiogram. Within the ICU, there will still be susceptibility differences in isolates from patients with community-acquired infections and those with health care–associated or nosocomial infections. An ICU-specific antibiogram may also be insufficient for choosing empiric therapy for MDR pathogens, as it does not provide information about cross-resistance. A combination antibiogram provides information on cross-resistance patterns in those isolates already resistant to one agent, and has been used to improve empiric initial therapy for late-onset HAP.[184] Antibiogram data can also be incorporated into empiric antibiotic selections in treatment guidelines for common infections. Properly implemented treatment guidelines that recognize patient-specific risks for resistant pathogens and incorporate local resistance data can increase the likelihood of appropriate initial therapy and improve outcome.[59,184,185] In addition to choice of antimicrobial regimens, treatment guidelines should address issues of obtaining appropriate cultures, which are critical to the subsequent process of revising and de-escalating therapy.

The choice of initial therapy is a key determinant of infection outcome in critically ill patients, but it is subsequent antibiotic management decisions that will have more impact on curtailing unnecessary antibiotic usage and preventing emergence of resistance. De-escalation is the process of narrowing or discontinuing broad-spectrum antimicrobial therapy.[186] This process includes first determining if there is an infection that requires continued antibiotics, then defining the optimal drug and duration of therapy for the confirmed infection. De-escalation is more difficult than improving initial antibiotic selections, due to inadequate microbiologic data, physician concerns about undertreating infections, and the lack of criteria for determining presence of infection. Key components of the de-escalation process are obtaining appropriate culture data at onset of therapy, rapid identification of resistant pathogens in the laboratory, and use of objective criteria for defining presence of infection. In recent studies in VAP, use of clearly defined clinical and microbiologic criteria for narrowing or discontinuation of therapy led to fewer days of antibiotic usage and decrease in subsequent infection with antibiotic-resistant pathogens, without an increase in mortality.[185,187] Adjuvant biomarkers such as procalcitonin may also help support decisions to discontinue antibiotics in patients with suspected sepsis or severe pneumonia.[188,189]

Other components of improving antibiotic usage include optimization of dosing and duration of therapy. Individualized dosing regimens based on improved pharmacokinetic and pharmacodynamic modeling may include higher doses with modified intervals, prolonged infusion times, or continuous infusion. Preliminary but limited data suggest that such regimens may lead to improved outcomes, especially in gram-negative pneumonia, and to decreased emergence of resistance.[190] Clinical pharmacists can provide logistical support for the implementation of novel dosing regimens and can ensure appropriate monitoring and dosing adjustments in the presence of organ toxicity. Decreasing the total duration of therapy to decrease emergence of resistance is also an area of intense study.[191,192] In one elegant study of VAP, 8 days of therapy was comparable to 15 days for patients with VAP except for infection due to nonfermenting gram-negative rods.[191] Numerous studies have evaluated shorter regimens for treating a variety of infections, but few have involved critically ill patients.

Antibiotic stewardship programs may also regulate antibiotic usage by formulary restrictions on the use of specific antibiotics,[183,186] which may include up-front restriction policies or mandatory prospective review of therapy after a defined period of use, typically 48 to 72 hours. Up-front restriction policies improve adherence to institutional guidelines for empiric antibiotic selection and prevent exposure to unnecessary or more toxic agents, but do not facilitate the de-escalation process. Prospective reviews permit analysis of culture and susceptibility data and assessment of clinical response, organ dysfunction, and other factors that will impact on the decision to narrow or completely discontinue antibiotic therapy. Other antibiotic strategies evaluated for potentially decreasing resistance in ICUs include antibiotic cycling, although cycling programs have demonstrated only limited efficacy in recent studies.[193]

INFECTION PREVENTION IN THE ICU

Infection prevention policies impact on antimicrobial resistance in the ICU in several ways. One is by prevention of nosocomial infections, especially device-associated infections that are often caused by MDR pathogens. Much of the decrease in invasive health care associated MRSA infections in the United States is attributed to the decrease in line-associated bacteremias.[27] Decreased nosocomial infection rates should also translate into overall decreases in antibiotic use, and thus less selective pressure for emergence of resistance. Strategies for prevention of nosocomial infections, including line-related bacteremia, catheter-associated urinary tract infection, and VAP have been extensively reviewed.[194–196] The second impact of infection prevention is through screening, identification, and appropriate isolation of patients harboring resistant organisms to prevent the cross-transmission of resistant pathogens. This approach may also include topical or systemic decolonization of patients.

Infection prevention practices can be grouped into global measures that may impact on transmission of multiple resistant pathogens, and targeted interventions for specific pathogens.[81,197] Examples of global interventions include hand hygiene and universal precautions, optimizing staffing rations, environmental cleaning strategies, and universal patient decolonization strategies. Often global interventions are "bundled" together, making it more difficult to evaluate effectiveness of individual components of the bundle. Opportunities for hand hygiene are higher but rates of compliance are lower in ICUs than in other hospital units.[197] Increased hand hygiene compliance has consistently been shown to decrease rates of nosocomial infection and transmission of MRSA.[197,198] Many MDR pathogens survive for prolonged periods on inanimate surfaces, thus environmental cleaning policies need to ensure the routine and systematic cleaning of potentially contaminated surfaces. Universal topical decolonization by chlorhexidine bathing of all ICU patients is advocated as a potential intervention for VRE and MRSA. In recent studies in Medical ICUs, chlorhexidine bathing reduced VRE colonization and cross-transmission as well as VRE bacteremia, and also decreased MRSA transmission.[197,199,200]

All patients harboring MDR organisms should be placed in contact isolation, either in single rooms or cohorted with other colonized/infected patients.[81] The policies and procedures for identification of patients colonized with MDR pathogens, and even which pathogens to screen for, vary widely between facilities and between countries. Screening has been most extensively evaluated for MRSA and VRE. Patients with MRSA or VRE are passively identified from routine clinical cultures or identified through an active surveillance program. Active surveillance can identify 50% more MRSA carriers than is found by passive surveillance, and an even greater proportion of VRE carriers.[197,201] MRSA screening most commonly includes nasal swabs but may also include sampling wounds and other skin sites. Perirectal or stool samples are used for VRE screens. Samples can be processed on routine or specialized culture media or by molecular methods. Rapid molecular methods such as PCR provide results within 24 hours and often within a few hours, but add significantly to screening costs.[197,202] Increased costs may be offset by more rapid removal of patients from isolation. However, more rapid identification of MRSA carriers does not always result in decreased MRSA transmission.[202] Screening strategies include universal screening of all hospital or ICU admissions, or targeted screening of higher risk populations such as transfers from other hospitals and long-term care facilities. Several states in the United States have legislative mandates for hospital screening for MRSA.[177] Deciding who to screen, how to screen, and how often to screen has significant cost implications, and benefits of screening may vary considerably depending on ICU type and size, and rates of MRSA and VRE. Screening practices for MDR gram-negatives organisms are even more variable than for MRSA and VRE.

One step beyond identification and isolation is the more controversial approach of active decolonization of patients with MDR bacteria. The effectiveness of aggressive MRSA screening and decolonization policies in European countries with low MRSA incidence has been used to justify the wider use of these practices. MRSA decolonization, primarily with nasal mupirocin and topical chlorhexidine, has been evaluated in a variety of preoperative, inpatient, and outpatient settings, and is routine practice in many ICUs.[197,203,204] However, there is limited evidence that decolonization contributes to sustained decreases in MRSA infection and cross-transmission beyond the results from hand hygiene and isolation alone.[197] The addition of systemic therapy with doxycycline plus rifampin to an MRSA decolonization protocol resulted in more prolonged MRSA clearance, but such regimens are not currently recommended, because of the lack of evidence of effectiveness in the ICU setting and concern for promoting further resistance.[204,205] There are no proven effective regimens for clearing VRE from the gastrointestinal tract, or for decolonizing those with MDR gram-negative organisms. Chlorhexidine can decrease levels of skin colonization with MDR gram-negatives, though MICs to chlorhexidine are higher than for gram-positive organisms. Selective decontamination of the digestive tract in the ICU using nonabsorbable antibiotics such as polymyxins should be avoided, to help preserve the effectiveness of these agents for the treatment of MDR gram-negative infections.

REFERENCES

1. Boucher HW, Talbot GH, Bradley JS, et al. Bad bugs, no drugs: no ESKAPE! An update from the Infectious Diseases Society of America. Clin Infect Dis 2009; 48:1–12.
2. European Centre for Disease Prevention and Control/European Medicines Agency Joint Technical Report. The bacterial challenge: time to react. Available at: http://www.emea.europa.eu/pdfs/human/antimicrobial_resistance/EMEA-576176-2009.pdf. Accessed September 9, 2009.
3. Livermore DM. Has the era of untreatable infections arrived? J Antimicrob Chemother 2009;64:i29–36.
4. Esposito S, Leone S. Antimicrobial treatment for intensive care unit (ICU) infections including the role of the infectious disease specialist. Int J Antimicrob Agents 2007;29:494–500.
5. International Organization for Standards. 15 November 2006, posting date. Susceptibility testing of infectious agents and evaluation of performance of antimicrobial susceptibility testing devices. 1. Reference method for testing the in vitro activity of antimicrobial agents against rapidly growing aerobic bacteria involved in infectious diseases. ISO 20776–1. International Organization for Standardization (ISO). Geneva, Switzerland.
6. Woodford N, Sundsfjord A. Molecular detection of antibiotic resistance: when and where? J Antimicrob Chemother 2005;56:259–61.
7. Martínez JL, Baquero F, Andersson DI. Predicting antibiotic resistance. Nat Rev Microbiol 2007;5:958–65.
8. Plesiat P. Biochemistry of resistance. In: Courvalin P, Leclercq R, Rice LB, editors. Antibiogram. Portland (OR): Eska Publishing, ASM Press; 2010. p. 17–24.
9. Jacoby GA, Munoz-Price LS. The new β-lactamases. N Engl J Med 2005;352: 380–91.
10. Andersson DI, Hughes D. Antibiotic resistance and its cost: is it possible to reverse resistance? Nat Rev Microbiol 2010;8:260–71.
11. Rice LB. Genetics of resistance. In: Courvalin P, Leclercq R, Rice LB, editors. Antibiogram. Portland (OR): Eska Publishing, ASM Press; 2010. p. 25–36.
12. Périchon B, Courvalin P. VanA-type vancomycin-resistant Staphylococcus aureus. Antimicrob Agents Chemother 2009;53:4580–7.
13. Poole K. Efflux-mediated antimicrobial resistance. J Antimicrob Chemother 2005;56:20–51.
14. Falagas ME, Koletsi PK, Bliziotis IA. The diversity of definitions of multidrug-resistant and pandrug-resistant Acinetobacter baumannii and Pseudomonas aeruginosa. J Med Microbiol 2006;55:1619–29.
15. Chambers HF, Deleo FR. Waves of resistance: Staphylococcus aureus in the antibiotic era. Nat Rev Microbiol 2009;7:629–41.
16. Boyce JM, Causey WA. Increasing occurrence of methicillin-resistant Staphylococcus aureus in the United States. Infect Control 1982;3:377–83.
17. Klevens RM, Edwards JR, Tenover FC, et al, National Nosocomial Infections Surveillance System. Changes in the epidemiology of methicillin-resistant

Staphylococcus aureus in intensive care units in US hospitals, 1992–2003. Clin Infect Dis 2006;42:389–91.

18. Boucher HW, Corey RG. Epidemiology of methicillin-resistant *Staphylococcus aureus*. Clin Infect Dis 2008;46:S344–9.

19. Moran GJ, Krishnadasan A, Gorwitz RJ, et al. Methicillin-resistant *S. aureus* infections among patients in the emergency department. N Engl J Med 2006; 355:666–74.

20. Seybold U, Kourbatova EV, Johnson JG, et al. Emergence of community asso- ciated methicillin-resistant *Staphylococcus aureus* USA300 genotype as a major cause of health care-associated blood stream infections. Clin Infect Dis 2006; 42:647–56.

21. Hiramatsu K. Vancomycin-resistant *Staphylococcus aureus*: a new model of antibiotic resistance. Lancet Infect Dis 2001;1:147–55.

22. Sánchez García M, De la Torre MA, Morales G, et al. Clinical outbreak of linezol- id-resistant *Staphylococcus aureus* in an intensive care unit. JAMA 2010;303: 2260–4.

23. Boucher HW, Sakoulas G. Perspectives on daptomycin resistance, with emphasis on resistance in *Staphylococcus aureus*. Clin Infect Dis 2007;45: 601–8.

24. Klevens RM, Morrison MA, Nadle J, et al, Active Bacterial Core Surveillance (ABCs) MRSA Investigators. Invasive methicillin-resistant *Staphylococcus aureus* infections in the United States. JAMA 2007;298:1763–71.

25. Cosgrove SE, Qi Y, Kaye KS, et al. The impact of methicillin resistance in *Staph- ylococcus aureus* bacteremia on patient outcomes: mortality, length of stay, and hospital charges. Infect Control Hosp Epidemiol 2005;26:166–74.

26. Filice GA, Nyman JA, Lexau C, et al. Excess costs and utilization associated with methicillin resistance for patients with *Staphylococcus aureus* infection. Infect Control Hosp Epidemiol 2010;31:365–73.

27. Kallen AJ, Mu Y, Bulens S, et al. Health care-associated Invasive MRSA infec- tions, 2005–2008. JAMA 2010;304:641–8.

28. US Department of Health and Human Services. HHS action plan to prevent health- care-associated infections. Avaialble at: http://www.hhs.gov/ophs/initiatives/hai/ infection.html. Accessed September 7, 2010.

29. Burton DC, Edwards JR, Horan TC, et al. Methicillin-resistant *Staphylococcus aureus* central line-associated bloodstream infections in US intensive care units, 1997–2007. JAMA 2009;301:727–36.

30. Perencevich EN, Dikema DJ. Decline in invasive MRSA infection: Where to go from here? JAMA 2010;304:687–9.

31. European Antimicrobial Resistance Surveillance System (EARSS) Annual Report 2008. Vol 2010. Bilthoven (the Netherlands): EARSS; 2008. Available at: http:// www.rivm.nl/earss/Images/EARSS%202008_final_tcm61-65020.pdf. Accessed September 7, 2010.

32. Herold BC, Immergluck LC, Maranan MC, et al. Community-acquired methicillin resistant *Staphylococcus aureus* in children with no identified predisposing risk. JAMA 1998;279:593–8.

33. Centers for Disease Control and Prevention. Four pediatric deaths from commu- nity-acquired methicillin-resistant *Staphylococcus aureus*—Minnesota and North Dakota, 1997–1999. JAMA 1999;282:1123–5.

34. Udo EE, Pearman JW, Grubb WB. Genetic analysis of community isolates of methicillin-resistant *Staphylococcus aureus* in Western Australia. J Hosp Infect 1993;25:97–108.

35. Martinez-Aguilar G, Avalos-Mishaan A, Hulten K, et al. Community-acquired, methicillin-resistant and methicillin-susceptible *Staphylococcus aureus* musculoskeletal infections in children. Pediatr Infect Dis J 2004;23:701–6.

36. David MZ, Daum RS. Community-associated methicillin-resistant *Staphylococcus aureus*: epidemiology and clinical consequences of an emerging epidemic. Clin Microbiol Rev 2010;23:616–87.

37. Gordon RJ, Lowy FD. Pathogenesis of methicillin-resistant *Staphylococcus aureus* infection. Clin Infect Dis 2008;46:S350–9.

38. Kirst HA, Thompson DG, Nicas TI. Historical yearly usage of vancomycin. Antimicrob Agents Chemother 1998;42:1303–4.

39. Howden BP, Davies JK, Johnson PD, et al. Reduced vancomycin susceptibility in *Staphylococcus aureus*, including vancomycin-intermediate and heterogeneous vancomycin-intermediate strains: resistance mechanisms, laboratory detection, and clinical implications. Clin Microbiol Rev 2010;23:99–139.

40. Tenover FC, Moellering RC. The rationale for revising the Clinical and Laboratory Standards Institute vancomycin minimal inhibitory concentration interpretive criteria for *Staphylococcus aureus*. Clin Infect Dis 2007;44:1208–15.

41. Clinical and Laboratory Standards Institute. Performance standards for antimicrobial susceptibility testing; Twentieth informational supplement. CLSI document M100–S20. Wayne (PA): Clinical and Laboratory Standards Institute; 2010.

42. Liu C, Chambers HF. *Staphylococcus aureus* with heterogeneous resistance to vancomycin: epidemiology, clinical significance, and critical assessment of diagnostic methods. Antimicrob Agents Chemother 2003;47:3040–5.

43. Wang G, Hindler JF, Ward KW, et al. Increased vancomycin MICs for *Staphylococcus aureus* clinical isolates from a university hospital during a 5-year period. J Clin Microbiol 2006;44:3883–6.

44. Rybak MJ, Lomaestro BM, Rotschafer JC, et al. Vancomycin therapeutic guidelines: a summary of consensus recommendations from the infectious diseases Society of America, the American Society of Health-System Pharmacists, and the Society of Infectious Diseases Pharmacists. Clin Infect Dis 2009;49:325–7.

45. Lodise TP, Graves J, Graffunder E, et al. Relationship between vancomycin MIC and failure among patients with methicillin-resistant *Staphylococcus aureus* bacteremia treated with vancomycin. Antimicrob Agents Chemother 2008;52: 3315–20.

46. Lodise TP, Lomaestro B, Graves J, et al. Larger vancomycin doses ($\geq$4 grams/day) are associated with an increased incidence of nephrotoxicity. Antimicrob Agents Chemother 2008;52:1330–6.

47. Farrell DJ, Mendes RE, Ross JE, et al. Linezolid surveillance program results for 2008 (LEADER Program for 2008). Diagn Microbiol Infect Dis 2009;65:392–403.

48. Long KS, Poehlsgaard J, Kehrenberg C, et al. The Cfr rRNA methyltransferase confers resistance to phenicols, lincosamides, oxazolidinones, pleuromutilins, and streptogramin A antibiotics. Antimicrob Agents Chemother 2006;50:2500–5.

49. Fraimow HS. Lipopeptides, lipoglycopeptides and glycolipodepsipeptides. In: Courvalin P, Leclercq R, Rice LB, editors. Antibiogram. Portland (OR): Eska Publishing, ASM Press; 2010. p. 295–304.

50. Moise PA, North D, Steenbergen JN, et al. Susceptibility relationship between vancomycin and daptomycin in *Staphylococcus aureus*: facts and assumptions. Lancet Infect Dis 2009;9:617–24.

51. Moise PA, Hershberger E, Amodio-Groton MI, et al. Safety and clinical outcomes when utilizing high-dose (> or = 8 mg/kg) daptomycin therapy. Ann Pharmacother 2009;43:1211–9.

52. Putnam SD, Sader HS, Farrell DJ, et al. Sustained antimicrobial activity of tige-cycline against methicillin-resistant *Staphylococcus aureus* (MRSA) from United States Medical Centers from 2004 through 2008. J Chemother 2010;22:13–6.
53. Gardiner D, Dukart G, Cooper A, et al. Safety and efficacy of intravenous tige-cycline in subjects with secondary bacteremia: pooled results from 8 phase III clinical trials. Clin Infect Dis 2010;50:229–38.
54. Nace H, Lorber B. Successful treatment of methicillin-resistant *Staphylococcus aureus* endocarditis with telavancin. J Antimicrob Chemother 2010;65:1315–6.
55. Fowler VG Jr, Boucher HW, Corey GR, et al. Daptomycin versus standard therapy for bacteremia and endocarditis caused by *Staphylococcus aureus*. N Engl J Med 2006;355:653–65.
56. Falagas ME, Manta KG, Ntziora F, et al. Linezolid for the treatment of patients with endocarditis: a systematic review of the published evidence. J Antimicrob Chemother 2006;58:273–80.
57. Baddour LM, Wilson WR, Bayer AS, et al. Infective endocarditis: diagnosis, anti-microbial therapy, and management of complications: a statement for health-care professionals. Circulation 2005;11:e394–434.
58. Hawkey PM. Pre-clinical experience with daptomycin. J Antimicrob Chemother 2008;62(Suppl 3):7–14.
59. American Thoracic Society, Infectious Diseases Society of America. Guidelines for the management of adults with hospital-acquired, ventilator-associated, and healthcare-associated pneumonia. Am J Respir Crit Care Med 2005;17: 388–416.
60. Wunderink RG, Rello J, Cammarata SK, et al. Linezolid vs vancomycin: analysis of two double-blind studies of patients with methicillin-resistant *Staphylococcus aureus* nosocomial pneumonia. Chest 2003;124:1789–97.
61. Wiersma P, Tobin D'Angelo M, Daley WR, et al. Surveillance for severe commu-nity-associated methicillin-resistant *Staphylococcus aureus* infection. Epidemiol Infect 2009;137:1674–8.
62. Stevens DL, Ma Y, Salmi DB, et al. Impact of antibiotics on the expression of virulence-associated exotoxin genes in methicillin-sensitive and in methicillin-resistant *Staphylococcus aureus*. J Infect Dis 2007;195:202–11.
63. Nathwani D, Morgan M, Masterson RG, et al. Guidelines for UK practice for the diagnosis and management of methicillin-resistant *Staphylococcus aureus* (MRSA) infections presenting in the community. J Antimicrob Chemother 2008;61:976–94.
64. Weigelt J, Itani K, Stevens D, et al. Linezolid versus vancomycin in the treatment of complicated skin and soft tissue infections. Antimicrob Agents Chemother 2005;49:2260–6.
65. Arbeit RD, Maki D, Tally FP, et al. The safety and efficacy of daptomycin for the treatment of complicated skin and soft tissue infection. Clin Infect Dis 2004;38: 1673–81.
66. Florescu I, Beuran M, Dimov R, et al. Efficacy and safety of tigecycline compared with vancomycin or linezolid for treatment of serious infections with methicillin-resistant *Staphylococcus aureus* or vancomycin-resistant entero-cocci: a Phase 3, multicentre, double-blind, randomized study. J Antimicrob Chemother 2008;62(Suppl 1):i17–28.
67. Han LL, McDougal LK, Gorwitz RJ, et al. High frequencies of clindamycin and tetracycline resistance in methicillin-resistant *Staphylococcus aureus* pulsed-field type USA300 isolates collected at a Boston ambulatory health center. J Clin Microbiol 2007;45:1350–2.

68. Deresinski S. Vancomycin in combination with other antibiotics for the treatment of serious methicillin-resistant *Staphylococcus aureus* infections. Clin Infect Dis 2009;49:1072–9.
69. Cosgrove SE, Vigliani GA, Fowler VG Jr, et al. Initial low-dose gentamicin for *Staphylococcus aureus* bacteremia and endocarditis is nephrotoxic. Clin Infect Dis 2009;48:713–21.
70. Perlroth J, Kuo M, Tan J, et al. Adjunctive use of rifampin for the treatment of *Staphylococcus aureus* infections: a systematic review of the literature. Arch Intern Med 2008;168:805–19.
71. Jang HC, Kim SH, Kim KH, et al. Salvage treatment for persistent methicillin-resistant *Staphylococcus aureus* bacteremia: efficacy of linezolid with or without carbapenem. Clin Infect Dis 2009;49:395–401.
72. Steenbergen JN, Mohr JF, Thorne GM. Effects of daptomycin in combination with other antimicrobial agents: a review of in vitro and animal model studies. J Antimicrob Chemother 2009;64:1130–8.
73. Hidron AI, Edwards JR, Patel J, et al, National Healthcare Safety Network Team, Participating National Healthcare Safety Network Facilities. NHSN annual update: antimicrobial-resistant pathogens associated with healthcare-associated infections: annual summary of data reported to the National Healthcare Safety Network at the Centers for Disease Control and Prevention, 2006–2007. Infect Control Hosp Epidemiol 2008;29:996–1011.
74. Donskey CJ, Chowdhry TK, Hecker MT, et al. Effect of antibiotic therapy on the density of vancomycin-resistant enterococci in the stool of colonized patients. N Engl J Med 2000;343:1925–32.
75. Arias CA, Murray BE. Emergence and management of drug-resistant enterococcal infections. Expert Rev Anti Infect Ther 2008;6:637–55.
76. Murray BE. Beta-lactamase-producing enterococci. Antimicrob Agents Chemother 1992;36:2355–9.
77. Rybkine T, Mainardi JL, Sougakoff W, et al. Penicillin-binding protein 5 sequence alterations in clinical isolates of *Enterococcus faecium* with different levels of beta-lactam resistance. J Infect Dis 1998;178:159–63.
78. Rice LB, Carias LL, Rudin S, et al. *Enterococcus faecium* low-affinity pbp5 is a transferable determinant. Antimicrob Agents Chemother 2005;49:5007–12.
79. National Nosocomial Infections Surveillance System. National Nosocomial Infections Surveillance (NNIS) system report, data summary from January 1992 through June 2004, issued October 2004. Am J Infect Control 2004;32: 470–85.
80. Recommendations for preventing the spread of vancomycin resistance: recommendations of the Hospital Infection Control Practices Advisory Committee (HICPAC) Centers for Disease Control and Prevention. MMWR Morb Mortal Wkly Rep 1995;44(RR–12):1–13.
81. Siegel JD, Rhinehart E, Jackson M, et al, Healthcare Infection Control Practices Advisory Committee. Management of multidrug-resistant organisms in healthcare settings. Atlanta (GA): Centers for Disease Control and Prevention; 2006.
82. Fraimow HS, Courvalin P. Resistance to glycopeptides in gram-positive pathogens. In: Fischetti VA, Novick RP, Ferretti JJ, et al, editors. Gram positive pathogens. 2nd edition. Washington, DC: ASM Press; 2006. p. 782–800.
83. Arias CA, Contreras GA, Murray BE. Management of multidrug-resistant enterococcal infections. Clin Microbiol Infect 2010;16:555–62.
84. Herrero IA, Issa NC, Patel R. Nosocomial spread of linezolid-resistant, vancomycin-resistant *Enterococcus faecium*. N Engl J Med 2002;346:867–9.

85. Scheetz MH, Knechtel SA, Malczynski M, et al. Increasing incidence of linezolid-intermediate or -resistant, vancomycin-resistant *Enterococcus faecium* strains parallels increasing linezolid consumption. Antimicrobial Agents Chemother 2008;52:2256–9.

86. Eliopolous GM. Aminoglycoside resistant enterococcal endocarditis. Infect Dis Clin North Am 1993;7:117–33.

87. Gavaldà J, Len O, Miró JM, et al. Brief communication: treatment of *Enterococcus faecalis* endocarditis with ampicillin plus ceftriaxone. Ann Intern Med 2007;146:574–9.

88. Centers for Disease Control and Prevention. Active Bacterial Core Surveillance Report, Emerging Infections Program Network, Streptococcus pneumoniae, provisional-2009. 2010. Available at: http://www.cdc.gov/abcs/reports-findings/survreports/spneu09.pdf. Accessed September 9, 2010.

89. Liñares J, Ardanuy C, Pallares R, et al. Changes in antimicrobial resistance, serotypes and genotypes in *Streptococcus pneumoniae* over a 30-year period. Clin Microbiol Infect 2010;16:402–10.

90. Reinert RR. The antimicrobial resistance profile of *Streptococcus pneumoniae*. Clin Microbiol Infect 2009;15:S7–11.

91. Dagan R, Klugman KP. Impact of conjugate pneumococcal vaccines on antibiotic resistance. Lancet Infect Dis 2008;8:785–95.

92. Canton R, Morosini M, Enright MC, et al. Worldwide incidence, molecular epidemiology and mutations implicated in fluoroquinolone-resistant *Streptococcus pneumoniae*: data from the global PROTEKT surveillance programme. J Antimicrob Chemother 2003;2:944–52.

93. Delcour AH. Outer membrane permeability and antibiotic resistance. Biochim Biophys Acta 2009;1794:808–16.

94. Donnenberg MS. Enterobacteriaceae. In: Mandell GL, Bennett JE, Dolin R, editors. Mandell, Douglas, and Bennett's principles and practice of infectious diseases. 7th edition. Philadelphia: Churchill Livingstone Elsevier; 2010. p. 2815–7.

95. Hooper DC. Efflux pumps and nosocomial antibiotic resistance: a primer for hospital epidemiologists. Clin Infect Dis 2005;40:1811–7.

96. Chambers HF. Penicillins and β-lactam inhibitors. In: Mandell GL, Bennett JE, Dolin R, editors. Mandell, Douglas, and Bennett's principles and practice of infectious diseases. 7th edition. Philadelphia: Churchill Livingstone Elsevier; 2010. p. 309–22.

97. Poole K. Resistance to beta-lactam antibiotics. Cell Mol Life Sci 2004;61:2200–2.

98. Bush K, Jacoby GA. Updated functional classification of beta-lactamases. Antimicrob Agents Chemother 2010;54:969–76.

99. Paterson DL. Resistance in gram-negative bacteria: enterobacteriaceae. Am J Med 2006;119:S20–8.

100. Livermore DM. Defining an extended-spectrum beta-lactamase. Clin Microbiol Infect 2008;14:S3–10.

101. Paterson DL, Bonomo RA. Extended-spectrum beta-lactamases: a clinical update. Clin Microbiol Rev 2005;18:657–86.

102. Queenan AM, Bush K. Carbapenemases: the versatile beta-lactamases. Clin Microbiol Rev 2007;20:440–58.

103. Jacoby GA. AmpC beta-lactamases. Clin Microbiol Rev 2009;22:161–82.

104. Robicsek A, Jacoby GA, Hooper DC. The worldwide emergence of plasmid-mediated quinolone resistance. Lancet Infect Dis 2006;6:629–40.

105. Jacoby GA. Mechanisms of resistance to quinolones. Clin Infect Dis 2005;41: S120–6.
106. Strahilevitz J, Jacoby GA, Hooper DC, et al. Plasmid-mediated quinolone resistance: a multifaceted threat. Clin Microbiol Rev 2009;22:664–89.
107. Vakulenko SB, Mobashery S. Versatility of aminoglycosides and prospects for their future. Clin Microbiol Rev 2003;16:430–50.
108. Poole K. Aminoglycoside resistance in *Pseudomonas aeruginosa.* Antimicrob Agents Chemother 2005;49:479–87.
109. Michalopoulos A, Falagas ME. Colistin and polymyxin B in critical care. Crit Care Clin 2008;24:377–91.
110. Nation RL, Li J. Colistin in the 21st century. Curr Opin Infect Dis 2009;22:535–43.
111. Livermore DM. Tigecycline: what is it, and where should it be used? J Antimicrob Chemother 2005;56:611–4.
112. Giamarellou H, Poulakou G. Multidrug-resistant Gram-negative infections: what are the treatment options? Drugs 2009;69:1879–901.
113. Clinical and Laboratory Standards Institute. Performance standards for antimicrobial susceptibility testing; Ninth informational supplement, CLSI document M100–S9. Wayne (PA): Clinical and Laboratory Standards Institute; 1999.
114. Moland ES, Hanson ND, Black JA, et al. Prevalence of newer beta-lactamases in gram-negative clinical isolates collected in the United States from 2001 to 2002. J Clin Microbiol 2006;44:3318–24.
115. Rosenthal VD, Maki DG, Jamulitrat S, et al, INICC Members. International Nosocomial Infection Control Consortium (INICC) report, data summary for 2003–2008, issued June 2009. Am J Infect Control 2010;38:95–104, e2.
116. Zhanel GG, Decorby M, Nichol KA, et al. Characterization of methicillin-resistant *Staphylococcus aureus,* vancomycin-resistant enterococci and extended-spectrum beta-lactamase-producing *Escherichia coli* in intensive care units in Canada: results of the Canadian National Intensive Care Unit Study (2005–2006). Can J Infect Dis Med Microbiol 2008;19:243–9.
117. Zhanel GG, DeCorby M, Laing N, et al, Canadian Antimicrobial Resistance Alliance (CARA). Antimicrobial-resistant pathogens in intensive care units in Canada: results of the Canadian National Intensive Care Unit (CAN-ICU) study, 2005–2006. Antimicrob Agents Chemother 2008;52(7):1430.
118. Pitout JD. Infections with extended-spectrum beta-lactamase-producing enterobacteriaceae: changing epidemiology and drug treatment choices. Drugs 2010;70:313–33.
119. Paterson DL, Ko WC, Von Gottberg A, et al. Antibiotic therapy for *Klebsiella pneumoniae* bacteremia: implications of production of extended-spectrum beta-lactamases. Clin Infect Dis 2004;39:31–7.
120. Endimiani A, Luzzaro F, Perilli M, et al. Bacteremia due to *Klebsiella pneumoniae* isolates producing the TEM-52 extended-spectrum beta-lactamase: treatment outcome of patients receiving imipenem or ciprofloxacin. Clin Infect Dis 2004; 38:243–51.
121. Kang CI, Kim SH, Park WB, et al. Bloodstream infections due to extended-spectrum beta-lactamase producing *Escherichia coli* and *Klebsiella pneumoniae*: risk factors for mortality and treatment outcome, with special emphasis on antimicrobial therapy. Antimicrob Agents Chemother 2004;48:4574–81.
122. Zanetti G, Bally F, Greub G, et al, Cefepime Study Group. Cefepime versus imipenem-cilastatin for treatment of nosocomial pneumonia in intensive care unit patients: a multicenter, evaluator-blind, prospective, randomized study. Antimicrob Agents Chemother 2003;47:3442–7.

123. Peterson LR. Antibiotic policy and prescribing strategies for therapy of extended-spectrum beta-lactamase-producing Enterobacteriaceae; the role of piperacillin-tazobactam. Clin Microbiol Infect 2008;14:S181–4.

124. Gavin PJ, Suseno MT, Thomson RB Jr, et al. Clinical correlation of the CLSI susceptibility breakpoint for piperacillin- tazobactam against extended-spectrum-beta-lactamase-producing *Escherichia coli* and *Klebsiella* species. Antimicrob Agents Chemother 2006;50:2244–7.

125. Rodríguez-Baño J, Navarro MD, Romero L, et al. Bacteremia due to extended-spectrum beta -lactamase-producing *Escherichia coli* in the CTX-M era: a new clinical challenge. Clin Infect Dis 2006;43:1407–14.

126. Tumbarello M, Spanu T, Sanguinetti M, et al. Bloodstream infections caused by extended-spectrum-beta-lactamase-producing *Klebsiella pneumoniae*: risk factors, molecular epidemiology, and clinical outcome. Antimicrob Agents Chemother 2006;50:498–504.

127. Paterson DL, Ko WC, Von Gottberg A, et al. Outcome of cephalosporin treatment for serious infections due to apparently susceptible organisms producing extended-spectrum beta-lactamases: implications for the clinical microbiology laboratory. J Clin Microbiol 2001;39:2206–12.

128. Kotapati S, Kuti JL, Nightingale CH, et al. Clinical implications of extended spectrum beta-lactamase producing *Klebsiella* species and *Escherichia coli* on cefepime effectiveness. J Infect 2005;51:211–7.

129. Wong-Beringer A, Hindler J, Loeloff M, et al. Molecular correlation for the treatment outcomes in bloodstream infections caused by *Escherichia coli* and *Klebsiella pneumoniae* with reduced susceptibility to ceftazidime. Clin Infect Dis 2002;34:135–46.

130. Goethaert K, Van Looveren M, Lammens C, et al. High-dose cefepime as an alternative treatment for infections caused by TEM-24 ESBL-producing *Enterobacter aerogenes* in severely-ill patients. Clin Microbiol Infect 2006;12:56–62.

131. Labombardi VJ, Rojtman A, Tran K. Use of cefepime for the treatment of infections caused by extended spectrum beta-lactamase-producing *Klebsiella pneumoniae* and *Escherichia coli*. Diagn Microbiol Infect Dis 2006;56:313–5.

132. Bin C, Hui W, Renyuan Z, et al. Outcome of cephalosporin treatment of bacteremia due to CTX-M-type extended-spectrum beta-lactamase-producing *Escherichia coli*. Diagn Microbiol Infect Dis 2006;56:351–7.

133. Bhat SV, Peleg AY, Lodise TP Jr, et al. Failure of current cefepime breakpoints to predict clinical outcomes of bacteremia caused by gram-negative organisms. Antimicrob Agents Chemother 2007;51:4390–5.

134. Lee SY, Kuti JL, Nicolau DP. Cefepime pharmacodynamics in patients with extended spectrum beta-lactamase (ESBL) and non-ESBL infections. J Infect 2007;54:463–8.

135. Endimiani A, Perez F, Bonomo RA. Cefepime: a reappraisal in an era of increasing antimicrobial resistance. Expert Rev Anti Infect Ther 2008;6:805–24.

136. Thomson KS, Moland ES. Cefepime, piperacillin-tazobactam, and the inoculum effect in tests with extended-spectrum beta-lactamase-producing Enterobacteriaceae. Antimicrob Agents Chemother 2001;45:3548–54.

137. Craig WA, Bhavnani SM, Ambrose PG. The inoculum effect: fact or artifact? Diagn Microbiol Infect Dis 2004;50:229–30.

138. Kim YK, Pai H, Lee HJ, et al. Bloodstream infections by extended-spectrum beta-lactamase-producing *Escherichia coli* and *Klebsiella pneumoniae* in children: epidemiology and clinical outcome. Antimicrob Agents Chemother 2002;46:1481–91.

139. Kaye KS, Cosgrove S, Harris A, et al. Risk factors for emergence of resistance to broad-spectrum cephalosporins among *Enterobacter* spp. Antimicrob Agents Chemother 2001;45:2628–30.

140. Chow JW, Fine MJ, Shlaes DM, et al. *Enterobacter* bacteremia: clinical features and emergence of antibiotic resistance during therapy. Ann Intern Med 1991; 115:585–90.

141. Choi SH, Lee JE, Park SJ, et al. Emergence of antibiotic resistance during therapy for infections caused by Enterobacteriaceae producing AmpC beta-lactamase: implications for antibiotic use. Antimicrob Agents Chemother 2008; 52:995–1000.

142. Nordmann P, Cuzon G, Naas T. The real threat of *Klebsiella pneumoniae* carbapenemase-producing bacteria. Lancet Infect Dis 2009;9:228–36.

143. Bratu S, Tolaney P, Karumudi U, et al. Carbapenemase producing *Klebsiella pneumoniae* in Brooklyn, NY: molecular epidemiology and *in vitro* activity of polymyxin B and other agents. J Antimicrob Chemother 2005;56:128–32.

144. Yong D, Toleman MA, Giske CG, et al. Characterization of a new metallo-beta-lactamase gene, bla(NDM-1), and a novel erythromycin esterase gene carried on a unique genetic structure in *Klebsiella pneumoniae* sequence type 14 from India. Antimicrob Agents Chemother 2009;53:5046–54.

145. Kumarasamy KK, Toleman MA, Walsh TR, et al. Emergence of a new antibiotic resistance mechanism in India, Pakistan, and the UK: a molecular, biological, and epidemiological study. Lancet Infect Dis 2010;10:597–602.

146. Centers for Disease Control and Prevention (CDC). Detection of Enterobacteriaceae isolates carrying metallo-beta-lactamase-United States, 2010. MMWR Morb Mortal Wkly Rep 2010;59:750.

147. Rolain JM, Parola P, Cornaglia G. New Delhi metallo-beta-lactamase (NDM-1): towards a new pandemia? Clin Microbiol Infect 2010 Sep 27. DOI: 10.1111/j.1469-0691.2010.03385.x.

148. Peleg AY, Hooper DC. Hospital-acquired infections due to gram-negative bacteria. N Engl J Med 2010;362:1804–13.

149. Elemam A, Rahimian J, Mandell W. Infection with panresistant *Klebsiella pneumoniae*: a report of 2 cases and a brief review of the literature. Clin Infect Dis 2009;49:271–4.

150. Endimiani A, Hujer AM, Perez F, et al. Characterization of blaKPC-containing *Klebsiella pneumoniae* isolates detected in different institutions in the Eastern USA. J Antimicrob Chemother 2009;63:427–37.

151. Lee J, Patel G, Huprikar S, et al. Decreased susceptibility to polymyxin B during treatment for carbapenem-resistant *Klebsiella pneumoniae* infection. J Clin Microbiol 2009;47:1611–2.

152. Walkty A, DeCorby M, Nichol K, et al. In vitro activity of colistin (polymyxin E) against 3,480 isolates of gram-negative bacilli obtained from patients in Canadian hospitals in the CANWARD study, 2007-2008. Antimicrob Agents Chemother 2009;53:4924–6.

153. Daly MW, Riddle DJ, Ledeboer NA, et al. Tigecycline for treatment of pneumonia and empyema caused by carbapenemase-producing *Klebsiella pneumoniae*. Pharmacotherapy 2007;27:1052–7.

154. Anthony KB, Fishman NO, Linkin DR, et al. Clinical and microbiological outcomes of serious infections with multidrug-resistant gram-negative organisms treated with tigecycline. Clin Infect Dis 2008;46:567–70.

155. Castanheira M, Sader HS, Deshpande LM, et al. Antimicrobial activities of tigecycline and other broad-spectrum antimicrobials tested against serine

carbapenemase- and metallo-beta-lactamase-producing Enterobacteriaceae: report from the SENTRY Antimicrobial Surveillance Program. Antimicrob Agents Chemother 2008;52:570–3.

156. Kelesidis T, Karageorgopoulos DE, Kelesidis I, et al. Tigecycline for the treatment of multidrug-resistant Enterobacteriaceae: a systematic review of the evidence from microbiological and clinical studies. J Antimicrob Chemother 2008;62:895–904.

157. McGowan JE Jr. Resistance in nonfermenting gram-negative bacteria: multidrug resistance to the maximum. Am J Med 2006;119(6 Suppl 1):S29–36.

158. Lister PD, Wolter DJ, Hanson ND. Antibacterial-resistant *Pseudomonas aeruginosa*: clinical impact and complex regulation of chromosomally encoded resistance mechanisms. Clin Microbiol Rev 2009;22:582–610.

159. Peleg AY, Seifert H, Paterson DL. *Acinetobacter baumannii*: emergence of a successful pathogen. Clin Microbiol Rev 2008;21:538–82.

160. Denton M, Kerr KG. Microbiological and clinical aspects of infection associated with *Stenotrophomonas maltophilia*. Clin Microbiol Rev 1998;11:57–80.

161. Streit JM, Jones RN, Sader HS, et al. Assessment of pathogen occurrences and resistance profiles among infected patients in the intensive care unit: report from the SENTRY Antimicrobial Surveillance Program (North America, 2001). Int J Antimicrob Agents 2004;24:111–8.

162. Livermore DM. Of *Pseudomonas*, porins, pumps and carbapenems. J Antimicrob Chemother 2001;47:247–50.

163. Bonomo RA, Szabo D. Mechanisms of multidrug resistance in *Acinetobacter* species and *Pseudomonas aeruginosa*. Clin Infect Dis 2006;43:S49–56.

164. Toleman MA, Bennett PM, Bennett DM, et al. Global emergence of trimethoprim/ sulfamethoxazole resistance in *Stenotrophomonas maltophilia* mediated by acquisition of *sul* genes. Emerg Infect Dis 2007;13:559–65.

165. Kallen AJ, Hidron AI, Patel J, et al. Multidrug resistance among gram-negative pathogens that caused healthcare-associated infections reported to the National Healthcare Safety Network, 2006–2008. Infect Control Hosp Epidemiol 2010;31:528–31.

166. Mandell L. Doripenem: a new carbapenem in the treatment of nosocomial infection. Clin Infect Dis 2009;49:S1–3.

167. Peleg AY, Potoski BA, Rea R, et al. *Acinetobacter baumannii* bloodstream infection while receiving tigecycline: a cautionary report. J Antimicrob Chemother 2007;59:128–31.

168. Fishbain J, Peleg AY. Treatment of *Acinetobacter* infections. Clin Infect Dis 2010; 51:79–84.

169. Petrosillo N, Ioannidou E, Falagas ME. Colistin monotherapy vs. combination therapy: evidence from microbiological, animal and clinical studies. Clin Microbiol Infect 2008;14:816–27.

170. Nicodemo AC, Paez JI. Antimicrobial therapy for *Stenotrophomonas maltophilia* infections. Eur J Clin Microbiol Infect Dis 2007;26:229–37.

171. Falagas ME, Valkimadi PE, Huang YT, et al. Therapeutic options for *Stenotrophomonas maltophilia* infections beyond co-trimoxazole: a systematic review. J Antimicrob Chemother 2008;62:889–94.

172. Insa R, Cercenado E, Goyanes MJ, et al. In vitro activity of tigecycline against clinical isolates of *Acinetobacter baumannii* and *Stenotrophomonas maltophilia*. J Antimicrob Chemother 2007;59:583–5.

173. Wexler HM. *Bacteroides*: the good, the bad, and the nitty-gritty. Clin Microbiol Rev 2007;20:593–621.

174. Garrett WS, Onderdonk AB. Bacteroides, Prevotella, Porphyromonas, and *Fusobacterium* species (and other medically important anaerobic gram-negative bacilli). In: Mandell GL, Bennett JE, Dolin R, editors. Mandell, Douglas, and Bennett's principles and practice of infectious diseases. 7th edition. Philadelphia: Churchill Livingstone Elsevier; 2010. p. 3111–9.

175. Snydman DR, Jacobus NV, McDermott LA, et al. Lessons learned from the anaerobe survey: historical perspective and review of the most recent data (2005–2007). Clin Infect Dis 2010;50:S26–33.

176. Nagy E, Urbán E, Carl Erik Nord on behalf of the ESCMID Study Group on Antimicrobial Resistance in Anaerobic Bacteria*. Antimicrobial susceptibility of *Bacteroides fragilis* group isolates in Europe: 20 years of experience. Clin Microbiol Infect 2010. [Epub ahead of print].

177. National Conference of State Legislatures. Healthcare-Associated Infections Homepage Healthcare-Associated Infections Homepage. Available at: http://www.ncsl.org/default.aspx?tabid=14084. Accessed September 10, 2010.

178. CDC. Campaign to prevent antimicrobial resistance in healthcare settings. Available at: http://www.cdc.gov/drugresistance/healthcare/ha/12steps_HA.htm. Accessed September 10, 2010.

179. Fridkin SK, Steward CD, Edwards JR, et al. Surveillance of antimicrobial use and antimicrobial resistance in United States hospitals: project ICARE phase 2. Clin Infect Dis 1999;29:245–52.

180. Rogues AM, Dumartin C, Amado B, et al. Relationship between rates of antimicrobial consumption and the incidence of antimicrobial resistance in *Staphylococcus aureus* and *Pseudomonas aeruginosa* isolates from 47 French hospitals. Infect Control Hosp Epidemiol 2007;28:1389–95.

181. Kumar A, Roberts D, Wood KE, et al. Duration of hypotension before initiation of effective antimicrobial therapy is the critical determinant of survival in human septic shock. Crit Care Med 2006;34:1589–96.

182. Kollef MH, Sherman G, Ward S, et al. Inadequate antimicrobial treatment of infections: a risk factor for hospital mortality among critically ill patients. Chest 1999;115:462–74.

183. Dellit TH, Owens RC, McGowan JE Jr, et al. Infectious Diseases Society of America and the Society for Healthcare Epidemiology of America: guidelines for developing an institutional program to enhance antimicrobial stewardship. Clin Infect Dis 2007;44:159–77.

184. Beardsley J, Williamson J, Johnson J, et al. Using local microbiologic data to develop institution-specific guidelines for the treatment of hospital acquired pneumonia. Chest 2006;130:787–93.

185. Ibrahim EH, Ward S, Sherman G, et al. Experience with a clinical guideline for the treatment of ventilator associated pneumonia. Crit Care Med 2001;29:1109–15.

186. Gandhi TN, DePestel DD, Collins CD, et al. Managing antimicrobial resistance in intensive care units. Crit Care Med 2010;38:S315–23.

187. Singh N, Rogers P, Atwood CW, et al. Short-course empiric antibiotic therapy for patients with pulmonary infiltrates in the intensive care unit. A proposed solution for indiscriminate antibiotic prescription. Am J Respir Crit Care Med 2000;162: 505–11.

188. Bouadma L, Luyt CE, Tubach F, et al. Use of procalcitonin to reduce patients' exposure to antibiotics in intensive care units (PRORATA trial): a multicentre randomised controlled trial. Lancet 2010;375:463–74.

189. Schuetz P, Christ-Crain M, Thomann R, et al. Effect of procalcitonin-based guidelines vs standard guidelines on antibiotic use in lower respiratory tract

infections: the ProHOSP randomized controlled trial. JAMA 2009;302: 1059–66.

190. Lodise TP, Lomaestro BM, Drusano GL. Application of antimicrobial pharmaco-dynamic concepts into clinical practice: focus on beta-lactam antibiotics: insights from the Society of Infectious Diseases Pharmacists. Pharmacotherapy 2006;26:1320–32.

191. Chastre J, Wolff M, Fagon JY, et al. Comparison of 8 vs. 15 days of antibiotic therapy for ventilator-associated pneumonia in adults: a randomized trial. JAMA 2003;290:2588–98.

192. Niederman MS. Use of broad-spectrum antimicrobials for treatment of pneu-monia in seriously ill patients: maximizing clinical outcomes and minimizing selection of resistant organisms. Clin Infect Dis 2006;42:S72–81.

193. Kollef MH. Is antibiotic cycling the answer to preventing the emergence of bacterial resistance in the intensive care unit? Clin Infect Dis 2006;43:S82–8.

194. Chittick P, Sherertz RJ. Recognition and prevention of nosocomial vascular device and related bloodstream infections in the intensive care unit. Crit Care Med 2010;38:S363–72.

195. Shuman EK, Chenoweth CE. Recognition and prevention of healthcare-associ-ated urinary tract infections in the intensive care unit. Crit Care Med 2010;38: S373–9.

196. Gastmeier P. Evidence-based infection control in the ICU (except catheters). Curr Opin Crit Care 2007;13:557–62.

197. Lin MY, Hayden MK. Methicillin-resistant Staphylococcus aureus and vancomy-cin-resistant enterococcus: recognition and prevention in intensive care units. Crit Care Med 2010;38:S335–44.

198. Tschudin-Sutter S, Pargger H, Widmer AF. Hand hygiene in the intensive care unit. Crit Care Med 2010;38:S299–305.

199. Vernon MO, Hayden MK, Trick WE, et al. Chlorhexidine gluconate to cleanse patients in a medical intensive care unit: the effectiveness of source control to reduce the bioburden of vancomycin-resistant enterococci. Arch Intern Med 2006;166:306–12.

200. Climo MW, Sepkowitz KA, Zuccotti G, et al. The effect of daily bathing with chlo-rhexidine on the acquisition of methicillin-resistant Staphylococcus aureus, van-comycin-resistant enterococcus, and healthcare associated bloodstream infections: results of a quasi-experimental multicenter trial. Crit Care Med 2009;37:1858–65.

201. Huskins WC. Interventions to prevent transmission of antimicrobial-resistant bacteria in the intensive care unit. Curr Opin Crit Care 2007;13:572–7.

202. Tacconelli E, De Angelis G, de Waure C, et al. Rapid screening tests for meth-icillin-resistant Staphylococcus aureus at hospital admission: systematic review and meta-analysis. Lancet Infect Dis 2009;9:546–54.

203. Lucet JC, Regnier B. Screening and decolonization: does methicillin-suscep-tible Staphylococcus aureus hold lessons for methicillin-resistant S. aureus? Clin Infect Dis 2010;51:585–90.

204. Ammerlaan HS, Kluytmans JA, Wertheim HF, et al. Eradication of methicillin-resistant Staphylococcus aureus carriage: a systematic review. Clin Infect Dis 2009;48:922–30.

205. Simor AE, Phillips E, McGeer A, et al. Randomized controlled trial of chlorhexi-dine gluconate for washing, intranasal mupirocin, and rifampin and doxycycline versus no treatment for the eradication of methicillin-resistant Staphylococcus aureus colonization. Clin Infect Dis 2007;44:178–85.

Index

Note: Page numbers of article titles are in **boldface** type.

Moving?

Make sure your subscription moves with you!

To notify us of your new address, find your **Clinics Account Number** (located on your mailing label above your name), and contact customer service at:

Email: journalscustomerservice-usa@elsevier.com

800-654-2452 (subscribers in the U.S. & Canada)
314-447-8871 (subscribers outside of the U.S. & Canada)

Fax number: 314-447-8029

Elsevier Health Sciences Division
Subscription Customer Service
3251 Riverport Lane
Maryland Heights, MO 63043

Printed and bound by CPI Group (UK) Ltd, Croydon, CR0 4YY

03/10/2024

01040456-0003